The Animal Desk Reference II

Essential Oils for Animals

Melissa Shelton DVM
Holistic Veterinarian

Copyright March 2018
Melissa Shelton DVM

www.OilyVet.com
www.AnimalDeskReference.com

Copyright 2018. All rights reserved. No part of this text may be reproduced or transmitted in any form or by any means, electronic or mechanical, including photocopying, recording, or by any information storage and retrieval system, without permission in writing from the author.

The information contained within this book is for educational purposes only, and only represents a guideline for your use of essential oils and products for animals. The author will assume no liability for any loss or damage of any nature, by the use of any information contained within this publication.

As medical knowledge is constantly changing, new information becomes available. Treatment recommendations and suggestions may change and techniques advance with time. The author has taken care as far as possible, to ensure that the information given in this text is accurate and up to date. However, readers are strongly advised to work in cooperation with a veterinarian, and to use common sense in how to proceed with any illness or administration of natural remedies.

Dedication:

This second edition of the ADR book is dedicated to all those who have shared my passion of essential oils, especially for their animal family members. And, naturally to my amazing family; my husband Winston, my daughter Ramie, and my son Reiker.

My wish is that each and every one of you, know how special your support, comments, case studies, and encouragement has been to me!

With love, joy, and a bit of humor,

Melissa Shelton DVM

TABLE OF CONTENTS

PREFACE 11
ACKNOWLEDGEMENTS 17

VETERINARY AROMATIC MEDICINE 18

ESSENTIAL OILS 19
ESSENTIAL OIL CONSTITUENTS 24
CO_2 EXTRACTS 30

METABOLISM THEORY 34
JUST THE SCIENCE 38
METABOLIC PATHWAYS 54
DETOXIFICATION 58
EXCRETION 60
ABSORPTION 62
SENSITIZATION 71
DRUG INTERACTIONS 74
CARRIER OILS 77
DMSO 94

OIL COLLECTION METHODS 95
HYDROSOLS 97
INSTRUCTIONS FROM THE AUTHOR 98
THE SAFE USE OF OILS 102

TABLE OF CONTENTS

OIL SELECTION 106
ORGANOLEPTICS 110
GRAS STATUS 112
GAS CHROMATOGRAPHY & MASS SPECTROMETRY 115

ESSENTIAL OIL DILUTION RATES 117
USE OF NEAT OIL 127
FORMS OF DILUTION 130
DROPS & MEASUREMENTS 133

OILS & REPRODUCTION 136
SENSITIVITY TO OILS 140
PHOTOSENSITIVITY 143
ESSENTIAL OIL AVERSIONS 144

METHODS OF APPLICATION 146
DIFFUSION 147
INGESTION OF OILS 152
ADDING OILS TO DRINKING WATER 157
MIXING OILS INTO FOODS 162
ORAL ADMINISTRATION 165

THREE PART BLENDS 167
TOPICAL APPLICATIONS 174

ESSENTIAL OILS & EYES 184
ESSENTIAL OILS & EARS 187

TABLE OF CONTENTS

RECTAL INSTILLATION 191
HOW MUCH, HOW OFTEN 193
PREVIOUS TECHNIQUES 196
DRIP & RUB TECHNIQUES 199
BODY SUPPORTIVE BLENDS 204
EMOTIONAL WORK WITH OILS 207
ZOOPHARMACOGNOSY 212

ADVANCED TECHNIQUES 214
INJECTIONS & IV'S 217
INTO THE FUTURE 219
FUTURE RESEARCH 222

ESSENTIAL OIL SINGLES 223
ESSENTIAL OIL BLENDS 337

ESSENTIAL OILS: AVIAN 343
AVIAN CONDITIONS 348

ESSENTIAL OILS: FERRETS 371

ESSENTIAL OILS: RABBITS 375

ESSENTIAL OILS: EXOTIC ANIMALS 382

ESSENTIAL OILS: FELINE 397
FELINE SUPPORTIVE BLEND 402
FELINE CONDITIONS 405

TABLE OF CONTENTS

CANINE SUPPORTIVE BLEND 445
CANINE CONDITIONS 446

EQUINE SUPPORTIVE BLEND 518
EQUINE CONDITIONS 519

LARGE ANIMAL TECHNIQUES 561

REFERENCES 571

INDEX 573

PREFACE

It is hard for me to believe, that my first edition of *The Animal Desk Reference: Essential Oils for Animals* was written in 2011, and published in 2012! So much has changed in this timeframe – and not only do I know so much more about essential oil use with animals, but I have come to change some stances drastically.

I used to feel that if I found one great company or supplier of essential oils that I could just recommend that everyone uses their oils. Securing a known quality level, or guarantee of safety. But, that was not a truth. I guess I know it for all parts of the world, and especially in the animal industry. A great new and natural dog food will be created, and it becomes a booming business. It then can be sold to a larger conglomerate, and voila! The food now becomes sourced to make profit margins wider. The passion that originally went into the food being developed is replaced by "suits". That is what I feel is happening within the essential oil world as well.

So many people love essential oils. It bonds us together, but can also create a huge divide. Companies are pitted against company. Don't use brand "X" and you are labeled and ridiculed. Use brand "Y" and you are instantly a non-caring or naive person who has had the wool pulled over their eyes. The truth of the matter is that no company will likely ever be perfect. And many companies will not uphold the original goals a small company had in mind, as growth starts to consume them.

So yes, you will notice that since writing the first edition of this book, I have left my association with a major player in the essential oil market. To end a bit of confusion, I never worked "for them". I was a distributor just like anyone else. I never wrote the first book "for them" nor was I asked by the company to write it. It merely came out of my huge desire for a similar reference to be available to me when I started using essential oils in my veterinary practice. If I was going to accumulate all of that information and data, I might as well share it with the world. At that time, that brand of essential oils was all I knew, and all I felt comfortable with. And until 2012, I did feel they were the superior oils on the market.

PREFACE

The first edition of this book was self-published, and a completely independent investment on my part, as is this second edition. This edition will not include any proprietary recommendations. This way the knowledge will pertain more to the current information at hand, instead of formulations that can change with time.

If you are new to this book in its second edition form – WELCOME! And please allow me to explain a little bit about myself, so you know who you will be learning from as you read the following pages.

In 2008, after actually using essential oils several times in the past, my human family created the additional encouragement I needed to find more powerful natural health options. My children just could not tolerate artificial dyes, flavorings, or sugaring agents in cough syrups, etc. So, I needed something else. A community education class offering sparked my interest on natural remedies for colds, coughs, flus…and the rest is history as they say.

After that initial introduction to essential oils, I went to class after class to learn more. Naturally as a veterinarian, when you are around a lot of other people and they learn that you are a vet, you get a lot of stories about animals. It just so happens that when you are at essential oil classes, these talks then tend to gravitate towards their animals and their experiences with essential oils with them. I became known as the veterinarian who did not shun the owner for using essential oils with their animal companions. So many had negative experiences when their veterinarian found out they were using essential oils, that they just stopped even telling them. It is a sad situation when your health care professional does not get the full information.

Word started to spread. People started to travel to our veterinary hospital from all around. Driving hours to our clinic to see the "oily vet" – and even from neighboring states. And essential oils, were truly amazing! I was having so much fun in an integrative, holistic practice, with true and powerful tools that I have great passion and love for. Each and every case for the following years, ALWAYS included essential oils in their protocols. It became what I was known for. Diffusion during a spay or neuter. Emotional support before, during, and after procedures. And difficult cases, for which there was no answer other than euthanasia…actually responded to essential oil use! I can honestly say, essential oils were a game changer for how I practiced medicine and surgery.

Requests started to come in for me to also teach classes. I found a new passion I loved – writing books, teaching classes, and all the while getting to also join those things with essential oils, animals, and veterinary medicine. And these new passions also allowed me more family time and structure. It was an instant hit!

I couldn't be blessed more to be able to do all of the things I love, and rotate which one is at the forefront at any one time. If I am a bit tired of writing, I'll teach a class. If I miss clinical work, hospital ICU care seems only a rescue cat away! Since 2011, I had dedicated my veterinary hospital to the advancement of veterinary aromatic medicine. And as other engagements drew my time, I realized that I would have to close our veterinary hospital to traditional appointments and care, even if they did include essential oils. I did not even have enough time to complete and follow up with the many consultations that were being requested. So, I made the difficult decision to "retire" from routine clinical work, and solely dedicate myself to essential oil research, education, and product evaluation and development.

It didn't happen overnight, but by the end of 2012, I had fully stopped taking appointments, even for my most loved clients. To say that I *actually* retired, would almost be laughable. What I found, is that by not taking spay and neuter surgeries, or dental procedures, I was focusing on only very difficult cases with the goal of using veterinary aromatic medicine. I was able to "cherry pick" some very interesting cases to work with; including zoos and animal rescues, to elephant sanctuaries in Brazil. I think retirement, actually challenged my veterinary brain more! I was called upon to help with the most difficult of difficult cases. And I loved it!

It was also during 2012 that I had the stark realization that what I thought to be true about the sources of essential oils I had selected, was changing. The fact of the matter is, I was the "go to" person for almost anyone and everyone to contact for essential oil advice with animals. From even large candy bar companies hoping to create a product for dental health with essential oils in it, to every single "member" of several essential oil companies who had questions they could not have answered by the company itself. So when things started to change for the company I previously used, there was no one to contact for animal help except for me I guess. And the emails started to flood in. Being honest is not a popular position in a sales related industry. But I would never put an animal at undue risk just to protect a sale, a company, or my own previous recommendations from being found untrue.

PREFACE

What was being reported varied from previously effective essential oils becoming ineffective, to actual chemical irritations and burns occurring to the skin of animals. The chemical irritations had not been present in the same past use of identical oils, but then all of a sudden, when you get multiple emails reporting the same problem – your concern grows. I had sent out an email to all of my "downline" stating to avoid certain products until we knew more about what was happening. And, I also gave alternative sources for a known high quality replacement. Oops. I guess that is a big no-no. Honesty. So, I was contacted fairly quickly in an attempt to "muzzle" me. Let's just say, this was the beginning of the end. I will always put animals first. There is nothing, even my own pride, revenues…nothing…that I would put before an animals well-being. Throughout 2012, and into 2013, it was not limited to one event or product. And by the end of 2013, I knew I had to make my exit.

It is an odd situation to be in, when others use your name and reputation to sell their products and promote their company. It becomes a bit uncomfortable, and actually a bit "icky". No one else will ever care for my name, license, and reputation – as much as I will. So removing that opportunity from the hands of others, was very important to me.

But now what? I love essential oils. I teach other veterinarians how to use essential oils in practice, but also realize that the quality of these oils were highly important to obtaining results and avoiding ill effects. How do I leave my modality of choice, my passion, behind? I couldn't. But, how do I find other high quality oils? Was the propaganda true? Are they out there?

Thankfully, the answer is yes! High quality oils are truly out there! And hopefully this book can help to teach others how I became able to evaluate sources on my own, and how you can too. The sad part is, it is a bit of a time and money investment. Even when I started purchasing one brand of oils in 2008, I had always been buying other oils "on the side". I am a curious person. So it never made sense to me that "only XYZ" could be high quality. After all, even though I might have my favorite dog foods, there is never only one. And my favorite cannot be perfect for every individual. What you learn by comparing hundreds of essential oils side by side – is priceless.

I do have to say that unfortunately, I have never met a retailer, supplier, distiller, or other company in the essential oil world, in which I love each and every one of their essential oils they carry and offer. It's like a fine restaurant. You're likely to have your favorite dishes, but you may not love everything on the menu. And in terms of veterinary medicine, sometimes even a certain high quality essential oil, is still not what I would select for animal use. This comes with years of experience, but there are just some selections between high quality oils, that I prefer for one reason or another for veterinary aromatic medicine. It sometimes cannot be explained other than "I see more results clinically."

To be able to teach essential oil use to veterinarians and others interested in this modality, I felt a huge commitment to making sure that a pure and high quality source, one that I felt was appropriate for clinical use, was available to others. And therefore, I really had to be a part of the selection and screening process – for my own peace of mind. At first, I relied on industry experts who I feel honored enough to call friends. And after a bit of hand-holding, I did grow to realize that I could evaluate a distiller, supplier, or lot of oils myself. But more importantly, to use those oils with animals, and monitor them with the eyes, hands, and laboratory tools of a veterinarian, is irreplaceable.

In 2014, I was able to release animalEO® Essential Oils for Animals to the public. These are blends and single essential oils that are screened specifically by me, for their appropriateness for use with animals. This book is not about trying to sell you my oils, it is still for education. But if you are not confident that you have the knowledge base to select which oils you would like to use, you can rest on my evaluation and selections. This is also a great place to mention "grades" and how little they actually mean.

There are many marketing phrases in the essential oil world. From certified this, to pure that, to therapeutic grade, etc... These all truly mean nothing. There is no standardization. There are no regulations. There is nothing that actually dictates what it means to call an essential oil these things. The grade is only as good as the person grading it. So yes, you will find that animalEO essential oils are "veterinary grade". Again, it means nothing except for the fact that I am a veterinarian. And I would use these essential oils in veterinary applications. And if you trust me as your person to evaluate oils for you, then there you go. Veterinary grade essential oils are for you!

animalEO® Essential Oils are available to you as a resource. You are most certainly not required to use them, and I do not contest that "my oils" are the only oils you can ever use with animals. They are a tool, and an ability for you to know that I feel 100% confident with the oils I have screened, to recommend that you can use them within your personal creations, or with your precious animals. However, you will still need to make sure that you use even the best quality essential oils with proper methods, techniques, and care. With poor advice or recommendations, any essential oil can be dangerous.

PREFACE

When this second edition is released, it will be 2018! It is hard to believe that there will be SEVEN years of knowledge to impart into these pages. There is so much to add, and there is still so much more beyond what I can include within this book. I hope that you enjoy this new information, and continue to learn in love, light, and truth.

Melissa Shelton DVM
Holistic & Integrative Veterinarian, Mom, &
Animal Lover

ACKNOWLEDGEMENTS

To the millions of people out there, who love their animals, and seek the truth in health. I thank you! You make my job so enjoyable, and I can't wait to share this portion of knowledge with you!

To all of the aromatherapists, of whom are too numerous to count. Even when we have to "agree to disagree" – I appreciate those of you with a willingness to listen, and to not judge me for my past associations.

To the chemists, suppliers, and industry experts who have taught me so much. I thank you for sharing your knowledge with me.

VETERINARY AROMATIC MEDICINE

Do not be alarmed by this phrase. You do not have to be a veterinarian, nor do you have to have medical knowledge to practice the safe and effective use of essential oils with animals. However, I do believe that the practice does need to have a bit more respect for the knowledge placed within essential oil use, and especially within the animal kingdom. Veterinary refers to the fact that this knowledge is treated with great respect, and has been looked at critically by veterinarians and the field of veterinary medicine. Aromatic refers to the essential oils, not in a fragrance manner, but in the sense that they are volatile substances – often classified in chemistry as "aromatic". And Medicine denotes the purpose and art that essential oils may have when you use them with animals. Essential oils need to be regarded similarly to how we use drugs and herbs. There are species considerations, dosing considerations, and interval considerations. This is normal. This is Veterinary Aromatic Medicine.

Veterinary Aromatic Medicine is for everyone. There certainly is the ability for veterinarians to use essential oils in much more profound ways, and with much more profound knowledge and monitoring, but truly – anyone with a diffuser in their home, or utilizing high quality essential oils within their home or on their human person – may indeed be experiencing Veterinary Aromatic Medicine.

ESSENTIAL OILS

What are essential oils you ask? To me, they are one of the most amazing plant based items on earth. I won't focus on the intricate details of essential oils, but will include a list of my favorite learning tools in the reference section of this book. You will learn enough in this chapter, to create a basic understanding necessary to start your journey with veterinary aromatic medicine.

Essential oils are not "oils" at all actually. Not in the sense that we think of oil. Many veterinarians have been concerned at their clients diffusing essential oils, thinking more along the lines of a fatty oil (like mineral oil) – which we know to be incredibly harmful if inhaled and present in the lungs. But essential oils are a bit misnamed due to history. Thought of as essential due to the fact that they were considered the "quintessence" of the plant, and labeled as an "oil" – they in fact are the aromatic and volatile chemicals contained within certain aromatic plant species.

Not all plants are aromatic, or amenable to collection of the volatile essential oils. It is estimated that approximately 1% of plant species on earth are aromatic in nature. Essential oils are considered a secondary metabolite to the plant. While not critical to everyday life and growth, essential oils require energy from the plant to create, therefore must serve some important function. Mother Nature would not waste energy in the creation of secondary metabolites, if there were not good purposes behind the process.

Essential oils are created in the plant by several processes. There are biosynthetic pathways in which the plant constructs a variety of building blocks into the desired end product. The essential oil. The most common biosynthetic pathways involved in essential oil creation in the plant are the Mevalonate, Shikimic Acid, and Pyruvate pathways. Plants and humans (animals) share the Mevalonate Pathway in common, while the other pathways are recognized only in plants, bacteria, or other organisms.

The Mevalonate Pathway is largely responsible for the creation of isoprene units, which are the building blocks of essential oils. The Pyruvate Pathway also makes isoprene units, but is present in plants and bacteria, and not humans (animals). The Shikimate Pathway creates "aromatic" or circular molecules such as benzene rings. These facts are not critical to know, in all honesty, when you are exploring the use of essential oils with animals. However, for those with a science and biology interest, it can be fascinating.

The take away from the biosynthesis paragraphs is this. We (animals in general) share some common things with plants, making their secondary metabolites valuable to our own body systems.

Once these pathways have created the essential oil compounds, they will be stored in specialized cells in the plant. These cells can be located in different parts of the plant; flowers, roots, rhizomes, bark, leaves, fruit, seeds, etc. Depending on the aromatic plant, different parts of the plant can be collected and "processed" in an attempt to collect this precious essential oil. Each plant will generally have a different requirement or protocol for when to harvest, how to harvest, how to handle the plant matter (dried, fresh, chipped, etc...) as well as different methods of distillation or collection that best suit that plant.

Some plants may create a different essential oil based on which portion of the plant is collected and distilled. For instance, Clove can be from the bud or from the leaf. Cinnamon can be from the bark or the leaf. Even though from the same plant, the essential oil can be quite different.

The secondary metabolites (essential oils) are involved in several helpful biological functions for the plant. The essential oils may act as a defense against insects, or could even attract beneficial insects. Those who might eat offensive insects when they start chewing on a plant, may be attracted to the "meal" by the essential oils released by the plant. We also recognize that many essential oils are made to be helpful to the plant in healing an injury, such as a torn leaf or damaged bark. When we crush aromatic plant matter, we obviously detect the volatile essential oils quite readily.

Another large and important function of the essential oils for a plant is defense against bacteria, fungi, and other pathogens. Plants have been on this Earth, longer than human beings. In all of their time, they have learned how to avoid pathogen resistance, unlike our "advanced" pharmacology and science that makes the same exact chemical every time – allowing bacteria to modify and compensate around the killing mechanism. Plants have the wonderful ability to create a slightly different essential oil based on environmental conditions and stressors. And this fact gives them amazing ability to vary the components created within the essential oil, even if just slightly enough to baffle a strong bacteria.

Essential oils are made up of what we call constituents. These are chemical molecules that are basically the ingredients of Mother Nature's soup. There are different categories to consider when we want to talk about the chemical constituents of essential oils.

First, we can focus on broad categories. This might be Monoterpenes, Sesquiterpenes, Phenols, Terpenoids, Phenylpropanoids, Alcohols, Ketones, etc... There are many variations in between that also describe the chemical foundation of a component, such as Monoterpene Phenol. Yes, you are correct, a bit on the boring side and confusing. But again, thankfully, you will not have to know this information to perfection in order to use essential oils! However, it is nice sometimes to recognize the word, and know what it pertains to. So I will just provide a brief overview.

These constituent categories can be helpful in knowing the characteristics of a given essential oil. For example, Monoterpenes in general tend to be highly lipid soluble. There are other attributes often related to these categories, such as the fact that Phenols are often excellent antimicrobial agents, but also tend to be a bit on the "hot" side. A hot oil is one that generally may create a burning feeling, such as Cinnamon oil on your tongue or Oregano oil on your face…not something you are likely to do twice.

It is important to not get caught up in the "rules" of these components. Although in general we can view basic attributes, it is definitely not a constant that all Ketones or all Esters will carry the same properties.

After the basic chemical descriptions of the constituent categories, comes the actual name of some of the compounds. So this might sound a bit more familiar like Linalool, Limonene, Carvacrol, Menthol, Nepatalactone, etc. Again, these individual constituents may have consistent characteristic functions; however Linalool within Lavender may reveal a bit different overall contribution than the Linalool in Basil. For me, it is not about the single constituent or "fraction" of the essential oil, but the synergy and magic that the entire plant creates with its own individual "soup recipe". It is more of a pharmacological mindset to extract only Linalool, and to use it for aromatic medicine or for research. For me, plant based medicine will always involve that which we gather from the entire plant.

See the chapter Oil Collection Methods for more on the different techniques used to collect essential oils from the plant.

Another thing you may note in the names of chemical constituents is letters. So this may look like D-Limonene or L-Limonene. These indicators are representative of the way the molecule reflects light, and these different molecules are called isomers. While very similar, they are also very different. Levo-rotary is denoted as an upper or lower case "L" or [-]. In college organic chemistry, we remembered that "L" meant to the left, or counter-clockwise. Dextro-rotary is denoted by an upper or lower case "D" or [+] sign. This designation means the light is refracted to the "right" or clockwise. Organic chemistry quick tip – since I am "positively right-handed", I am the most dexterous with my right hand, or a positive spin. Therefore, dextro-rotary meant to the "right" and was also designated with the [+} sign. I am also "negatively" impacted when using my left hand – so the levo-rotary again was to the left and denoted by the [-} sign. While it may not be the most important factor for you to have a grasp of, there is one important fact regarding levo and dextro rotary molecules.

First, the isomers, also called enantiomers, while having all of the same chemical atoms, can be quite different in smell and action. A common example of this variation is d-carvone and l-carvone. D-carvone is found in dill oil, and gives that characteristic pickle smell. L-carvone is found in spearmint, and smells minty. These isomers are basically identical, but are more similar to a mirror image of each other – much like our right and left hand. And here is the kicker, only Mother Nature (or the plant) has the ability to make only one version of this chemical. So, while a dill plant will only produce 100% of d-carvone and a spearmint plant will only produce 100% of l-carvone – we would find that if we would try to create carvone in a laboratory, we would get both levo and dextro molecules. Humans are just not as good as nature. So when evaluating essential oils, we can use facts such as this to occasionally detect adulterations or synthetics.

Another term you may see is *cis-* or *trans-* before an isomer name. This also designates a variation on how the molecule is put together. Again, a bit too involved for what is needed to understand about essential oils for our purposes, but at least you have a slight understanding of what this means in front of a name.

And finally, there are whole bunches of Greek letters. You will see these commonly in front of constituent names. Basically, they are just part of the name for our purposes. β-Myrcene, α-Pinene, γ-Terpinene are a few common ones. Just know that we generally say "beta", "alpha", or "gamma" – and you'll be just fine. Although, when other letters of the Greek alphabet start to come into play – you may hear both versions of the letter. ρ-Cymene is most commonly going to be said "P" Cymene, mainly because we all forget that ρ is the Greek letter rho. Some do say Rho-Cymene, but even I had to google what it was again.

When there are numbers in front of a chemical constituent, such as 1,8-Cineole, we just say "one eight cineole". These numbers designate where on the molecule the oxygen atom is bonded. So in 1,8-Cineole the oxygen molecule is bonded to the first and eighth carbon atoms.

And now, you know just enough to sound well informed! Kudos!

ESSENTIAL OIL CONSTITUENTS

While I do not feel that we should focus all of our attention to an individual constituent, I will cover the basics of the common categories. This stuff makes my brain hurt, so I will go over it in the basic ways that make sense to me. I like things simple, and easy to convert into one of my favorite subjects, FOOD!

So, essential oils are hydrocarbon based. This means they are mainly built of carbon and hydrogen. Different numbers of carbons and different numbers of hydrogens are put together in a variety of ways, to make different molecules. This gives us our base structure to work from. The hydrocarbon base is like your noodles at a pasta bar. You start with a base, and what you add to it next, makes your meal. Of course, there are a few versions of pasta. Rotini, spaghetti, fettuccini, and all will hold the pasta sauces a bit differently, or give you a bit of a different experience.

The pasta sauces, vegetables, or "adds" that you put to your pasta, those are the "functional groups". Do you add a cream sauce, or a tomato sauce? Do you add mushrooms, cheese, or other vegetables? All of these things drastically change the pasta dish you are finally served; however, they are all still based in pasta.

Hydrocarbons in general are very lipid soluble, meaning they mix with fatty substances readily – also called lipophilic. As the functional groups start being added to the "pasta" – this can change the solubility characteristics a bit. So some molecules will be more or less soluble in lipids, and some will be more or less soluble in aqueous or water solutions. Aromatic hydrocarbons are a class that is defined by having a benzene ring – or a special structure within the molecule.

An isoprene unit is the base unit of most essential oil compounds. An isoprene unit contains 5 carbon units. The most common type of compound found in essential oils is the monoterpene. A monoterpene consists of TWO isoprene units put together in its simplest form. One way to remember how many isoprene units are in a compound, is to double the "base word" meaning. So "mono" would typically mean "one" – however it really means one pair of isoprene units. So a monoterpene has 10 carbon molecules, or 2 isoprene units. A sesquiterpene contains 3 isoprene units, or 15 carbon molecules. "sesqui" is the Latin for one and a half – so again if we double this we get the "3" isoprene units – which means three times five carbons. Then you may occasionally hear about diterpenes within essential oils, which are an even larger molecule. "Di" meaning two, this doubles into 4 pairs of isoprene units, or 20 carbon atoms. Diterpenes rarely cross over into steam distillation, as they are a bit too heavy and less volatile in nature. There are only a few steam distilled essential oils containing diterpenes. Molecules larger than diterpenes are not found in steam distilled essential oils.

The most common essential oil drawing talk of diterpenes currently is Copaiba. This oil is actually available in a steam distilled and a resin form. Copaiba is unique in that it can be tapped from the tree, much like the liquid collected to make maple syrup. The sap or resin directly from the tree contains these diterpenes, and the steam distilled essential oil generally does not. There are various benefits being reported to the presence of the diterpenes, although clinically we may see different responses to the oleoresin versus the steam distilled version.

Research being cited to support the importance of diterpenes, also seems to support that steam distilled Copaiba is still remarkably effective, despite the apparent lack of diterpenes. Steam distilled Copaiba, is generally higher in β-Caryophyllene which is another constituent with considerable research and popularity. While I do believe there may be reasons for the use of both Copaiba forms, the oleoresin is more natural and representative of the tree itself. See more about Copaiba under its single oil information and description.

If you are fascinated with diterpenes, the diterpenes found within some species of Copaiba are kaurenoic, hardwichiic, kovalenic, polyalthic, and copalic acids. Copalic acid and kaurenoic acid are likely the most prevalent and talked about. Certainly more information will come to the forefront, however just remember, most research can be slanted to support whatever version you wish to promote and sell. So if I like sustainability and presence of diterpenes, I'll report these as the most beneficial reason to use the oleoresin. And if I want to promote that the steam distilled contains more β-caryophyllene and so that is more beneficial, I can likewise show you parts of research to support that. The truth is, the best version is the one that works best for the patient. I continue to monitor and research the differences noted clinically between the two – but a clear realization that both may be completely appropriate and effective is encouraged.

Once we have monoterpenes, sesquiterpenes, and diterpenes – we can now discuss the meaning of *–terpenoid*. When we see monoterpenoid, this just means that it is a terpene that has now be modified, so it is "monoterpene-like" by definition. Most modification is by the addition of those functional groups (or pasta adds) which we mentioned earlier.

Another phrase you may come across is "folding". This is often seen with citrus oils such as Orange, and from some bulk suppliers you may see "Orange 10-fold" or "Orange 5-fold". This is a term pertaining to de-terpination – or the removal of less stable terpenes from the essential oil. This is done to improve shelf life, and is often done for the food and fragrance industry more than for medical applications. This process is fractionation of the oil, and results in a more concentrated citrus oil. Therefore 10-fold oil will be stronger than 5-fold citrus oil. For example – 5-fold Orange oil may have an aldehyde percent of 4.48% while 10-fold Orange will have 8.52% aldehydes. Folded oils are generally left to the flavor and fragrance world, and are not used for therapeutic purposes.

Let's discuss the functional groups. It's no lie. I sort of hate chemistry. Well, I sort of love it. Then go back to "disliking it strongly" pretty fast. Quite honestly, it makes my brain hurt. So, in an effort to not make your brain hurt (there are plenty of books and courses that can achieve that if you are into that sort of thing) – I will present the simple and easy version for you.

Below are the functional groups (pasta sauce and other ingredients) we can add to your hydrocarbons (pasta). Remember, your base hydrocarbon might be a monoterpene (let's call this rotini), or a sesquiterpene (spaghetti seems in order), a diterpene, or even an aromatic hydrocarbon (which we also call phenylpropanoids). Add your other menu items, and you're on your way to creating certain types of essential oil constituents.

Alkenes. These are quite common in essential oils, and result when another hydrocarbon is added to our hydrocarbon base (have a little pasta with your pasta!). Typically they may end in the *-ene* suffix but not always. Common alkenes include α-pinene, chamazulene, α-humulene, β-myrcene, and anethole. In general, most alkenes carry properties such as anti-inflammatory, analgesic, antifungal, antimicrobial, and anticancer.

Alcohols. Add a hydroxyl group (-OH) and you now have an alcohol. Alcohols are reported to be relatively non-toxic and non-irritating. They tend to have properties such as antiviral, antifungal, antiseptic, and uplifting (think getting drunk with ethanol). Common alcohols include linalool, santalol, citronellol, geraniol, eudesmol, and bisabolol. Sometimes you will note some compounds with and without their Greek letters or other designations (+) – such as with α-bisabolol. For the most part, this will still be the same chemical. Sometimes we just get a bit lazy. Alcohols generally end in the suffix "-ol".

Phenols. Phenols often strike fear into the heart of aromatherapists especially when considering cats. This essential oil group also has a hydroxyl group added to it (-OH), but it is added to a benzene ring. This combination makes them more acidic, and a bit more reactive in nature (think getting heartburn from adding a tomato-based sauce to your pasta instead of creamy). This classification of oils, is one most commonly reported to be afraid of in cats. However, much of the information is based on very old research, with very little attention to current and updated veterinary knowledge. Please see the chapter Metabolism Theory for more information. Examples of phenols are carvacrol, eugenol, thymol, and chavicol. Phenols are often considered "hot" oils, and appropriate dilution is almost always recommended. Characteristics associated with phenols include that they are powerful antibacterial and antifungal agents, are often used in disinfecting, support and stimulate the immune system, decrease inflammation, are anti-parasitic, anti-tumoral, and so much more. When used properly, phenols can be an important part of veterinary aromatic medicine.

Aldehydes. Add a (-CHO) and you have an aldehyde. Often described as fruity in odor, common aldehydes include cinnamaldehyde, geranial (note the –al instead of –ol), citronellal, citral, and neral. Aldehydes are known to be more irritating to the skin and may cause sensitization. Aldehydes are also more prone to oxidation damage, which is linked to skin irritations and sensitization even more so. They are reported to have properties such as antiseptic, anti-inflammatory, immune-supportive, and calming.

Ketones. Similar to Aldehydes, however much more stable. In general, ketones are thought to be excreted from the body (usually in the urine) in an unchanged state – so less metabolized. These compounds generally end in "-one". Certain ketones are thought to have neurotoxic properties, so care should be taken with oils high in ketones, especially in cases of decreased urine output or kidney function. The neurotoxic concern is likely to be related to overwhelming the body's ability to excrete the unchanged ketones adequately in the urine. Again, making the dosing and frequency of administration of oils the most important factor in their use. Ketones are reported to aid in digestion, reduce scar tissue, facilitate tissue repair and regeneration, are anti-inflammatory, relaxing and calming. Common ketones of interest include camphor, carvone, menthone, and thymoquinone. Thujone is possibly the more discussed ketone, in terms of toxicity concerns.

Carboxylic Acids. When Aldehydes become oxidized, they form Carboxylic Acids (-COOH). These substances are poorly volatile, but are highly reactive. They should not normally be contained in essential oils.

Esters. Also sometimes called Carboxylic Esters, esters are fruity and sweet in smell, and generally end in the suffix (-ate). Esters are reported to be very antispasmodic, anti-inflammatory, calming and relaxing, and antimicrobial. Common Esters include neryl acetate, linalyl acetate, and methyl salicylate.

Ethers. These may also be called oxides when in their cyclic form, and when we think of items that are "oxygen added" we should consider them to be stronger in nature. Much like "oxidation" of an oil will make it more likely to irritate skin; molecules containing oxygen tend to be a bit more powerful. Even laundry additives are now "powered by oxygen" - to remove stubborn stains. One way to remember the difference between Esters and Ethers is that in "Ether" there is the dominant letter "t" immediately after the "E". In college organic chemistry, we determined that the "t" would stand for "two" – as in O_2. This gave us at least some way to remember that the Ether contained more oxygen or O_2 bonds than the Esters. Ethers also have "two" carbon bonds to the oxygen molecule. Again, using that theme – then we realize that the oxygen molecule could also be within the carbon ring, making this form a cyclic ester (or oxide). Ethers generally end in (-ole) and are reported to possess properties such as anti-inflammatory, antiseptic, diuretic, expectorant, calming and stimulating, and helpful for nerve issues. Common ethers include anethole, estragole, myristicin, and the famous 1,8-cineole (which is an oxide).

Lactones. Lactones are cyclic esters. They have a higher molecular size and weight, so are therefore less volatile. These compounds include nepetalactone and coumarin. Lactones have many properties reported for them, including anti-inflammatory, antiviral, antimicrobial, analgesic, relaxing and in the case of nepetalactone – immense anti-bug properties.

Furanocoumarins. These are important to recognize, as they are the compounds often found within citrus oils which give them their photosensitizing nature.

Known as "phototoxic" compounds, they can include bergapten, angelicin, and methoxsalen. While some types of furanocoumarins are the basis of concern with eating grapefruit or consuming the juice with medications, these chemicals are not present within grapefruit essential oil to any level that would be likely to cause drug interactions (Tisserand and Young, Essential Oil Safety).

While this is indeed an abbreviated version of chemistry – it does get you an insight into the terminology and properties reported to be common. However, it remains vastly important to evaluate an essential oil as a whole, and not as a vision of a few dominant chemical constituents.

CO_2 EXTRACTS

CO_2 extracts bear their own chapter as a new identity in the world of Veterinary Aromatic Medicine. In some ways, they are a completely different beast. While, I am sure I will not move over towards their use completely, there are some magical differences within these extracts that make their notice worthwhile. First let's explain why and how they are different from "essential oils".

The technology to extract plant components with Carbon Dioxide (CO_2) has been around since the 1950's. It started in the Russian food industry mainly, and since the 1970's Russia has almost exclusively used CO_2's for these purposes. When Russia shared this technology with England and the U.S. – naturally it was bound for "improvements" where bigger is always better. So we now see a lot of "Super Critical" CO_2 extraction terms, where higher pressure is used to extract even more, even faster. Not always the most ideal situation, but I digress.

CO_2 extracts have had a distinct minus to their reputation, as historically there were "bad" extraction techniques involving hydrocarbons such as butane, propane, pentane or hexane. However, now days, most CO_2 extracts are produced for the food and flavor industry, and safe practices are more likely. However, it is always wise to double check.

In short, CO_2 is used as a solvent for the extraction of plant substances (instead of steam with average distillation). CO_2 is known for low toxicity, has the properties to be used as a gas or liquid based on temperature and pressure variations, and is relatively inert as a chemical – so does not mix with or alter the compounds it extracts. Once the CO_2 liquid passes through the plant material collecting the substances we desire, it is converted back to its gas state, and is drawn off of the end product. CO_2 extraction does not denature or chemically alter constituents found within the plant, as can happen with steam distillation. CO_2 extraction is generally more efficient than steam distillation, resulting in a higher yield from the same amount of plant material. Extracts from plants derived from CO_2 extraction, are considered more identical to what is found within the living plant, without any solvent residue.

There are several versions within CO_2 extraction, and you are likely to come across the phrase "Supercritical" or sCO_2. A basic CO_2 uses liquid CO_2 (also called Subcritical) for its extraction process, and a Supercritical uses both liquid and gas. Within these processes, you can also get a few variations on the type of extraction that is selected to occur.

Liquid Subcritical CO_2 extraction generally extracts compounds with 5-20 carbon molecules. So, the molecules are smaller in size and more aromatic in nature. These extracts are often more similar in nature to steam distilled essential oils.

Select Supercritical CO_2 extractions vary temperature and pressure to extract more plant compounds, generally ranging between 5-25 carbon molecules. I most commonly hear this version referred to as a Select CO_2, and these can be greatly varied by the extraction technician or desires of a practitioner or flavorist. Basically a Select is able to be customized to a wide degree – "selecting" your temperature and pressure settings, in order to "select" a distinct version of an extract.

Total (Complete) Supercritical CO_2 extracts contain the volatile and non-volatile components of a plant. This will include lipids, colors, waxes, and resins. These are often very thick, colored, or solid in nature. Total CO_2 extracts are much more akin to working with herbal medicine, spiked with essential oils. Compounds with 5-60 carbon molecules may be found in Total extracts.

Steam distillation of a plant, will generally yield compounds with only 5-15 carbon molecules in size. And very rarely are diterpenes (Carbon 20) found within steam distilled products. CO_2 extraction remains a very efficient alternative for some essential oils. In the case of an oil like Sandalwood, steam distillation takes 7 days, but only 1 ½ hours with CO_2 extraction.

There was still a natural question of if CO_2 is left behind within the extract, and if that was cause for concern. There is some residual CO_2 left behind within an extract, and it is reported that approximately 3% of the CO_2 used during a distillation is "lost" during the process. This indicates that it is within the extract somewhere. However, we are reassured that with time, the CO_2 leaves the extract. It can take a couple of weeks to do so, and until it does, the extract may look cloudy.

A more real concern with CO_2 extraction is that if the plant material is not organic, and contains pesticides, pollutants or chemicals these will carry over into the final extract. Because so much extraction occurs with the CO_2 process, the larger molecules (even bad ones) will be carried over; more so than with steam distillation. While tests can be done for contaminants, and procedures (fractionation) can be performed on extracts to remove the contaminants, it is a concern we need to be aware of.

CO_2 extracts will often be reported to have varying percentages of volatile components. Those with a volatile content of 75% or more, often behave more like a steam distilled essential oil, and can be considered for diffusion purposes. Other extracts will be very heavy, waxy and will require special handling in their use. Because of the plant compounds contained within CO_2 extracts, we must consider them more closely to herbal medicine in nature. Specialist in CO_2 extracts, Mark Webb, describes CO_2 extracts as "herbal medicine on steroids". It is clearly concentrated herbal medicine!

In my own evaluation of CO_2 extracts, there are clear advantages and disadvantages in my eyes. First, I do rather like the artistry of essential oils. After taking a 2 day course on CO_2's I came to this conclusion. CO_2 extraction felt a bit more like a C-Section. A bit sterile, controlled, and highly technical – still a very wonderful medical event, but different. While essential oils are like natural childbirth. Each of my children's births were different, with a bit of a story and emotion to it. Certainly, variation and nature came into play. And the end result was not as "clinical" and was certainly filled with a different sort of love and emotion. Naturally, my veterinary mind explains a lot of things in a medical manner. But I do truly find this a wonderful comparison between CO_2 extracts and steam distilled essential oils.

There are certainly CO_2 extracts I wish to use in my practice. And they will be noted in the single descriptions if I feel they should have notice. CO_2 extracts may be more stable, contain beneficial plant compounds that essential oils do not, and be able to be used as oral herbal medicine in ways we could never imagine. However, I will still use essential oils along with them.

CO_2 extracts to take specific note of are Black Cumin, Black Pepper, Calendula, German Chamomile, Ginger, Juniper, Lavender, Oregano, Rosemary Extract for antioxidant and preservation (not the essential oil), and Turmeric. Carrier oils are also reported to be of much higher quality when CO_2 extracted, especially oils such as Evening Primrose, which is notorious for "going bad" – however the CO_2 extract of Primrose oil is much more stable.

Scott Johnson also has a large reference book called *Supercritical Essential Oils: A Companion Resource to Medicinal Essential Oils*. In his book, he also refers to Supercritical CO_2 extracts as "SFE" or Supercritical Fluid Extraction. This is an excellent reference if you are more interested in CO_2 extracts, and the book includes comparisons in the constituents found between SFE and steam distilled oils.

The main reason I will be reluctant to move towards total use of CO_2 extracts in my practice, is for the simple fact that I will have to strictly adhere to herbal medicine risks and interactions that go along with more plant chemicals being present in the extract. More simply stated, I do not have to worry about herb to herb, or herb to drug interactions with the use of steam distilled essential oils. And while I love botanical medicine, I am not an herbalist, and could never quite get as excited about herbs as I felt passionate about essential oils.

However, when I consider an item such as German (blue) Chamomile; the CO_2 is truly different than the steam distilled essential oil. With steam distillation of this plant, chamazulene is produced, which gives it its gorgeous blue color. However, this is indeed a byproduct of distillation, and not the chemical that is found within the plant itself. Chamazulene is found in little to no amounts within the CO_2, while Matricin (the original chemical) is. Matricin is normally changed by the distillation process, to form chamazulene. While chamazulene is known to have its own beneficial properties, matricin is reported to have 10 times the anti-inflammatory action as chamazulene. So for some purposes, we could place a preference on the CO_2 extract of German Chamomile.

The preference for CO_2 extracts will also be noteworthy when we are making balms, creams, ointments, or shampoos of sorts. By having some of the beneficial plant waxes, lipids, anti-oxidants, and heavier plant compounds within the extract, we can see prevention of evaporation and a fixative and sealant sort of action. In this way, applications may last longer, or form a helpful and healing barrier to infection or other damages. The presence of more plant materials and waxes, are likely to prove highly beneficial for bug repellant actions.

Certain oils for ingestion also shine as CO_2 extracts. Black Pepper CO_2 contains the valuable piperine, which is why Black Pepper (ground) is often used in combination with turmeric paste recipes. Piperine aids in bio-availability of curcumin (one of the active compounds in turmeric), as well as having its own anti-oxidant properties. While the essential oil of Black Pepper does not contain piperine, the Select and Total CO_2 extracts do. And when considering Turmeric, the CO_2 extract is also a wonderful way to concentrate the beneficial compounds found within the spice. Most herbal supplements containing Turmeric extracts, are indeed CO_2 extracts. CO_2 extracts are likely to become more and more popular as concentrated and convenient ways to provide herbal medicine.

METABOLISM THEORY

Essential oils are not metabolized by the body as a whole unit. Each individual constituent will have its own specific enzymatic pathways that are used by a body to process and eliminate the chemical. This is not a known process for all constituents, and since there are thousands upon thousands of constituents, it is unlikely that this information will be available any time soon.

There are some well-known constituents that have been mapped by research. Limonene is known to utilize the CYP_2C_9 and CYP_2C_{19} enzymes. These enzymes are part of the famous Cytochrome P450 or CYP_{450} pathways. While this information may be necessary in the advanced pharmacology of essential oils, thankfully, you do not need to understand it fully on your journey of the use of essential oils. However, as there are a few misconceptions about essential oil metabolism, excretion, and its importance in animals, I will teach you what you need to know to fully understand the controversy, and the apparent truth behind it.

There is a lot of confusion regarding the metabolism of essential oils, especially in regards to cats. It is not uncommon that someone who is using essential oils with a certain species, will be ridiculed and ostracized. However, those who carry the biggest stick in the complaint, rarely have any animal physiology or pharmacology training. It is not that being safe is wrong; I value those who would like to take the cautionary path and avoid all use of essential oils with species of concern. However, to say that no one can do it, is just like saying that cats cannot have Morphine in veterinary medicine. It is just out of date information, and although you are welcome to practice the safest of safe protocols, we need to change the informational tide of what we truly know to be accurate in the animal field.

Where does this controversy come from? Let's take cats as our example. They are commonly reported as being "deficient" in their liver enzymes. That they just cannot metabolize essential oils, and that they will build up over time, creating horrible side effects and potential death. I would like to think that cats are not deficient, they are just cats. Just like saying that we are deficient in fur, or that Australians drive on the "wrong" side of the road from Americans, it is a point of view type of statement. We are comparing a completely different animal species, with a completely different metabolism set up, to completely unrelated species such as dogs and humans. Let's let cats be cats. And just enjoy them for the unique creatures they are.

Where did our misconception about cats come from? One main research article that is used to support that phenols are toxic to cats is from 1972. This is very, very old in the medical field. And if one reads further into the research, it has nothing to do with natural essential oils, and everything to do with benzyl alcohol being injected, added to meat products as a preservative, or used as a bacteriostatic in drug or biological products. Sure, if you only read the headline of "Toxicosis in cats from the use of benzyl alcohol in lactated Ringer's solution" in the Journal of American Veterinary Medical Association in 1983, you may worry also about the use of any phenol. However, we really need to evaluate apples to apples. If you knew nothing of veterinary medicine, feline physiology, or the vast difference between a chemical benzene ring and a natural substance containing a benzene ring, you would err on the side of caution. Which seems to be the case for most of the aromatherapy world at this time.

And sadly, more current information is out there. Even in the November 1984 edition of *Veterinary Clinics of North America: Small Animal Practice – Vol. 14, No. 6*; titled *Symposium on Advances in Feline Medicine II*, there is an incredibly profound statement by Jeff R. Wilcke DVM, MS. "Even drugs known for toxicity in cats can be used safely if we are aware of and compensate for certain peculiarities." That basically says it all. And that is 1984! Here we are – some 33 years later, still questioning if essential oils are killing cats, and reporting all over the place that it is a huge area of concern.

Cats would be dropping over dead all over the world, if essential oils were truly as toxic as those reports imply. With the amazing amount of essential oil use in households containing all sorts of animals, I am impressed at the level of safety actually witnessed. Just like with the phenol research, it will matter what quality of essential oil is used. I do not think that synthetics or altered essential oils should be in the same category at all with true and natural essential oils.

Certainly, any essential oil that would be more towards a "fragrance-grade" oil – will have the potential to cause long term problems. Just as we documented cases of liver value elevation in homes with a lot of air freshener and artificial fragrance use, these lesser essential oils are akin to spraying perfume on your cat and wondering why that didn't bode well. And it is just unfortunate in the current market of essential oils that there are so many poor grade essential oils being sold as high quality. If you are purchasing an essential oil based on cost, or because it is easily available at the health food or grocery store – you have likely already selected some of the poorer grade oils on the market. But hype does not also guarantee quality. Marketing is just marketing, no matter how convincing it may sound. It is best to consider if your essential oil source is truly "on the line" at the end of the day for the results and quality that you obtain. If they say you can use an oil with your cat, and you experience an adverse event, is that person or product truly held accountable? If not, proceed with caution.

Can cats metabolize essential oils? Yes, they can. And no, they will not build up over time, although cats can have what we refer to as a different half-life for a chemical, or elimination time. In a study of plasma half-lives for sodium salicylate it was discovered that ponies, swine, goats, dogs, and cats had drastically different elimination times. Ponies had a 1.0 hour half-life, while the others displayed 5.9, 0.78, 8.6, and 37.6 hours respectively. A cat actually took almost 38 hours to eliminate the drug, while a dog took just under 9. Does this mean the cat is deficient? No, it means the cat is not a dog, and the cat is not a goat, and the cat is not a pony! And look at how fast a goat eliminated the drug – we do not call the other species deficient in the goats shadow – we just accept that there are species differences. And that my friend, is how drug doses are created.

Essential oils need to be regarded similarly to how we use drugs. There are species considerations, dosing considerations, and interval considerations. This is normal.

What really is the case with cat metabolism? The actual science behind the specific differences in cat metabolism is as follows. When cats are compared to other species, it appears that they have less ability to conjugate xenobiotics with glucuronic acid. There appears to be a lack of UDP-glucuronyltransferase activity towards certain substrates. However UDP-glucose dyhydrogenase and glucouronic acid are present in amounts consistent with normal activity in other species. Glucuronides of endogenous body compounds such as bilirubin, are formed in normal rates in cats. However, when glucuronides are formed for phenols, it may be a smaller percentage of the total drug eliminated. There is a variation in some of the enzyme affinity for different "drug molecules", and so we need to allow this to influence our therapeutic protocols for everything we expose a cat to.

The nature of the chemical the cat is exposed to, and the presence of alternative pathways for metabolism, need to be considered in feline pharmacokinetics of essential oils. How efficient the alternative pathways are, and what metabolite they might produce in the process, also must be considered. Some metabolites can indeed be viewed as toxic in their own right, but in some instances the metabolite is the more biologically active or beneficial molecule to the body. To quote Dr. Wilcke, "Alternative metabolic pathways may produce compounds that are as toxic, if not more so, than the parent compound, and in greater quantities than expected for other species. This situation is very difficult to predict until the drug is actually used in cats."

So we need to be careful about our extrapolation of generalities to cats and other animals of concern, such as ferrets. The wealth of information present to show that cats are tolerating proper use of essential oils is far more current, and overwhelming in amount. When we consider that there are several essential oil distribution companies with several million people each within them. And all of those members are using essential oils almost daily in their home, and that 63% of all homes contain animals...I think we need a check and balance of how toxic this situation really is. The simple evidence is that in the absence of gross misuse and overdose of essential oils, they really are quite safe.

The subject of First Pass Metabolism of essential oils will be discussed in the chapter of Absorption, as this is highly dependent on the route in which the essential oil enters the body.

JUST THE SCIENCE

During the completion of this book, a report of a cat becoming ill from the use of essential oils went "viral" on Facebook. This chapter was created in response, as it was incredibly clear, that even those known as aromatherapy experts – were unable to cite references and display knowledge behind what they were taught.

The data and research behind cats.

The following research articles appear to be much of the basis for our concern with cats, but also what is ignored in terms of continuing advancement of our education and knowledge base. I will start with the oldest first. And this is not even close to all relevant material.

1963. Larson, EJ: Toxicity of low doses of aspirin in the cat. J. Am. Vet. Med. Assoc., 143:837-840.

1965. Jones, LM (ed): Veterinary Pharmacology and Therapeutics. Edition 3. Ames, Iowa State University Press.

1965. Roe FJ, Field WE. Chronic toxicity of essential oils and certain other products of natural origin. Food Cosmet. Toxicol. 3(2):311-23.

1966. Dutton, GJ (ed): Glucuronic Acid: Free and Combined Chemistry, Biochemistry, Pharmacology, and Medicine. New York, Academic Press.

1967. Herrgesell, JD.: Aspirin poisoning in the cat. J. Am. Vet. Med. Assoc., 151:452-455.

1968. Davis LE, Donnelly EJ: Analgesic drugs in the cat. J. Am. Vet. Med. Assoc., 153:1161-1167.

1969. Zontine, WJ, Uno, T: Acute aspirin toxicity in a cat. Vet. Med. Small Anim. Clin., 64:680-682.

1971. Yeh SY, Chernov HI, Woods LA. Metabolism of morphine by cats. J. Pharm. Sci. 60(3):469-471.

1972. Davis LE, Westfall BA: Species differences in biotransformation and excretion of salicylate. Am. J. Vet. Res., 33:1253-1262.

1972. Jansen PL, Henderson PT. Influence of phenobarbital treatment on p-nitrophenol and bilirubin glucuronidation in Wistar rat, Gunn rat and cat. Biochem. Pharmacol. 15;21(18):2457-62.

1972. Bedford, PGC, and Clarke, EGC: Experimental benzoic acid poisoning in the cat. Vet. Rec., 90:53-58.

1973. Yeary, RA, and Swanson, W: Aspirin dosages for the cat. J. Am. Vet. Med. Assoc., 163:1177-1178.

1973. Hietanen E, Vainio H. Interspecies variations in small intestinal and hepatic drug hydroxylation and glucuronidation. Acta. Pharmacol. Toxicol. (Copenh). 33(1):57-64.

1974. Fertziger AP, Stein EA, Lynch JJ. Letter: Suppression of morphine-induced mania in cats. Psychopharmacologia. 8;36(2):185-7.

1974. Capel ID, Millburn P, Williams RT. The Conjugation of 1- and 2-Naphthols and other Phenols in the Cat and Pig. Xenobiotica. 4(10):601-615.

1975. Finco, DR, Duncan JR, Schall, WD, et. al.: Acetaminophen toxicosis in the cat. J. Am. Vet. Med. Assoc., 166:469-472.

1975. Schillings RT, Sisenwine SF, Schwartz MH, Ruelius HW. Lorazepam: glucuronide formation in the cat. Drug Metab. Dispos. 3(2):85-8.

1978. Erichsen, DF, Harris SG, and Upson DW: Plasma levels of digoxin in the cat: Some clinical applications. J. Am. Anim. Hosp. Assoc., 14:734-737.

1980. Erichsen, DF, Harris, SG, and Upson DW: Therapeutic and toxic plasma concentrations of digoxin in the cat. Am. J. Vet. Res., 41:2049-2058.

1980. Davis, LE: Clinical pharmacology of salicylates. J. Am. Vet. Med. Assoc., 176:65-66.

1982. Federal Drug Administration Bureau of Veterinary Medicine: Benzyl alcohol hazardous as a parenteral preservative. J. Am. Vet. Med. Assoc., 181:641.

1982. Schleifer, JH and Carson TL: Toxicity of benzyl alcohol preservative. Letter. J. Am. Vet. Med Assoc., 181:853.

1982. Bolton, G. R., and Powell, W.: Plasma kinetics of digoxin in the cat. Am. J. Vet. Res., 43:1994-1999.

1982. Akesson, C. E. and Linero, P.E.: Effect of chloramphenicol on serum salicylate concentrations in cats and dogs. Am. J. Vet. Res., 43:1471-1472.

1982. Gaunt, SD, Baker DC, and Green RA.: Clinicopathologic evaluation of N-acetylcysteine therapy in acetaminophen toxicosis in the cat. Am. J. Vet. Res., 42-1981.

1982. Schmoldt A, von der Eldern-Dellbrügge U, Benthe HF. On the glucuronidation of digitalis compounds in different species. Arch. Int. Pharmacodyn. Ther. 255(2):180-90.

1983. Cullison, R. F., Menard, P.D., and Buck W.B.: Toxicosis in cats from the use of benzyl alcohol in lactated Ringer's solution. J. Am. Vet. Med. Assoc., 182:61.

1983. Prasuhn, LW: Tylenol poisoning in the cat. Letter. J. Am. Vet. Med. Assoc., 182:4.

1984. Wilcke, JR: Idiosyncracies of Drug Metabolism in Cats: Effects on Pharmacotherapeutics in Feline Practice. Symposium on Advances in Feline Medicine II. Vet. Clin. North Am. Small Anim. Pract., 14(6):1345-1354.

1984. Hassell TM, Maguire JH, Cooper CG, Johnson PT. Phenytoin metabolism in the cat after long-term oral administration. Epilepsia. 25(5):556-63.

1984. Savides MC, Oehme FW, Nash SL, Leipold HW. The toxicity and biotransformation of single doses of acetaminophen in dogs and cats. Toxicol. Appl. Pharmacol. 5;74(1):26-34.

1984. Smith GS, Watkins JB, Thompson TN, Rozman K, Klaassen CD. Oxidative and conjugative metabolism of xenobiotics by livers of cattle, sheep, swine and rats. J. Anim. Sci. 58(2):386-95.

1985. Vollmer KO, von Hodenberg A. Metabolism of thymoxamine. III. Structure elucidation of the metabolites and interspecies comparison. Eur. J. Drug Metab. Pharmacokinet. 10(2):139-45.

1986. Watkins JB 3rd, Klaassen CD. Xenobiotic biotransformation in livestock: comparison to other species commonly used in toxicity testing. J. Anim. Sci. 63(3):933-42.

1986. Rousseaux CG, Smith RA, Nicholson S. Acute Pinesol toxicity in a domestic cat. Vet. Hum. Toxicol. 28(4):316-7.

1986. Elegbede JA, Maltzman TH, Verma AK, Tanner MA, Elson CE, Gould MN. Mouse skin tumor promoting activity of orange peel oil and d-limonene: a re-evaluation. Carcinogenesis. 7(12):2047-9.

1986. Hink WF, Fee BJ. Toxicity of D-limonene, the major component of citrus peel oil, to all life stages of the cat flea, Ctenocephalides felis (Siphonaptera: Pulicidae). J. Med. Entomol. Jul 28;23(4):400-4.

1986. Hooser SB, Beasley VR, Everitt JI. Effects of an insecticidal dip containing d-limonene in the cat. J. Am. Vet. Med. Assoc. Oct 15;189(8):905-8.

1988. Powers KA, Hooser SB, Sundberg JP, Beasley VR. An evaluation of the acute toxicity of an insecticidal spray containing linalool, d-limonene, and piperonyl butoxide applied topically to domestic cats. Vet Hum Toxicol. Jun;30(3):206-10.

1988. Hink WF, Liberati TA, Collart MG. Toxicity of linalool to life stages of the cat flea, Ctenocephalides felis (Siphonaptera: Pulicidae), and its efficacy in carpet and on animals. J. Med. Entomol. Jan;25(1):1-4.

1990. Magdalou J, Chajes V, Lafaurie C, Siest G. Glucuronidation of 2-arylpropionic acids pirprofen, flurbiprofen, and ibuprofen by liver microsomes. Drug Metab. Dispos. 18(5):692-7.

1990. Webb DR, Kanerva RL, Hysell DK, Alden CL, Lehman-McKeeman LD. Assessment of the subchronic oral toxicity of d-limonene in dogs. Food Chem Toxicol. Oct;28(10):669-75.

1990. Hooser SB. Toxicology of selected pesticides, drugs, and chemicals. D-limonene, linalool, and crude citrus oil extracts. Vet. Clin North Am Small Anim. Pract. Mar;20(2):383-5. Review.

1992. Frank AA, Ross JL, Sawvell BK. Toxic epidermal necrolysis associated with flea dips. Vet. Hum. Toxicol. Feb;34(1):57-61.

1994. Villar D, Knight MJ, Hansen SR, Buck WB. Toxicity of melaleuca oil and related essential oils applied topically on dogs and cats. Vet. Hum. Toxicol. 36(2):139-42.

1994. Grosjean, Nelly. Veterinary Aromatherapy: Natural remedies for cats, dogs, horses, birds & for the rearing of farm animals. St. Edmundsbury Press, England.

1995. Rosenbaum MR, Kerlin RL. Erythema multiforme major and disseminated intravascular coagulation in a dog following application of a d-limonene-based insecticidal dip. J. Am. Vet. Med. Assoc. Nov 15;207(10):1315-9.

1995. Nicholson SS. Toxicity of Insecticides and Skin Care Products of Botanical Origin. Veterinary Dermatology 6(3).

1997. Court MH and Greenblatt, DJ: Biochemical Basis for Deficient Paracetamol Glucuronidation in Cats: an Interspecies Comparison of Enzyme Constraint in Liver Microsomes. J. Pharm. Pharmacol., 49:466-449.

1997. Court MH, Greenblatt DJ. Molecular basis for deficient acetaminophen glucuronidation in cats. An interspecies comparison of enzyme kinetics in liver microsomes. Biochem. Pharmacol. 53(7):1041-7.

1997. Chauret N, Gauthier A, Martin J, Nicoll-Griffith DA. In vitro comparison of cytochrome P450-mediated metabolic activities in human, dog, cat, and horse. Drug Metab. Dispos. 25(10):1130-6.

1998. Bischoff K, Guale FJ. Australian tea tree (Melaleuca alternifolia) oil poisoning in three purebred cats. Vet. Diagn. Invest. 10(2):208-10.

1999. Guitart R, Manosa S, Guerrero X, Mateo R. Animal poisonings: the 10-year experience of a veterinary analytical toxicology laboratory. Vet. Hum. Toxicol. 41(5):331-5.

2000. Castro E, Soraci A, Fogel F, Tapia O. Chiral inversion of R(-) fenoprofen and ketoprofen enantiomers in cats. J. Vet. Pharmacol. Ther. 23(5):265-71.

2000. Court MH, Greenblatt DJ. Molecular genetic basis for deficient acetaminophen glucuronidation by cats: UGT1A6 is a pseudogene, and evidence for reduced diversity of expressed hepatic UGT1A isoforms. Pharmacogenetics. 10(4):355-69.

2001. Castro EF, Soraci AL, Franci R, Fogel FA, Tapia MO. Disposition of suprofen enantiomers in the cat. Vet. J. 162(1):38-43.

2002. Lee JA, Budgin JB, Mauldin EA. Acute necrotizing dermatitis and septicemia after application of a d-limonene-based insecticidal shampoo in a cat. J Am Vet Med Assoc. Jul 15;221(2):258-62, 239-40.

2002. Leigh Bell, Kristen. Holistic Aromatherapy for Animals: A Comprehensive Guide to the Use of Essential Oils & Hydrosols with Animals. Findhorn Press, Scotland, UK.

2003. Wynn, SG and Marsden, S. Manual of Natural Veterinary Medicine: Science and Tradition. Mosby/Elsevier.

2004. Krishnaswamy S, Hao Q, Von Moltke LL, Greenblatt DJ, Court MH. Evaluation of 5-hydroxytryptophol and other endogenous serotonin (5-hydroxytryptamine) analogs as substrates for UDP-glucuronosyltransferase 1A6. Drug Metab. Dispos. 32(8):862-9.

2005. Robertson, SA. Managing pain in feline patients. Vet. Clin. North Am. Small Anim. Pract. 35(1):129-146.

2006. Tanaka N, Miyasho T, Shinkyo R, Sakaki T, Yokota H. cDNA cloning and characterization of feline CYP1A1 and CYP1A2. Life Sci. 25;79(26):2463-73.

2007. Lascelles BD, Court MH, Hardie EM, Robertson SA. Nonsteroidal anti-inflammatory drugs in cats: a review. Vet. Anaesth. Analg. 34(4):228-50.

2007. Sun J. D-Limonene: safety and clinical applications. Altern. Med. Rev. 12(3):259-64.

2008. Hovda LR. Toxin exposures in small animals. in: Bonagura Jd and Twedt dC (eds). Kirk's current veterinary therapy XIV. Philadelphia: Elsevier Saunders, 2008, pp 92–94

2010. Grave TW, Boag AK. Feline toxicological emergencies: when to suspect and what to do. J. Feline Med. Surg. Nov;12(11):849-60.

2010. Poppenga R. Toxicological Emergencies In: Drobatz KJaC, Merilee F, ed. Feline Emergency and Critical Care Medicine. Aimes, Iowa: Blackwell Publishing, Ltd, 2010.

2011. Rishniw M, Wynn SG. Azodyl, a synbiotic, fails to alter azotemia in cats with chronic kidney disease when sprinkled onto food. J. Fel. Med. Surg. 13(6): 405-409.

2011. Shrestha B1, Reed JM, Starks PT, Kaufman GE, Goldstone JV, Roelke ME, O'Brien SJ, Koepfli KP, Frank LG, Court MH. Evolution of a major drug metabolizing enzyme defect in the domestic cat and other felidae: phylogenetic timing and the role of hypercarnivory. PLoS One. Mar 28;6(3):e18046.

2012. Norrgran J, Jones B, Lindquist NG, Bergman A. Decabromobiphenyl, polybrominated diphenyl ethers, and brominated phenolic compounds in serum of cats diagnosed with the endocrine disease feline hyperthyroidism. Arch. Environ. Contam. Toxicol. 63(1):161-8.

2012. Genovese AG, McLean MK, Khan SA. Adverse reactions from essential oil-containing natural flea products exempted from Environmental Protection Agency regulations in dogs and cats. J. Vet. Emerg. Crit. Care (San Antonio). 22(4):470-5.

2012. McLean MK, Hansen SR. An overview of trends in animal poisoning cases in the United States: 2002-2010. Vet. Clin. North Am. Small Anim. Pract. 42: 219-228.

2012. Caloni F, Cortinovis C, Rivolta M, Davanzo F. Animal poisoning in Italy: 10 years of epidemiological data from the Poison Control Centre of Milan. Vet. Rec. 21;170(16):415.

2013. Moraes TM, Rozza AL, Kushima H, Pellizzon CH, Rocha LR, Hiruma-Lima CA. Healing actions of essential oils from Citrus aurantium and d-limonene in the gastric mucosa: the roles of VEGF, PCNA, and COX-2 in cell proliferation. J. Med. Food. 16(12):1162-7.

2013. Court, MH: Feline drug metabolism and disposition: pharmacokinetic evidence for species differences and molecular mechanisms. Vet. Clin. North Am. Small Anim. Pract., 43(5):1039-1054.

2013. Ebner T, Schänzle G, Weber W, Sent U, Elliott J. In vitro glucuronidation of the angiotensin II receptor antagonist telmisartan in the cat: a comparison with other species. J. Vet. Pharmacol. Ther. 36(2):154-60.

2013. Kim YW, Kim MJ, Chung BY, Bang du Y, Lim SK, Choi SM, Lim DS, Cho MC, Yoon K, Kim HS, Kim KB, Kim YS, Kwack SJ, Lee BM. Safety evaluation and risk assessment of d-Limonene. J. Toxicol. Environ. Health B Crit Rev. 16(1):17-38.

2014. Khan SA, McLean MK, Slater MR. Concentrated tea tree oil toxicosis in dogs and cats: 443 cases (2002-2012). J. Am. Vet. Med. Assoc. 1;244(1):95-99.

2014. Saengtienchai A, Ikenaka Y, Nakayama SM, Mizukawa H, Kakehi M, Bortey-Sam N, Darwish WS, Tsubota T, Terasaki M, Poapolathep A, Ishizuka M. Identification of interspecific differences in phase II reactions: determination of metabolites in the urine of 16 mammalian species exposed to environmental pyrene. Environ. Toxicol. Chem. 33(9):2062-2069.

2014. Van Beusekom CD, Fink-Gremmels J, Schrickx JA. Comparing the glucuronidation capacity of the feline liver with substrate-specific glucuronidation in dogs. J. Vet. Pharmacol. Ther. 37(1):18-24.

2014. Dhibi S, Mbarki S, Elfeki A, Hfaiedh N. Eucalyptus globulus extract protects upon acetaminophen-induced kidney damages in male rat. Bosn J Basic Med Sci. May;14(2):99-104.

2014. McDonnel SJ, Tell LA, Murphy BG. Pharmacokinetics and pharmacodynamics of suberoylanilide hydroxamic acid in cats. J. Vet. Pharmacol. Ther. 37(2):196-200.

2014. Caloni F, Cortinovis C, Pizzo F, Rivolta M, Davanzo F. Epidemiological study (2006-2012) on the poisoning of small animals by human and veterinary drugs. Vet Rec. 1;174(9):222.

2014. Audrain H, Kenward C, Lovell CR, Green C, Ormerod AD, Sansom J, Chowdhury MM, Cooper SM, Johnston GA, Wilkinson M, King C, Stone N, Horne HL, Holden CR, Wakelin S, Buckley DA. Allergy to oxidized limonene and linalool is frequent in the U.K. Br J Dermatol. Aug;171(2):292-7.

2015. Van Beusekom CD, van den Heuvel JJ, Koenderink JB, Russel FG, Schrickx JA. Feline hepatic biotransformation of diazepam: Differences between cats and dogs. Res. Vet. Sci. 103:119-25.

2015. Kakehi M, Ikenaka Y, Nakayama SM, Kawai YK, Watanabe KP, Mizukawa H, Nomiyama K, Tanabe S, Ishizuka M. Uridine Diphosphate-Glucuronosyltransferase (UGT) Xenobiotic Metabolizing Activity and Genetic Evolution in Pinniped Species. Toxicol. Sci. 147(2):360-9.

2015. Addie DD, Boucraut-Baralon C, Egberink H, Frymus T, Gruffydd-Jones T, Hartmann K, Horzinek MC, Hosie MJ, Lloret A, Lutz H, Marsilio F, Pennisi MG, Radford AD, Thiry E, Truyen U, Möstl K. European Advisory Board on Cat Diseases. Disinfectant choices in veterinary practices, shelters and households: ABCD guidelines on safe and effective disinfection for feline environments. J. Fel. Med. Surg. 17(7):594-605.

2015. Ramos CAF, Sá RCDS, Alves MF, Benedito RB, de Sousa DP, Diniz MFFM, Araújo MST, de Almeida RN. Histopathological and biochemical assessment of d-limonene-induced liver injury in rats. Toxicol. Rep. 9;2:482-488.

2016. Redmon JM, Shrestha B, Cerundolo R, Court MH. Soy isoflavone metabolism in cats compared with other species: urinary metabolite concentrations and glucuronidation by liver microsomes. Xenobiotica. 46(5):406-15.

2017. Slovak JE, Mealey K, Court MH: Comparative metabolism of mycophenolic acid by glucuronic acid and glucose conjugation in human, dog, and cat liver microsomes. J. Vet. Pharmacol. Ther. 40(2):123-129.

2017. Mizukawa H, Ikenaka Y, Kakehi M, Nakayama S, Ishizuka M. Characterization of Species Differences in Xenobiotic Metabolism in Non-experimental Animals. Yakugaku Zasshi. 137(3):257-263.

2017. Burnett K, Puschner B, Ramsey JJ, Lin Y, Wei A, Fascetti AJ. Lack of glucuronidation products of trans-resveratrol in plasma and urine of cats. J. Anim. Physiol. Anim. Nutr. (Berl). 101(2):284-292.

Science shows – cats do possess less of the enzymes required for the metabolism of many items. Why do we state specific oils as cautionary for cats? Let's tackle a few.

Citrus oils. These are often listed as toxic to cats for a variety of reasons. A Google search reveals many of these theories, however very little link to any actual data or research. Among claims I found the following statements.
- *Citrus oils contain monoterpene hydrocarbons (limonene) which can be toxic to cats.*
- *d-Limonene and linalool are citrus oils with insecticidal properties. These are metabolized in the liver resulting in liver damage or failure.*
- *Cats are uniquely sensitive to phenolics and other compounds containing benzene rings. Compounds preserved in benzyl alcohol are toxic to cats.*
- *My cat had to be euthanized last January with the symptoms of Essential Oil poisoning, because I had no idea that the Citrus and Pine Oils I was diffusing near her litter box were causing her harm. Until I purchased this book recently, I had no idea that these seemingly harmless oils could be fatal to cats.*
- *Limonene is a terpene that leads to the citrus scent of lemons. D-limonene has been used in dog shampoos and fragrances. The small amount present in dog products is safe for most sizes of dogs. For cats, it can prove lethal. Limonene is also used in flavoring compounds, cosmetic products, and cleaning products. Keep all of these away from your feline.*
- *Citrus Oils: d-limonene and linalool are common citrus oils that be found in a variety of household products, including household and personal fragrances, cleansers, insect repellants, and even pet dips. These oils acts as irritants to the skin and gastric mucosa and commonly cause skin lesions and gastrointestinal upset. Exposure via the dermal or oral route can cause toxicity.*

In actuality – it was pretty difficult to find cases of citrus toxicity in cats. The main toxicity report regarding felines was for d-limonene. With a search PubMed for "limonene toxicity feline" – only three articles were found. One of these articles focused on the toxicity of d-limonene *against* the cat flea, and not actually as toxic to a cat. The other two articles (from 1986 and 1988) related to an insecticidal spray or dip containing d-limonene being applied to cats in high concentrations.

From *"Effects of an insecticidal dip containing d-limonene in the cat"* Journal of the American Veterinary Medical Association, 1986 – the following abstract is quoted:

"A study was undertaken to determine the effects of a single dermal application of a commercial insecticidal dip containing 78.2% d-limonene in cats. At the manufacturer's recommended concentration of 1.5 oz/gal of water, no clinical signs or lesions of toxicosis were seen. At 5 times the recommended concentration, clinical signs were mild and consisted of hypersalivation of short duration, ataxia, and muscle tremors resembling shivering. At 15 times the recommended concentration, clinical signs included hypersalivation lasting 15 to 30 minutes, moderate-to-severe ataxia lasting 1 to 5 hours, muscle tremors resembling shivering lasting 1 to 4 hours, and severe hypothermia beginning soon after treatment and lasting 5 hours. Gross lesions were confined to excoriation of the scrotal and perineal areas of the treated male cats at the 15 X concentration. No deaths or other lasting effects were seen at any dosage."

In general, all cases reported of citrus oil toxicity in cats also maintained that there was dermal exposure to the cats, at 5-10 times the normal concentrations. These were mainly within the dip and spray formulations.

Not related to the metabolism of d-limonene were articles on necrotizing dermatitis and severe skin reactions to the application of products (mainly for fleas) containing d-limonene. This was certainly not the only ingredient within the product, and certainly not obtained directly as an essential oil.

Please see the article from 2007 *"D-Limonene: safety and clinical applications"* for more complete information on safety data regarding d-limonene.

Linalool. In a search for "linalool toxicity feline" only two articles were found. Only one article (shared in the 1988 article *An evaluation of the acute toxicity of an insecticidal spray containing linalool, d-limonene, and piperonyl butoxide applied topically to domestic cats.*) referenced toxicity to cats. While the other article was in regards to linalool having toxic effects against the cat flea again, and not the cat itself.

It would appear, that based on research that linalool and limonene were effective against cat fleas, that someone created a product which did not possibly bode well for the feline population experiencing it. However, it would seem that these articles were taken as a blanket statement to say "no citrus oil, ever" for cats.

Eucalyptus. This oil is often reported as toxic to cats. While the essential oil and eucalyptol (1,8-cineole) is reported as toxic on the ASPCA Toxic and Non-Toxic Plants list, it does not give any further references or information as to why this might be. A search on PubMed does not reveal any associations directly with eucalyptus and animals. It is likely that gross misuse with topical applications or ingestion of the plant has resulted in this listing. Also, no information on species of eucalyptus is provided. While some may show concern for the high 1,8-cineole content of most eucalyptus oil, without gross and toxic misuse of the oil, it does not appear to have extreme toxicity concerns. Research even indicates it being protective against hepatotoxicity (2014 *Eucalyptus globulus extract protects upon acetaminophen-induced kidney damages in male rat.*) Research would appear to support that while topical and oral administrations of this oil should be done with care, diffusion is likely to hold no harm. More information can be found on eucalyptus safety within Tisserand and Young's *Essential Oil Safety* second edition.

Phenols. While research shows that cats have a decreased ability to metabolize phenols, this does not mean that they are completely unable. In the November 1984 edition of *Veterinary Clinics of North America: Small Animal Practice* – Vol. 14, No. 6; titled *Symposium on Advances in Feline Medicine II*, Jeff R. Wilcke DVM, MS states, "Even drugs known for toxicity in cats can be used safely if we are aware of and compensate for certain peculiarities."

In the 2011 article *Azodyl, a synbiotic, fails to alter azotemia in cats with chronic kidney disease when sprinkled onto food.;* Doctors Rishniw and Wynn state the following: "Recently, investigators have examined the ability of probiotic-prebiotic combination (known as 'synbiotic') therapy to aid in reducing azotemia – a process called 'enteric dialysis'. Specific bacteria capable of metabolizing urea, creatinine, indoles, phenol and nitrosamine into non-toxic metabolites, have been selected for this purpose." The statement would indicate that there are alternative methods for phenol metabolism, than simply the liver enzyme pathways that cats possess.

With logical and appropriate use of essential oils containing natural phenol compounds, cats clearly compensate for any reduction in metabolism speed. It again, is all dependent on the dose and frequency of administration. While it may seem logical that cats have lost their ability to metabolize plant related chemicals due to their "hypercarnivory" (2011 Shrestha et.al.) - it is interesting to consider these statements from 2017 *Comparative metabolism of mycophenolic acid by glucuronic acid and glucose conjugation in human, dog, and cat liver microsomes.*

"However, given the major role for glucuronidation...metabolism in humans, there are concerns that the known deficiencies of UGT1A9 (and other UGTs) in cats could also cause deficient MPA glucuronidation, potentially delaying MPA clearance and leading to MPA accumulation and toxicity. Without a good understanding of MPA clearance in cats, it is not possible to determine the dose required to achieve an effective and safe blood concentration in the feline species....we did find significantly slower formation of the MPA phenol glucuronide in cats vs. dogs and humans. However, we also found a much smaller difference in overall metabolism...by conjugation when comparing cat liver microsomes with dog and human liver microsomes despite significantly reduced MPA pheno glucuronide formation in cats. This occurred in large part because of the substantially higher relative contribution of glucosidation to total MPA conjugation in cat liver microsomes (60%) when compared to the dog (34%) and especially the human (2%) liver microsomes."

"Although glucosidation is the major pathway for conjugative metabolism of xenobiotics in nonvertebrate species (including insects and plants), glucuronidation is the dominant conjugative clearance mechanism in all vertebrates studied to date."

"In future studies, one should consider the potential for glucosidation (vs. glucuronidation) as a major alternate clearance pathway for drugs used in cats."

"Our results indicate that cats may express a UGT that has a higher catalytic efficiency for glucosidation of MPA than those expressed by humans and dogs."

These statements would seem to indicate, that while cats are "deficient" in one respect, they excel in others. And the fact that they perform glucosidation so much more efficiently when compared to humans or dogs, shows that they have other pathways of metabolism – even those that are normally more prevalent in insects and plants.

Benzene Rings, Benzyl Alcohol. These are also often listed as toxic to cats, and often are linked with phenol toxicity explanations. The main research that supports this claim is from 1982, when the FDA issued a statement finally claiming *Benzyl alcohol hazardous as a parenteral preservative*. While this substance is related to other chemicals found within essential oils, it is noteworthy that this is a synthetic compound, which was being used as a preservative in intravenous fluids. A much different situation than the proper use within aromatherapy applications. Benzyl alcohol is mainly found in "essential oils" that are not recommended for use with animals – these include Benzoin and other absolutes such as hyacinth, narcissus, violet leaf, champaca, bakul, and jasmine.

Pinene. An alkene hydrocarbon, this constituent is found in over 400 essential oils (Tisserand and Young 2014). While there is a report on Pine-sol toxicity (1986 Acute Pinesol toxicity in a domestic cat) it does appear that possibly this listing is more related to the increased potential of α-pinene containing oils to oxidize and cause increased rates of sensitization and reaction. While again, we should be careful to use fresh, non-damaged essential oils, and use them with proper dilutions and protocols, there did not appear to be an overt reason to avoid the chemical pinene in cats specifically.

Terpineol. Also found listed as contraindicated for cats, it is also "found in a great many essential oils" according to Tisserand and Young. Terpineol does not appear to have basis to avoid in cats specifically.

Single essential oils are also included on lists to avoid with cats. I urge you to find further reading within the reference book *Essential Oil Safety*, second edition by Robert Tisserand and Rodney Young. This book will help you the most when deciphering toxicity concerns and cautions.

Lemon, lime, orange, grapefruit, bergamot, mandarin, tangerine, petitgrain, and neroli all are included on lists as they are in the Citrus class of oils.

Cinnamon, clove, thyme, oregano, savory, and cassia are all higher in Phenols.

Cajuput is high in 1,8-cineole and also contains terpineol.

Camphor is an essential oil, and a chemical constituent found in many essential oils. There is a lot of data contained within Tisserand and Young's Essential Oil Safety on camphor which I encourage you to read. Listings cautioning against the use of camphor, never qualify if it is the constituent or the essential oil they are referring to. In high concentrations, it can pose health risks, and is listed as toxic in regards to humans. Camphor (many species) essential oil is not recommended for use within Veterinary Aromatic Medicine. Camphor as a chemical constituent can be found in small percentages within many essential oils known to be safe for use with animals, however oils high in camphor content, are often not used (Spike Lavender).

Pine (while no species is ever mentioned) contains pinene and terpineol, but is also prone to oxidation issues that can cause increase of dermatitis issues. Fir, Cypress, Juniper, and Spruce are likely included in most of the tree oil or "pine-type" categories to avoid.

Peppermint is often included in lists of oils to be avoided with cats. But research reviews, and even the most respected conservative animal references, rarely list it. Most toxicity or adverse events are from gross misuse and over dosage situations (full undiluted applications).

Tansy is often included in lists to be avoided with cats, again with no apparent justification. While certain species may have shown signs of adverse reactions with gross overuse, Tisserand and Young, Essential Oil Safety list Tansy (Tanacetum vulgare) as "Slightly toxic (oral), non-toxic (dermal)" for animals. The β-Thujone presence in this oil is likely what earns its concern, and listing – which is regarded as moderately toxic. In general, this is an oil that is not recommended for use within Veterinary Aromatic Medicine.

Tea Tree (or Melaleuca alternifolia) is almost always found on cautionary lists, however almost every report of toxicity is gross misuse.

Birch and Wintergreen should be avoided for use with animals due to methyl salicylate content.

Rue often makes the list of oils to avoid, but in actuality it is considered safe by the FDA for human consumption according to Tisserand and Young. While this oil is not commonly used with animals, it has been used within reasonable guidelines. It actually has available safety data with animals, and shows quite safe levels in terms of LD50 measurements. Aromatherapy literature carries much caution for this ketone rich oil, which has been thought to be neurotoxic or cause seizures. However, according to Tisserand and Young "A convulsant effect for rue oil seems unlikely."

There are a few oils that make the list as contraindicated for cats – but truly remain listed as contraindicated for almost all of the aromatherapy world. Bitter Almond, Boldo, Calamus, Garlic, Horseradish, Mustard, Sassafras, Wormseed (Chemopodium), and Pennyroyal are likely to be found on anyone's list of oils that are not commonly used or recommended for use, even with humans.

Clearly, essential oils are not benign substances. They must be respected and used with care. However, when reports of toxicity occur, it is greatly important that further information is provided regarding the case. In veterinary medicine, and with pet poison control centers everywhere, it would be irresponsible and unheard of to not ask further questions about a potential poisoning. However, the questions regarding essential oils and their evaluation are usually not collected in a clinical case. If you called the poison control center about potential rodenticide ingestion, you will immediately be asked for the active ingredients, brand, amount consumed, etc…to help with the evaluation and treatment options.

With essential oil toxicity cases I rarely find that information on the species of oil used, brand, lot number, purchase date, dosage and route to have been collected. This is vastly important to accurate and truthful documentation of valid concerns for every animal lover. Complete blood work and a minimum data base, is also rarely collected, nor compared to earlier values. If someone reports a case of essential oil toxicity to you – please do ask for the medical information. At a minimum I would ask for the species and source of the essential oil, purchase date, how it was used, how long it was used for, prior health concerns for the animal, weight and species of the animal, prior blood work results and status, and current laboratory and physical exam findings. So often, essential oils are the obvious thing to blame when an animal all of a sudden appears ill. And the internet is an easy way to find support of this theory. However, in true clinical evaluation, I often find very poor cause and effect relationships. With the vast number of people using essential oils in their home, we can be quick to get into a trap of blaming any illness upon the presence of essential oils. And this, we need to be careful to avoid. I have consulted with many veterinarians who missed the true diagnosis for weeks, due to the assumption that the essential oils were at the root cause. While I will never say essential oils cannot hurt an animal, we also need to be realistic that when a Facebook post is shared over half a million times, all to animal loving people – the statistics are in the favor of someone also having an animal that falls sick at the time of reading it.

We should be required to obtain more information to prove cause and effect relationships. And I urge you to always look at each research article, Facebook post, reference book, blog, or what-have-you with a critical eye. I often say I need to know more than "My cat was dying, so I applied essential oils and my cat died!" – as proof to a toxicity concern. I greatly sympathize with all of those who are concerned that they have unknowingly injured their animal with the use of essential oils. However, let's not forget that there are many more animal guardians who have compromised the health of their animal with poor diet (causing crystals and stones in urine) or with chronic use of fabric softeners, air fresheners, or second hand smoke. I merely urge a stance of critical evaluation, instead of fear-based and poorly documented reports and concerns.

METABOLIC PATHWAYS

Metabolism occurs in almost every process in our body. The body performs metabolization to help eliminate substances that have entered the body. These substances leave our body (excretion) in the form of urine and stool most commonly. But getting your food from your mouth, into your urine or stool is the process that metabolism is responsible for.

To enter our urine via the kidneys, substances requiring excretion need to be made water soluble. Eat some asparagus, and you will know pretty quickly that some sort of metabolite has entered your urine. Some metabolic processes focus on elimination of metabolites in the bile, and thus the stool.

You may have heard of Phase 1 and Phase 2 metabolism. Phase 1 utilizes the Cytochrome P_{450} Enzymes to enable oxidation, reduction, hydrolysis, hydration, and dehalogenation reactions. Basically, the body is adding or subtracting from a molecule to make it easier to excrete, or to deactivate any toxicity that might be present for the item. CYP_{450} enzymes are found in many tissues of the body including the liver, gastrointestinal tract, and skin.

Some drugs, herbs, or other nutrients can in fact up-regulate (induce) or down-regulate (inhibit) these enzymatic reactions. These changes are not necessarily good or bad – some can be viewed from either side of the fence. Milk Thistle is often considered beneficial for the liver, and can induce CYP enzymes. It all depends on what we would like for the body to do, and how we would like metabolites to be processed and dealt with.

In veterinary medicine, grapefruit juice was intentionally utilized to reduce the drug metabolism of cyclosporine, lowering its dosage requirement and making it more cost effective to use. Furanocoumarins within grapefruit juice, inhibit the CYP_3A_4 enzymes found in the liver and gastrointestinal tract. Through this action, there are several ways that Furanocoumarins can act to increase the presence of a drug. First, if drug metabolism by these enzymes in the intestinal wall is slowed down, more of the drug can actually be absorbed via the intestines. Next, if the Furanocoumarins cause the enzymes in the liver to metabolize less of the drug, there can be increased blood levels of the drug for a longer period of time. This is embraced in some aspects of natural medicine, while in the human markets it is often avoided. Of course, what pharmacology company would want you to use LESS drug, based on the healthy fact that you drink Grapefruit juice!

Speaking of Grapefruit and Furanocoumarins, now is a great time to mention that essential oils do not carry enough Furanocoumarins to affect this process, which is actually unfortunate. I am certain that it would be an easier route to use than getting a dog to consume a lot of grapefruit or grapefruit juice!

Again, it is important to remember that the body does not metabolize the whole essential oil, but it metabolizes each individual component separately. There are several essential oil constituents that have been mapped for the CYP enzymes they utilize. Limonene uses CYP_2C_9 and CYP_2C_{19}. Camphor uses CYP_2A_6. Myristicin uses CYP_3A_4 and CYP_1A_2. Thujone uses CYP_2A_6. However, until a large "pharma" company is interested in the use of a constituent, it is unlikely to be fully mapped and evaluated in research settings. The cost benefit ratio of this knowledge, is just not there for general public information.

Phase 2 metabolism consists of the Conjugation Pathways; methylation, acetylation, amino acid conjugation, glutathione conjugation, glucuronidation, and sulfation. These processes help to make water-soluble wastes that will be eliminated via the urine, bile, or stool. Glucuronidation is the most common Phase 2 reaction used, and according to Robert Tisserand and Rodney Young in their book Essential Oil Safety (2nd Edition) – many essential oil constituents fall into the categories of molecules that will be eliminated from the body at least in part by glucuronides and the glucuronidation process. These substances, or conjugates, are often then excreted in the urine, or enter the gastrointestinal tract (via bile for example) to be eliminated from the body.

Sulfation is also an important Phase 2 metabolic reaction. Catalyzed by sulfotransferase enzymes in the liver and other organs, it creates more polar, water soluble type metabolites, which would then often be excreted in urine.

We can also hear a lot about Glutathione. This is a very popular pathway to talk about, and it is responsible for the elimination of many toxic substances from the body. Free radicals and damaging molecules are often eliminated by Glutathione conjugation. So Glutathione is considered a very protective agent for the body. The liver is the main organ that performs Glutathione conjugation. In many research articles, you may read of Glutathione induction or modulation. Glutathione S-transferase is also a common phrase you will encounter. When you see these references, it is important to note that Glutathione or Glutathione S-transferase "induction" means that we are increasing its efficiency or its rate of synthesis or turn over. In essence – this is a good thing. Offering more protection to the liver, and a higher clearance of potentially toxic substances from the body.

Constituents of essential oils that are known to induce Glutathione S-transferase include Anethofuran, Benzyl isothiocyanate, (+)-Carvone, β-Caryophyllene, β-Caryophyllene oxide, Citral, Diallyl disulfide, Diallyl trisulfide, Eugenol, Geraniol, α-Humulene, (+)-Limonene, Methyl allyl trisulfide, Myristicin.

Essential oils which are known to induce Glutathione S-transferase (so these would be considered liver protective) include Ambrette, Angelica Root, Basil (multiple types), Bergamot, Caraway, Cardamom, Celery Seed, Chamomile, Coriander Seed, Cumin, Dill Weed, Eucalyptus, Fennel, Galangal, Garlic, Ginger, Grapefruit, Hop, Lemon, Lemongrass, Lime, Nutmeg, Orange, Oregano, Peppermint, Sandalwood, Spearmint, Tangerine, and Thyme. In research articles, it is often unspecified as to the direct species or chemotype of the essential oil used. Which is a huge frustration for medical research.

It is also important to recognize, that even if an essential oil or essential oil constituent is reported to be hepato (or liver) protective – it does not automatically guarantee that the essential oil is appropriate for use with animals. We should always strive to find and use the most animal appropriate oil for a situation, and hopefully one with a known use with animals and some clinical data in relation with it. When there is such a long list of potential essential oils available to help with a situation or condition we desire to benefit – we should always look at the list and filter out uncommon or more "harsh" oils. For example, for a cat, if I wanted to use the benefits of Glutathione induction – I would like to select the most feline appropriate oils from that above list, and also consider the routes of exposure that are appropriate for a feline, as well as if the cat would find it the most "cat-friendly". We do use Oregano and Thyme quite often in cats, in low concentrations. But there are likely not as many cats that would prefer a topical application of say Lime or Spearmint. Although, we may find that diffusion of some of these oils, could be attractive in the home, and still beneficial on some level.

There is also metabolism of essential oils within the skin. Dermal enzymes can perform both Phase 1 and Phase 2 reactions. In general the skin is less efficient, or metabolizes less, than the enzymes found in the liver. There are also species differences in the amount of dermal metabolism that may occur, so we need to consider this when generalizing research between species (humans included).

Compounds may have different isomers as well. And these isomers may utilize a different metabolic pathway from their "twin."

There are other considerations in metabolism as well. In humans, there has been note of different genetics possessing different enzyme abilities. Both ethnicity (some human European ancestry being deficient in CYP2D6 enzymes) and gender differences have been studied, and do not appear to be a rarity among the human population. This study is termed pharmacogenetics – and certainly it is likely to have an extension into the animal kingdom, not only in terms of species variations, but also with age, breed and sex.

DETOXIFICATION

What the heck is detoxification? This may just be one of the most overused and least understood term in the "aromatherapy" world today. Unfortunately, it has become a common phrase to explain why anyone (human or animal) may be having an adverse reaction or event regarding the use of essential oils. Did someone experience redness or a rash in relation to an essential oil application? Well then, GOOD FOR YOU! You are "detoxing" and you should be so happy! Well, not so much.

We often hear about a "healing crisis" in the world of natural medicine. But what does that mean, and should we have to experience it to promote health? I too, was lead to believe that this was a good thing, and evidence of the fact that we had initiated some sort of bodily reaction indicating that we were "moving" health in new direction. However, over time and with a ton of experience, you start to realize that we do not need to push the body to any sort of extreme, especially one that creates inflammation or displeasure to experience increased healing or health.

In the medical sense, detoxification would include things like the removal of toxic substances, the conversion of free radicals, or the repair of damaged tissues and cells. In a chemistry sense, detoxification may include the conversion of molecules to less toxic substances, which enable them to be eliminated or excreted from the body.

When people term an event "detoxing" – they are often referring to things like diarrhea, sweating, redness of the skin, rashes, blemishes, congestion, sneezing, headaches, etc. To me, these are all signs of the body's limited ability to excrete by-products of metabolism. For animals, these events could be similar. A common "detoxification event" that was considered beneficial in the past, was hives created on horses after topical applications of essential oils. While I did see clear clinical improvement in these horses that developed "welts" in response to an application, I also saw improvement in horses whose body was not overwhelmed with over-aggressive applications. And, while it did seem to hold true that once a horse gained better health, they created less welts or hives in response to essential oil use, it most certainly is not a "necessity" to create the hives, nor is it desirable when the end result is still the same.

Do not be fooled into the detoxification trap. It is not an event that we desire to go along with essential oil use. It is not necessary to gain health. And healing should never be an uncomfortable event. If we feel that we are having a "detoxification" reaction in response to oil use – it is most likely true that we should be using less essential oils, in lesser concentrations, or in different methods of application.

EXCRETION

After an essential oil constituent is metabolized, it is excreted in a variety of ways. The variation of which excretion pathway is utilized can be an important function in the effects of a particular essential oil.

Excretion will primarily occur from the kidneys, liver, lungs, and skin. The kidney is likely the most important organ of excretion when we consider essential oil metabolism. There can be variations based on the route of absorption of the essential oil as well. Essential oil constituents that are inhaled (diffusion) may use exhalation as the more common route of excretion, and some studies of essential oil constituent metabolism have shown no or minor presence of metabolites in feces or urine after inhalation.

Most excretion of essential oil metabolites will occur through the stool (in bile) and the urine. We can use some of these facts when we consider the target tissue we would like to expose to essential oil constituents. Carvacrol, found within Oregano oil for example, is rapidly excreted through the urine. As Carvacrol is also a potent antioxidant and strongly antibacterial, we can benefit from its presence in the urine as a therapeutic agent.

Elimination of essential oils however is quite fast. While there are not a lot of studies, it does appear that essential oil constituents are rapidly eliminated from the body. For constituents for which there is known data, elimination is recorded in terms of hours. In most research, almost all of the essential oils given (by a variety of routes including oral, intravenous, dermal) are eliminated completely from the body in under 72 hours, and often within 24 hours.

These times of elimination are often referred to as a "half-life". And it generally refers to the time it takes to eliminate, convert, or metabolize half of the substance that has been absorbed or administrated. What's important to recognize in terms of Veterinary Aromatic Medicine, is that the half-life of most essential oils is quite fast and efficient. It would be unusual for us to find significant levels of essential oil constituents within a body after 3 days (or 72 hours) of an application or administration.

Your take home points. Since the kidneys will be excreting a large portion of the metabolites of essential oil use, hydration is important. If you are administering essential oils to an already dehydrated animal, the likelihood of making them feel poorly, or cause a "healing crisis" will remain higher. If I am interested in treating a cat with renal (kidney) disease, that is already a bit compromised, not feeling well, and a bit dehydrated. My best course of action would be to hydrate the cat prior to introducing essential oil therapies. This would be a standard recommendation for all species. Hydration is important.

ABSORPTION

But how did the essential oil get into the body in the first place? There are actually several routes by which essential oils will enter the body.

The mildest method of absorption is likely inhalation. Although, I would not say that this is the least powerful. Inhalation can be from smelling from a bottle, from hands and other items such as diffuser necklaces or collar attachments, or by diffusion from some sort of apparatus. Diffusion to me, is the most important route of inhalation absorption.

Absorption can occur through many methods. Through the dermis or skin, through the buccal or mucous membranes, through the gastrointestinal (GI) tract (orally), through the lungs via inhalation, through the rectal tissues, through vaginal tissues, and essential oils have been injected or administered via intravenous solutions – which to some extent eliminate some of the need for absorption to actually occur. Although, even if an essential oil is injected into a cavity (intraperitoneal or IP injections are common in animal research), tissue, or directly into a vein, there is an amount of absorption that will occur within the surrounding tissues.

Absorption does not necessarily equate to the method of delivery however. Absorption is more about the presence of the essential oil in tissues after exposure to them. The amount of absorption that occurs, may depend greatly on the route of administration of the essential oil, the dose of the essential oil, how frequent the essential oil is given, and for how long the essential oil is given.

There are variables involved with the type of essential oil as well. Some essential oil constituents may be more readily absorbed through a certain route, such as inhalation versus dermal absorption. Other variables involve the subject (animal, skin, etc…) itself. So for instance, some species of animals may be more likely to absorb a higher amount of essential oils from a dermal (skin, fur) application than other species.

While skin that is heated or broken (open wounds) may absorb more essential oil than normal healed skin – hair follicle density in animals may play an important role in how much essential oil they absorb; and should factor into our calculations on dosages and exposure rates for certain species.

I was at a lecture discussing human transdermal absorption of essential oils when the light bulb clicked on in my head. The discussion was about hair follicles and how the sebum and sebaceous glands seem to have function in the distribution and absorption of fat soluble (lipophilic) essential oil constituents. In laymen's terms, the grease on our skin and in our hair follicles, is just what essential oils dissolve into better. They like fats, and so the fact that our skin and hair contains fatty sebum – will aid in the absorption of essential oils.

My light bulb involved the relation of the density and presence of hair follicles in different species. I leaned over to a colleague and whispered, "That's it! That's why Chinchillas are more sensitive to essential oil absorption than Horses, Cats, or Dogs!" Each animal species has a different number of hair follicles per square inch of skin. The fact that almost all animals have more hair follicles than humans, can help to explain why they may seem more sensitive to essential oil administration than humans. They simply can absorb more of it.

But when we look across the line of animal species, certainly we see that a horse or cow is much more tolerant and "less sensitive" to essential oil applications than a dog. And a dog more tolerant than a cat. And a cat more tolerant than a chinchilla or rabbit. The softer, more dense hair coats, have more hair follicles present in the skin. This means there are more "free-way on-ramps" for the essential oils to enter the body, through the skin. We simply need to take this into account when considering dosages, frequency of application, and routes of application or exposure.

For some of these much more sensitive species such as a chinchilla or rabbit, it can hold true that diffusion of the essential oil can indeed be absorbed through these multitudes of hair follicles. And so even essential oils present in the air can permeate fur, and be absorbed transdermally.

In general, we need to consider a few main factors regarding absorption when considering animals. The route of administration, the type or size of molecules of the essential oils, the carrier the essential oil may be within and the concentration of that solution, and the status, health, or hair follicle density of the animal skin in question. Then we need to consider the individual routes themselves.

Inhalation

I feel that this is one of the most important routes of absorption and essential oil exposure for animals. It is incredibly safe when high quality essential oils are used, and incredibly easy as we do not even have to touch the animal to administer. The lungs have a large surface area of exposure to the air and our blood supply. As their primary function is to absorb oxygen into our body, they obviously have efficient systems in place for the transfer of molecules.

The complication with inhalation of essential oils is the fact that we cannot always accurately determine the amount of essential oil present in the air, nor can we know for sure the amount inhaled and absorbed into the body. However, clinically we find that when essential oils are diffused through a diffusion system that utilizes water, and with a few rules and precautions in place – inhalation becomes a highly effective and highly safe method of exposure.

We do need to remain realistic about what inhalation can deliver however. Certainly inhalation of essential oils for nausea, can indeed result in less nausea. Inhalation of oils for stress and anxiety, can indeed lower blood pressure and result in a calmer state. But, when we start to wonder if diffusion of essential oils will help the aches and pains associated with chronic arthritis or more physical forms of pain – I do think we need to start to draw the line. Although the removal of the emotional and stress component of physical pain is still important and helpful, I would still default to the fact that oral or dermal administration of essential oils for more physical based musculoskeletal concerns (arthritis) is going to be far more consistent and effective.

The amount of essential oil absorbed into the blood stream or tissues of concern, after inhalation is not fully known. While there are several studies that look at this issue, there is not any hard data to state how we should be administering inhalation exactly. However, the truth remains that this route is useful, effective, and very, very safe when certain guidelines are followed (see the diffusion chapter).

My favorite part of inhalation of essential oils, relates to their metabolism and/or excretion from the lungs. In essence, certain essential oil constituents may be converted to more active molecules by enzymes contained directly within the lung tissue, and when the lung excretes the essential oils it was exposed to, we get a secondary therapeutic factor.

I call this…Therapeutic Mucus. Yep, you heard me. Sort of gross to think about, but I'll explain in simple terms. The essential oil is inhaled into the lungs. Some is absorbed into the blood stream, some is metabolized in different areas of the body including the lung, and most is likely exhaled or excreted at the lung location. Just like with a dust particle, when it is inhaled, it is trapped in mucous, and tiny little cilia (hairs) on the cells lining the respiratory tract move the particle up and out of the lungs and airways. Sort of a little conveyor belt of elimination. But, the glory of this conveyor belt… It is now exposing the surface of the respiratory tract to essential oils AGAIN! So the essential oils went in via inhalation, and then they are indeed coming back up! Then (try not to think about this too much) – when the mucus reaches the top…we tend to swallow it (animals and humans). And then we are ingesting the essential oil as well, in teeny tiny amounts. However, what I feel as still beneficial.

The avian species (birds) have an even more unique system. While they are less in the way of mucus producers, they have a different anatomical trait of air sacs. Basically, birds have different chambers throughout their body – and when they breathe – they basically breathe twice for each breath. While this system makes them lighter for flying, and is highly efficient for their high metabolism and absorption of oxygen, air sacs do lack certain qualities. Unfortunately, they are quite deficient in blood supply. So when a fungal or bacterial infection settles into an actual air sac chamber, it is difficult for traditional medications to penetrate to the location. With this fact, diffusion becomes even more beneficial for birds who are experiencing respiratory issues. We can get the essential oil into the air sac, where normal body circulation is less likely to reach.

When we consider all of the potential physical benefits of essential oils – anti-inflammatory, antifungal, antibacterial, reparative, mucolytic, antispasmodic, anti-viral – the ability for effects to be directly on the respiratory system is profound. Even in a situation such as collapsing trachea, while we do not expect to correct the physical issue of the weak and collapsing structural tissues, we most certainly can reduce the inflammation caused by the touching of tissues together, the spasm and irritation created, and promote better overall comfort by inhalation of essential oils.

The absorption of essential oils via inhalation, also bypasses what is known as First Pass Metabolism.

First Pass Metabolism

This is an important concept to understand regarding different routes of administration. First Pass Metabolism is the event in which the essential oil is exposed to metabolism in the liver, prior to ever reaching any sort of bodily destination. When you swallow an essential oil into the stomach – vessels in the stomach go directly to the liver first. Therefore, ingested essential oils are subjected to a large amount of first pass metabolism. This means that much less of the essential oil is available to benefit the body, and is already metabolized and beginning the excretion process before it was ever able to make an effect.

First pass metabolism decreases the bioavailability of the essential oil within the body, and will lower therapeutic effects. The oral route (swallowing) is one of the routes of administration most affected by first pass metabolism. However, buccal (oral absorption) through the mucous membranes is not the same. Sublingual (under the tongue) or buccal absorption from the mouth bypasses the first pass metabolism, resulting in more essential oil to be available for use within the body. It is unknown exactly how much essential oil is metabolized and how much reaches the intended tissues with oral ingestion of essential oils. While we do still see effects systemically with oral administration, we should strive for the use of other routes if they are effective.

Routes that avoid First Pass Metabolism include dermal absorption, inhalation, sublingual or buccal, and vaginal administration. Rectal administration has a variable amount of first pass metabolism based upon which rectal vein absorbs the essential oil. Essential oils absorbed into the Superior Rectal Vein are delivered directly to the liver first, and begin undergoing metabolism. The location in which the essential oils are instilled within a rectum, can affect how much of the essential oil is absorbed into that vein or not. Approximately two thirds (2/3) of the essential oils administered rectally avoid first pass metabolism. Or stated in another way, when infusing essential oils rectally, approximately 1/3 of the essential oil is lost to metabolism before it can act in the body.

With animals, we are most likely to use the routes of inhalation, topical absorption, oral ingestion, and buccal absorption to some extent. For most small animal care givers, infusions of essential oils into the rectum or vagina are less likely. For large animals such as cattle or horses, with vaginal infections or conditions, certainly infusion into the reproductive tracts is more common and likely to be highly beneficial. For small animals, I would caution to avoid vaginal administration unless under the distinct care of an experienced veterinarian. Rectal administrations can be given, and some people have found this easier than the oral route. The rectal route also carries with it some benefits for the lungs and respiratory system.

In summary – first pass metabolism occurs when an essential oil is directed to the liver prior to reaching other parts of the body. Both oral swallowing of essential oils, and rectal absorption of essential oils are subject to first pass metabolism, with oral swallowing to be the most affected. First pass metabolism reduces the amount of essential oil available to the rest of the body, and is dependent on the route of administration.

Buccal & Sublingual Absorption

This can be a bit harder to accomplish in some animals. Often in the veterinary hospital, we could drip an essential oil under the tongue or within the cheek of an animal awaking anesthesia with relative ease. However, in an awake animal, we may be limited to how much we can perform this absorption method. Several of the ways we utilize absorption through the mucous membranes of the mouth is through applying essential oils to the gums or inside of the mouth without the direct hope of them being swallowed.

For dogs, we may rub an essential oil onto the gums (in a carrier oil) or they could even lick essential oils from a drinking bowl, creating a coating of essential oil on their tongue. Even the use of essential oils with oral gels or toothpastes can result in some buccal absorption. With horses, we often pull out their bottom lip and deposit an amount of essential oil in the pocket created, to be absorbed through the buccal membrane. With cats, the act of grooming essential oils off of their hair coat, is likely to utilize absorption through the mucus membranes than it is with true ingestion.

Dermal Absorption

This pertains to any access an essential oil may have to the skin. Whether in a water mist, in a shampoo, gel, ointment, or carrier oil – any essential oil, including that which is diffused into the air – may have contact with the skin, hair, or hair follicles – and result in some absorption into the body.

Sometimes our hope for topical administration is more for a local effect. We may be trying to decrease inflammation or speed healing in the targeted tissue at the application site. But for many animals, we may be applying essential oils topically for a more systemic physical effect. So oils dripped onto the back, may indeed be with hopes of supporting liver health – and the oils were not required to be applied directly over the liver location. However, a sprain or ligament injury to a leg, may call for a direct application to that leg or area of injury. It is wonderful though, that applications of essential oils do not necessarily have to be at the site of the issue, to be effective.

Dermal application has several advantages to consider. One it is very convenient. Animals for the most part, are used to being touched, and so application by petting or dripping on and massaging in, are readily accepted and fairly easy to do. With dermal or topical application, we can see localized actions at the site of application, as well as throughout the body. Topical applications avoid first pass metabolism, and can also impart the benefits of "aromatherapy" or the effect of scent to emotions and even other aspects of inhalation exposure and absorption.

In some ways, dermal or topical applications can also have a negative aspect when we consider scent. Some animals or humans may be adverse to the odor. And in general, topical applications do have less systemic absorption than other routes. However, with animals, the act of grooming or licking, can greatly enhance the ability of a topical application to act systemically. Topical applications do have the potential for skin irritations, so we also must be mindful of this fact.

Oral Administration

This will generally consist of the consumption, or ingestion of essential oils. It can mean they are in a capsule, in a carrier, or even in foods. The essential oil enters the gastrointestinal tract to be absorbed, instead of being absorbed through the membranes of the mouth. Essential oils that enter the GI tract are subject to first pass metabolism by the liver. So much less of the essential oil is available to the body than via other routes of absorption. We don't exactly know how much of the essential oil is available intact after oral administration.

The odd part to consider of oral administration – is that a high percentage of the essential oil IS absorbed from this manner. However, it is absorbed then quickly taken directly to the liver. So there needs to be a bit of differentiation between absorption and bioavailability. One does not always equal the other. While it is typically assumed that 100% of an essential oil entering the GI tract is "absorbed" – that does not mean that 100% of that dose is active or available for the body to benefit from.

If we follow along the path of an orally given essential oil bolus (say a capsule) – we will see the following. The capsule is swallowed. The capsule breaks open in the stomach (usually) and the essential oil is released into the stomach. Some digestive enzymes may break down certain constituents, while other constituents are absorbed through the mucous membranes of the GI tract, into the blood stream, and then shuttled immediately to the liver for processing. In the liver, a significant portion of the molecules are deactivated or changed within the liver, and prepared for excretion into the urine (by the kidneys) or the bile (stool). This makes oral dosing a bit problematic, as we truly do not have accurate knowledge of how much essential oil remains to be active within the body after oral administration. Much more care should be given to this route of administration.

It has become a bit of a popular misconception that oral administration is necessary or superior in some way for animals, and likely this holds true on the human front as well. The actual use theory that I have become fond of – is to use the easiest and least problematic route of administration for each animal, until it shows that it is not effective enough. Basically, do not jump right to oral administration when topical application may do.

There are complications to oral administration of essential oils in animals. Gastrointestinal irritations are common, however rarely noted for what they truly are. I have witnessed so many cases of "GI burnout" due to the belief that a dog with cancer needed capsules upon capsules of Frankincense given orally. Sadly, many of these cases never even attempted to use the Frankincense in diffusion, topically, or through any of the mucous membranes prior to the excessive oral administration. In truth, it is more likely that these cases could have used less essential oil, and experienced even more benefits with fewer side effects with other routes of administration. Even rectal administration would be more beneficial in terms of bioavailability and lack of side effects.

The strong taste of essential oils is another aspect we need to consider when administering orally. Although there are a few essential oils that we add to foods regularly, in general the strong taste and smell require some consideration if they are to be added to items for ingestion. Most essential oils added into food should either use the food item as a "diluent" or carrier for the essential oil, or the essential oil should be added into an ingestible carrier oil (like raw or fractionated coconut oil) before it is mixed into the food. One drop placed directly into a bowl of dog food, will have a very strong "epicenter" of fragrance and taste. Causing most dogs to avoid the food.

However, if we mix the essential oil into some raw coconut oil, then mix that with a bone broth or other sort of soft, moist food item – it becomes diluted properly throughout the entire meal, and is much more likely to be consumed easily.

While there are certain essential oils which are more commonly given via the oral route, note that this route is likely to be less commonly used than we previously thought necessary. Those recommending oral use of essential oils as a first course of action, should be looked at with a cautious view.

Rectal administration

While this can be a viable route of administration of oils to animals, it has its draw backs for obvious reasons. Most animal care takers are not equipped to deal with the "rear entrance" of their animal. Without saying, it is certainly least appropriate for use with small animals such as cats, lizards, birds, and other critters. Dogs are likely the most common species in which we see rectal administration. Larger animals such as cattle or horses, have such large rectal areas, that instillation of a suppository would often be "lost" or passed quickly within the stool.

The rectal lining can become quite irritated from exposure to essential oils as well – so caution should be used. See the chapter on Rectal Instillation for more details on technique.

With Rectal administration approximately 1/3 (or more) of the administered essential oils will be subject to first pass metabolism before reaching the rest of the body, if it reaches the rest of the body.

Rectal administration is most commonly noted as being beneficial for lung conditions – as circulation from this route, will travel to the lungs prior to visiting the liver for considerable metabolism.

SENSITIZATION

There are some factors in absorption and use of essential oils, which can contribute to sensitization of humans to certain essential oils and essential oil constituents. To this date, I would say that the sensitization process appears to be more limited to the human animal species, than to our companions with fur, fins, or feathers. However, since humans will often be in contact with the essential oils their animals are using, we do need to have a clear understanding of sensitization.

For humans in contact with essential oils – the hands and feet actually carry the thickest layers of stratum corneum (skin) – making these surfaces less penetrable than other areas of skin. So basically, absorption through hands and feet is actually less – which may be why feet are often promoted as the "safer" location in which to apply essential oils to humans – especially oils noted to be "hot" in nature. Also present in the palms and soles of the feet – is a layer called the stratum lucidum – which likely provides an extra layer of resistance to penetration. Because most humans will be applying animal related products or blends with their hands – these factors make human exposure to blends, a bit less absorptive in nature, than the application to the animal.

Please read more on the application of essential oils to animal feet (especially paws of cats and dogs) – as they are not similar to our feet. Dog and cat paws contain sweat glands, and the nature of their tissues is more similar to our armpits. And so, if you have ever applied a "hot" essential oil into your armpit – you would sympathize why this route of application, is mainly frowned upon as a "good route" for animals.

Many people can confuse allergies with sensitization. Sensitization to a chemical is far different than an allergy to it. And a chemical irritation is also far different than a true sensitization or allergic response. What can be seen with certain essential oils, is that some individual chemicals can bind with hapten molecules within our body, to elicit a Type IV Hypersensitivity response. This is the similar response as our body has to Poison Ivy. It does not happen with the very first exposure, and may in fact take years to become evident. Then, the exposure tends to be dose related as to the severity of the reaction.

The reaction can be quite severe in some situations, and certainly some oils show more of a risk factor for eliciting a hapten reaction. Oxidized (older, poorly stored or handled essential oils), aldehydes, and absolutes seem to carry more risk in becoming a "hapten." Absolutes are derived by chemical means, and are not a true essential oil. Please see the chapter regarding Oil Collection Methods for more information on Absolutes.

Essential oils with a reputation for being more prone to causing Sensitization include: Cassia, Cinnamon Bark, Cinnamon Leaf, Clove Bud, Clove Leaf, Clove Stem, Holy Basil, Lemon Myrtle, Lemongrass, Lemon-Scented Tea Tree, Melissa, Opoponax (often an absolute), Peru Balsam, and Sage. Some may not be listed, while others are only listed due to their high citral or eugenol content, or other suspect constituents. Some of these oils have not had a clear link to a sensitization event, but are considered more likely. Most of the oils of caution, are more "intense" in nature, and can often be recognized for the caution they are due.

Limonene has been reported as a constituent that can actually decrease the effects of some sensitizing oils. Theories to this fact, are related somewhat into that Limonene is a dermal penetration enhancer. Anything that is brought through the skin faster, has less time to form compounds within the skin itself, or to be recognized. Therefore, decreasing its possible hapten complex and response. There are other molecules that enhance dermal absorption as well, and it may be this reason that the more full and complete essential oils, seem to cause less problems in terms of "reactions" than with chemically altered or laboratory created essential oils.

My curiosity is certainly piqued as to if sensitization will start to be seen as a larger "toxicity" issue in the animal world, especially as diffusion and use of synthetic and fragrance "essential oils" becomes more and more wide spread. In fact, I wonder if the "sensitization" and chemical irritation to poor grades will become almost one and the same. Imagine this – a chemical may indeed be able to act as a hapten, but it may also directly irritate the respiratory tract. If air freshener companies continue to market to the essential oil world, with their synthetic and obviously fragrance grade products – could we see even more irritations and thus sensitizations to these chemicals, which are certain to be labeled as toxicity? I think so.

Sensitization can apparently get better with time. The majority of humans I know who have become sensitized, actually include a larger portion of "careful" human aromatherapists and chemists. There is not always any known rhyme or reason to what, when, or how much is necessary for a sensitization situation to occur. I encourage you to read Tisserand & Young's Essential Oil Safety second edition for further information on sensitization, contact dermatitis, and other safety issues concerning essential oils and the science behind it. However, in work with animals, it appears that when we observe proper use methods for the animals, humans should well be within recommended safety dilutions and protocols with essential oils.

DRUG INTERACTIONS

We must always be concerned of the potential for essential oil use to interact with other medications that are being given to an animal. There is a wealth of information regarding this topic within Tisserand & Young's *Essential Oil Safety* – second edition.

While I respect the ability of some essential oils to alter the speed in which another drug may be metabolized, or to increase the expected effects of a drug we are using (wintergreen with anticoagulants) – the fact remains that with proper use of essential oils as described in this book – we have never witnessed a clinically significant adverse interaction with medications and essential oils.

I am not saying that with improper usage, we do not see issues. I have witnessed animals orally given inappropriate amounts of oil blends containing anti-coagulant oils – which have increased bleeding tendencies. However, you'll note that within this book – there is not an excessive recommendation towards certain administrations. The previous edition of this book focused on what had been used without causing harm, and so valuable information on "maximum" possible doses were included as the current knowledge.

As information grows and changes, we can change our approach to more of what is the "best" or more appropriate administration, route, or dosage – not just "we've given this much before and no one died!" As data is collected, we most certainly see this trend in veterinary medicine and all portions of medicine really, even human aromatherapy. LD50 measurements are certainly common in the human world – when any product or "chemical" may be introduced onto the market. Basically, it is a determination of how much of an essential oil may be necessary to kill (LD means Lethal Dose) 50% of your research subjects. What a horrible, horrible thing in actuality. Most of the time, it is done on rats, and this is supposed to give us valuable information on if Cinnamon oil is indeed safe to add to your toothpaste.

But, if we look at how knowledge evolves, then we notice that we often start with the information regarding a maximum dose that can be used, while still remaining safe. This really seems to exist for many traditional medications in the animal and human world. I remember seeing many new traditional drugs enter the veterinary market, which later went on to have dosing recommendations change drastically – usually lowering them. We find through experience, that lower doses may be safer or indeed still just as effective. I feel this is where the art of Veterinary Aromatic Medicine lies. Starting with reference point of what we have seen to be safe, but then modifying it to the "lowest effective dose" we can use.

Most certainly drug interactions will be more of a concern with oral administrations of essential oils, and with larger amounts of essential oil use. Most essential oils, such as wintergreen, which have a more accurate concern for drug interactions or even the worsening of certain conditions – are simply no longer recommended for use with animals.

There is some research now even showing that essential oils may act synergistically with traditional medications. In the research article *"Synergy between essential oil components and antibiotics: a review."* (Crit Rev Microbiol. 2014 Feb;40(1):76-94.) – Langeveld et al. state "EOs containing carvacrol, cinnamaldehyde, cinnamic acid, eugenol and thymol can have a synergistic effect in combination with antibiotics."

To me, I have always witnessed a synergistic result when I use essential oils properly with any traditional medication regime. Whether it is steroids, chemotherapy, thyroid medications, or antibiotics; I truly find that not only does the patient tolerate traditional medications better, but we may indeed be able to use less of the traditional medication. To me, this is not an adverse drug reaction. Any opportunity to decrease my need for potentially harmful medications with side effects, is a win in my book. However, in the human world, we are often made fearful of the fact that a drug may become more "powerful" while we use a natural substance.

I am just not one of those people. I can feel firsthand how diet affects me. If I eat sugar and gluten, my joints hurt horribly. I "could" continue to eat those things, and load myself up with a ton of anti-inflammatory drugs, as is the typical Band-Aid applied by traditionally minded doctors. Don't improve your life so you don't have fibromyalgia. No, instead just take this drug, and this drug, and this drug. To me, the addition of essential oils which may reduce my need to use traditional medications, will never be a drug interaction. It will be a huge benefit instead.

If you follow the instructions and suggestions for use within this book, I have no qualms that any medication your animal may be taking will create a concern. However, you may just find you will need less of it.

Caution and careful monitoring with a veterinarian is recommended whenever essential oils are used in animals receiving Insulin or oral hypoglycemic medications. Any essential oil intended to lower blood sugar, or support body functions may lower the need for these medications, so much so, that continued administration of prescribed insulin dosages, could prove dangerous. When working with a veterinarian, it is helpful to describe that you will be using a natural remedy that may reduce the required levels of Insulin or other diabetic medications. Most veterinarians are familiar with the careful monitoring and adjusting of Insulin doses in diabetic animals – especially when we are first introducing the therapy. In the case of essential oil use with diabetes, we basically monitor "in reverse," slowly exposing the animal to the natural remedy, while performing the same careful monitoring and blood glucose curves, at intervals determined by the veterinarian. Over time, Insulin and medication requirements may lessen, and a reduction in dosage can be made with your veterinarian.

For animals on Insulin already, I generally caution to use very small amounts of essential oils, and avoid multiple methods of application initially. We start extremely slowly when Insulin is already being given. Animals who are not receiving Insulin and have been newly diagnosed with Diabetes, seem much more able to utilize natural remedies in a more aggressive manner. Since we are not giving potentially dangerous injections of Insulin or medications that lower the blood sugar levels, we are able to expose the animal to more dietary changes, supplements, lifestyle improvements, and natural remedies without fear of correcting their condition "too quickly."

CARRIER OILS

Carrier oils are generally fatty or greasy oils, in which essential oils are combined for dilution. They may be called fixed oils or vegetable oils as well. They are used as one of the more effective ways to dilute and "carry" essential oils. Being that essential oils are "lipophilic" or capable of being combined within a fatty substance, fatty carrier oils are most often used to calm an intense essential oil experience or to dilute the essential oil for topical uses.

Please see the chapter on Forms of Dilution for more definitions and explanations of dilution, dispersment, solutions, emulsifiers, solvents, and surfactants.

A wonderful book all about carrier oils is *Power of the Seed: Your Guide to Oils for Health & Beauty* by Susan M. Parker. You can find this in our reference section as well.

Carrier oils themselves have different characteristics. Some carrier oils may be more effective for different conditions, and also duly noted is that some carrier oils become rancid more quickly. Some specialists report that even body heat could cause rancidity of a carrier oil!

Carrier oils include oils which are derived from plants, animals, and petrochemicals. In general, we should be focused on using plant derived carrier oils, however with urgent need, animal based fats can be used (such as butter). Petrochemicals should always be avoided for use with animals. Always. Carrier oils are non-volatile, and do not evaporate, and may also be referred to as fixed oils. Most plant-based carrier oils will be derived from the nut, grain, fruit, kernel, or seed of a plant. These items are most commonly exposed to great pressure to extract the oil, which is then filtered and refined. Some carrier oils are now being obtained by CO_2 Distillation as well.

It should be fully respected, that any carrier oil you use with an animal, will be coming in contact with a human. Whether in the application process, or by future petting and affection. It would be completely irresponsible to use a nut oil or oil with potential severe human allergy, on any animal that might come into contact with an unknown human population. Dogs visiting senior centers or performing therapy work of any sort, could encounter people with allergies. If any essential oil blend is to be made with public contact in mind, be well aware of potential human allergies before selecting your carriers.

Acai Oil (*Euterpe oleracea*) – an edible oil rich in nutrients. Used in human eczema, psoriasis, penetrates skin quickly and deeply, and is used with aromatherapy massage (human), and is especially good for swellings. Not commonly used with animals.

Almond Oil (*Amygdalus communis*) – also called Sweet Almond oil. Bitter or oil obtained from wild almonds should not be used. Sweet Almond oil is edible, and has a high ability to retain moisture and prevent water loss through the skin. As external use creates a protective film, it is not the most appropriate for use with fur, hair, and animal coats. It is often used for soap and salve making, and is quite appropriate in salves when support of the skin barrier is desired. As a general carrier oil for animals, it is not widely recommended. In Traditional Chinese Medicine Sweet Almond oil is a general oil for "Qi" issues, functional issues, and functional imbalances.

Aloe Vera Oil (*Aloe barbadensis*) – this is usually aloe extracts just added to soybean oil. Generally not recommended.

Andiroba Oil (*Carapa guianensis*) – this is a relative of Neem (in the same family *Meliaceae*), and carries similar properties. It is reported to have anti-inflammatory effects, promotes healing of cuts and wounds, is insecticidal, and has been used by Brazilian natives for treating all sorts of skin conditions. This oil is partially solid at room temperature and is not recommended for consumption, therefore generally not used with animals at this time. There are some reports of using this oil inside of ears, for ear mites and similar parasites.

Apricot Kernel Oil (*Prunus armeniaca*) – if you use this oil, make sure to use one listed as edible, not all are. This oil is reported to be nourishing to the skin, while carrying anti-inflammatory properties. Known for a high level of nitrilosides, these may have cancer preventive properties. The use in cancer salves and blends, may be beneficial. However, edible Apricot Kernel oil is not widely used with animals at this time.

Argan Oil (*Argania spinosa*) – originally argan nuts were harvested from the poop of goats who ate the fruit off of the tree! So yes, it is an edible oil. Increasing in popularity as "Moroccan Oil" for hair and beauty. It is reported to have protective properties for the skin, and seals in moisture. Used for problem skin in humans, it is not used with animals at this time.

Avocado Oil (*Persea gratissima*) – persin is a substance found within the leaves, bark, seeds, skin and pits of avocados. It is an oil-soluble fungicide, and while not toxic to humans, cats, or dogs; persin is toxic to birds, rabbits, horses and ruminants. For these reasons, Avocado oil should be eliminated when considering carrier oils for animal use.

Babassu Oil (*Orbignya oleifera*) – not widely used with animals at this time. Similar to coconut oil, it can be found in edible and non-edible forms.

Baobab Oil (*Adansonia digitata*) – not recommended for use with animals at this time. While some African natives reportedly use it for cooking, it appears to have some potentially toxic compounds of concern.

Blackberry Seed Oil (*Rubus fruticosus*) – an edible oil it is high in vitamin C. This is relatively new to the market with little information on use with animals as a carrier oil. With humans it is reported to be anti-inflammatory, scavenges free-radicals, soothing, and protective while nourishing the skin. It is not suggested for use with animals at this time.

Black Cumin Oil (*Nigella sativa*) – also called Nigella, or Black Seed oil. This edible oil has been used since ancient times, and is reported to support the immune system, promoting the activity of natural killer cells. For the respiratory system it is reported to dilate bronchioles, be antispasmodic, and have antihistamine actions. Therefore, it may be quite useful for cases of asthma. It is also antibacterial, antifungal, pain relieving, and sedating (calming). This oil is high in Essential Fatty Acids (EFA's), and internally is used for the treatment of digestive disorders, liver issues, intestinal parasites, headaches, and respiratory congestion and concerns. It is well reported to be of specific support to diabetics. Topically it is often used for treatment of eczema, psoriasis, sore joints, and dry skin. Truly an oil to marvel at. While this oil is a thicker oil, and not always the easiest to use as an animal carrier oil alone, it is a wonderful addition to blends created to support the above conditions and overall health. Ingestion of the oil by grooming, is likely to have wide benefits. My favorite quote regarding this oil is reported to be said by Mohamed, declaring black seed the remedy for "every disease except death".

Black Currant Seed Oil (*Ribes nigrum*) – an edible oil, it contains high levels of GLA (gamma-Linolenic acid), and also vitamin C. This oil is reported to have properties that improve elasticity of skin, calms inflammation, supports collagen regeneration, and also provides nutrients to joints and muscles. This oil is not widely used with animals at this time.

Blueberry Seed Oil (*Vaccinium corymbosum*) – an edible oil, it is a relatively newer addition to the carrier oil market. Reported to be highly antioxidant, it is helpful to deliver nutrients to the skin to help repair damage and scar tissue. This oil is not widely used with animals at this time.

Borage Seed Oil (*Borago officinalis*) – this edible oil contains the highest levels of GLA of any oil. The oil is likely to have anti-inflammatory actions that are helpful to support joint and soft tissue pain. It is not widely used with animals at this time.

Brazil Nut Oil (*Bertholletia excelsa*) – an edible oil, it is high in selenium. It is semi-solid and thick, and not used with animals at this time.

Broccoli Seed Oil (*Brassica oleracea italica*) – an edible oil, this oil contains a high level of very long-chain unsaturated fatty acids, which may be helpful in protection from sun damage. Sulforaphane within the oil, induces the production of Glutathione, which is protective to the body and cells on many levels. The oil can act to add luster and shine to hair and coat, although carries a bit of a sulfur smell. It is not widely used with animals at this time.

Buriti Oil (*Mauritia flexuosa*) – an orange/red edible oil, it is not used as a carrier oil with animals due to an array of staining issues. High in carotenoids and beta-carotene, it is reported to help heal wounds and prevent excessive scarring.

Camelina Oil (*Camelina sativa*) – an edible oil, it has a high nutritional value and has been used as a substitute for flax oil. It is high in omega-3 fatty acids, yet is surprisingly stable due to other antioxidants within the oil. It is absorbed readily into the skin, it is not commonly used with animals at this time.

Camellia Oil (*Camellia spp.*) – an edible oil, it has been used in Japan for thousands of years. It is a "drying" or astringent oil, so may be indicated for oily skin conditions. It is not commonly used as a carrier oil with animals at this time.

Canola Oil (*Brassica campestris*) – also called rapeseed. This oil generally originates from genetically modified crops, that are often highly sprayed with chemicals. Its use as a carrier oil is not recommended at this time.

Carrot Seed Oil (*Daucus carota*) – there is an essential oil distilled from Carrot Seed, and the carrier oil would be cold pressed or CO_2 extracted from the seed. These are quite different products. The fixed oil is dark green, and quite bitter. Staining of furniture and materials would be a concern for use on animals. However, the bitter property could have certain qualities we could exploit with wounds. Reported to have UV protective properties, it is also used for dry, cracked skin, restoring moisture to tissues. Carrot Seed oil as a carrier oil is not commonly used with animals at this time. However, addition to certain salves could be explored for its bitter qualities, possibly reducing the desire to lick a wound.

Carrot Root Oil (*Daucus carota*) – this preparation is usually a maceration of carrot root, within another carrier oil. There is also a CO_2 extract available, which also requires that it be mixed with another carrier oil to use. Also called Helio Carrot, it is also deep orange-yellow in color, and staining could be a concern. The high carotenoids within the oil are also shown to have some anti-cancer properties. This oil may also have UV protection, and is nourishing to the skin. This oil is not commonly used as a carrier oil with animals at this time.

Castor Oil (*Ricinus communis*) – this oil has been used for thousands of years, and orally it has laxative and purgative effects. There are many health benefits reported with this oil, and Castor oil packs have been used in humans over the liver region for a variety of benefits, including optimizing immune function. It is quite thick and viscous, so not an ideal carrier oil for animals topically. Its use as a general carrier oil is not commonly used with animals at this time. Because castor oil is well known to penetrate skin readily, it has also been reported to aide in other nutrients being absorbed into the body. However, the increase of external items that might be absorbed with the castor oil, includes pollutants and other chemicals that may be on an animal that we do not wish to carry into the body.

Cherry Kernel Oil (*Prunus avium*) – pressed from cherry pits, there would be some concern for certain animal species with the use of this oil. Animal research has shown the oil to be quite non-toxic, however birds are often cautioned away from cherry pits (as well as some other stones) due to their content of amygdalin (which can convert to cyanide) within the pit. It does not appear that cherry kernel oil will have toxicity concerns, and in some studies has been shown to reduce the rate of tumor growth in animals. This oil is not widely used with animals at this time.

Chia Seed Oil (*Salvia hispanica*) – this edible oil has been a superfood for hundreds of years. High in omega-3 fatty acids, natural antioxidants within the oil make it quite stable. It is reported to be anti-inflammatory, helpful with skin regeneration, and reduction of scarring. This oil is completely safe for use with animals, however is not widely used as a carrier oil at this time.

Cocoa Butter (*Theobroma cacao*) – this is a solid fat, which is not readily absorbed into the skin. It is often an ingredient for salves and homemade recipes. It creates more of a physical barrier to the skin, and is less likely to promote the absorption of essential oils into the skin. It also smells chocolate in nature, which should remind us that there are theobromine levels within it, making it inappropriate for ingestion by animals. Cocoa butter is not recommended for use with animals. Shea Butter is often considered as a replacement for Cocoa Butter.

Coconut Oil (*Cocos nucifera*) – no matter what, this should be your first selection when working with animals. There are several versions and names of coconut oil on the market including raw, virgin, fractionated, MCT, caprylic triglyceride, capric triglyceride, etc. For work with animals, we also have to consider the human coming into contact with our blends as well. If they have a nut allergy, and we create a blend with nut oils, while it may be safe for the animal, it could have obvious issues for the human. While there are some humans with coconut allergies, we have been impressed by the number of veterinarians with this allergy, willing to experiment on themselves to see if they are indeed also allergic to Fractionated Coconut Oil. The results. They were not! This is indeed a limited, and very experiential "study" but it was fairly dramatic to those involved.

One veterinarian cannot even touch a raw coconut oil, or use a lip balm that might contain it. However, she rubbed a high quality Fractionated Coconut Oil onto her lips, and nothing! While I am not suggesting that this is true for everyone, it does appear that the coconut allergy does require some of the actual coconut proteins, which would be present in raw or less refined coconut products.

Another consideration is that some coconut oil items are solvent extracted. This is where good quality and sourcing has to be known. It is regarded in the human massage industry, that reactions to the solvent extracted coconut oil is more common, and they urge the use of cold-extracted or cold-pressed oil.

What is the difference in coconut oils? Virgin or raw coconut oil will have a coconut scent, and is often solid at lower room temperatures. This is a wonderful oil for consumption, or ingredients in homemade salves and recipes. However, it is not liquid enough to use for an essential oil blend that is intended to drip out of a bottle. Allergies again must be considered with this version of coconut oil. It is usually extracted from the coconut milk and fresh meat.

Commercial coconut oil may be called "Coconut 76" meaning that it is liquid at 76 degrees Fahrenheit. This is extracted from the dried meat of the coconut and is less expensive. I do not recommend its use as a carrier oil.

Fractionated Coconut Oil generally begins with the Coconut 76, however the portion or "fraction" of the coconut oil that turns solid at lower temperatures is removed (the long-chain fatty acids). This "processing" results in a clear liquid, that does not harden, and has an incredibly long shelf life. It is well known to not stain the sheets or clothing for those working in the massage industry, and so is well liked in animal homes where the carrier oil may indeed get onto a couch or bedding.

MCT stands for medium-chain triglycerides, which include caprioc, caprylic, capric, and lauric acids depending on how many carbons the chain possesses. The MCT is a more concentrated form of these fatty acids, the name is often used interchangeably with Fractionated Coconut Oil. With MCT however, there are some reports of varying content of which medium-chain triglycerides are within it. Upon speaking to the wonderful people at CocoTherapy, who own their own coconut plantation and make coconut products for animals, I was interested to know that there were a variety of ways that Fractionated Coconut Oil could be made and "fractioned". Basically, certain percentages of the different fatty acids could be retained or added back into the Coconut Oil, making essentially custom formulations for certain needs. With the addition back of certain fatty acids, the fragrance of coconut could return to even a Fractionated Coconut Oil product.

For use with animals, and for a benign smell that will not affect essential oil blends, I prefer to use basic Fractionated Coconut Oil or MCT that does not have any scent. You should sample your carrier oils from any supplier you select, and determine for yourself if it is the best for your applications.

I also prefer Fractionated Coconut Oil for use with animals due to the fact that while it still may leave a bit of a greasy residue on fur, it doesn't seem to be as thick or goopy, and is very well tolerated with normal grooming practices. In fact, many cats actually enjoy licking Fractionated Coconut Oil off of their humans' legs.

In Traditional Chinese Medicine, coconut oil is noted to be ideal for Constitutional issues. Neurologic issues, brain, spine, genital, bone, and marrow issues would fall in this category. So, for example, in cases of arthritis, it would be indicated to make an essential oil blend within coconut oil.

Coffee Oil (*Coffea arabica*) – as coffee is not recommended for consumption by animals, this carrier oil is not recommended for use with animals.

Corn Oil (*Zea mays*) – the quintessential "vegetable oil" it is obviously edible. However, since this oil is greatly obtained from GMO crops, it is not recommended for use as a carrier oil with animals. However, in emergency situations where a fatty oil is needed to calm an abnormal exposure to essential oils (say in an eye) – this oil can be used to dilute the situation.

Cranberry Seed Oil (*Vaccinium macrocarpon*) – known as an excellent oil for skin conditioning, this oil contains nearly equal ratios of omega 3, 6, and 9 fatty acids. The oil is deeply yellow, and filled with phytonutrients and antioxidants. It is not widely used with animals at this time.

Cucumber Seed Oil (*Cucumis sativus*) – edible and high in phytosterols, this oil is reported to strengthen the skin barrier and promote regeneration of cells. This oil is quite stable, and highly moisturizing with anti-inflammatory and protective properties. It is not widely used as a carrier oil with animals at this time.

Daikon Radish Seed Oil (*Raphanus sativus*) – a relatively new oil, it is similar to broccoli seed oil, and most likely to be obtained by CO_2 extraction. It may do well for promoting smooth, glossy hair coat. Shelf life of this oil is shorter, only ranging from 6 months to a year. This oil is not used with animals at this time.

Evening Primrose Oil (*Oenothers biennis*) – also known by the initials EPO, this oil has been heralded for its content of gamma linolenic acid (GLA). An edible oil, it is found in many supplements and oral capsules in the natural market. GLA is touted to help maintain healthy skin, repair damage by the sun, and also help to control hormone-like prostaglandins. Other oils containing GLA include black currant and borage seed oil, which actually contain higher levels than EPO. As a rather expensive oil, it is also rich and thick, and not highly appropriate for use as a carrier oil solely. It is generally blended with other carrier oils at a 10% rate when use is desired. Evening Primrose oil also has quite a short shelf life, so is not highly practical for everyday use and is not commonly used as a carrier oil with animals at this time.

Flax Seed Oil (*Linum usitatissimum*) – a very common and edible oil, it oxidizes quickly and often goes rancid. While there are a lot of health benefits to this oil, it is rarely used as a carrier oil, especially as when it dries it tends to be sticky and solid. It is not recommended for use as a carrier oil.

Foraha – see Tamanu oil

Gevuina Oil (*Gevuina avellana*) – also called Chilean Hazelnut, it is more similar to macadamia nut oil. Known to be protective and repairing, Gevuina oil could be helpful for protection from weather such as in formulations for paw balms. Gevuina oil is also high in palmitoleic acid, which is a fatty acid found in skin sebum. This oil is a relatively stable oil, and is reported to last for 18 months with proper storage and care. This oil is not readily used with animals at this time.

Grape Seed Oil (*Vitis vinifera*) – pressed from the seeds of grapes, this oil is commonly used in the human markets. It is widely used in cooking, and is an edible oil. While grape pulp and skin has been reported as toxic to dogs and cats, the seed is not toxic. Grapeseed oil is well absorbed by the skin, and is reported to help strengthen collagen and support the health of connective tissues in skin and joints. Grapeseed oil should be kept refrigerated, so is not an ideal oil for use as a versatile carrier oil. In Traditional Chinese Medicine (TCM) Grapeseed oil is reported as a general oil for "Qi" issues, functional issues, and functional imbalances. This oil is not commonly used as a carrier oil for animals.

Hazelnut Oil (*Corylus aveliana*) – an edible oil, it is often used in foods and cooking. Paclitaxel found within the oil obtained from raw nuts, has been reported as a potent anti-cancer substance, and is also reported to be helpful for psoriasis, multiple sclerosis, Alzheimer's disease, and kidney diseases. Hazelnut oil readily penetrates the skin, and provides an astringent property while also stimulating skin circulation. It is a wonderful base oil when Calendula infusions are desired. Hazelnut oil is not widely used with animals at this time.

Hemp Seed Oil (*Cannabis indica*) – this oil is becoming increasingly popular. Hemp Seed oil is different from the CBD oil, and is quite reactive and prone to rancidity. As a carrier oil for essential oils, it is not commonly used for animals, however within salves and other recipes, it is soothing to the skin, anti-inflammatory, immune supporting, and may help heal burns.

Jojoba Oil (*Simmondsia chinensis*) – this oil is not technically an oil at all, but is a liquid wax, and will become solid at colder temperatures. Jojoba is reported to be very similar to the sebum on skin, and is reported to not clog pores. Most use Jojoba mixed with other carrier oils, at about a 10% concentration. This liquid wax is considered ingestible, but is not digestible, and may be passed through stool in a greasy form (steatorrhea). Overall, this liquid wax performs poorly with animal fur, and is not recommended for use as a carrier oil with animals.

Kiwi Seed Oil (*Actinidia chinesis*) – this edible oil is high in Vitamin C, and is absorbed readily into the skin. This oil is not commonly used with animals at this time.

Kukui Nut Oil (*Aleurtes moluccana*) – this oil is not edible, and not recommended for use as a carrier oil with animals.

Macadamia Nut Oil (*Macadamia ternifolia*) – an edible oil that is very similar to both mink oil and sebum. For products wishing to replace mink oil in their production, this oil should have been considered. This oil is one of the few high in Palmitoleic acid, which is reported to have anti-microbial actions as well as protecting against cellular breakdown. This oil would be especially protective against chapping and weather damage, and may be ideal for use in paw balms and similar recipes. The unrefined oil may smell nutty, which may encourage licking. Macadamia Nut oil is not widely used as a carrier oil with animals at this time.

Mango Butter (*Mangifera indica*) – often included in paw balm recipes, this oil is edible and solid at room temperature. It can be used as a replacement for cocoa butter. Mango Butter is reported to have rejuvenating and wound-healing properties, while being anti-fungal and anti-inflammatory. In paw balm recipes, it would lend moisturizing and repair to skin layers, while possibly being helpful in fighting topical fungal or yeast infections.

Meadowfoam Seed Oil (*Limnanthes alba*) – this is an edible oil, which is gaining popularity in human use. It contains a high percentage of vitamin E, and is thick. It will adhere to the skin and offer protection. For these reasons, it is not ideal for most use with animals as a carrier oil, but can be considered as an addition to salves, ointments or other recipes. It generally has a long shelf life, and may help to preserve other products. It is not widely used with animals at this time.

Milk Thistle Seed Oil (*Silybum marianum*) – silymarin or Milk Thistle is a common herb used to support the liver. The fatty oil of the seed of this plant, only retains some of the beneficial compounds of the herb, and the more refined the oil, the less of the beneficial compounds there are. Do not use this oil as a replacement for the herbal properties. The oil is high in Vitamin E, and is also reported to potentially be helpful for gastrointestinal ulcers when ingested. This oil is not commonly used with animals at this time.

Mineral Oil – No. Just No. This is a petroleum product, and not natural at all. Found in many human products, such as baby oil, Mineral Oil is not recommended for use with animals in any form.

Moringa Oil (*Moringa oleifera*) – this edible oil is also commercially known as Ben oil or Behen oil. It is incredibly stable, with a shelf life of up to 5 years. It is rich in vitamins and unsaturated fatty acids, and is reported to have antiseptic and anti-inflammatory properties – promoting healing of skin rashes, burns, cuts, bruises, and insect bites. It is a rather expensive oil, and often used in perfumery for enfleurage (the extraction of scents from flowers), as it helps to hold fragrances with the very-long-chain fatty acids it contains. Often reported to increase immunity when ingested in humans, this oil is not commonly used with animals at this time.

Neem Oil (*Azadirachta indica*) – an ancient healing oil, it might possibly be one of the most over-played oils in terms of desire to add into animal products. So many people focus on Neem as the "must have" addition for insect recipes, that they rarely consider that there are other more pleasant alternatives. Neem is wonderful, but is plagued with problems if ingested without true knowledge. As an oil, it is often semi-solid at room temperature, and dark in color. If you have obtained a very clear or liquid Neem oil, it may be that it is already cut into another carrier oil or highly refined.

While Neem oil is antibacterial, anti-fungal, antiviral, anti-parasitic, insect repelling, and healing – it is strong medicine, with a strong smell. This oil must certainly be diluted for use, and most who attempt to create products such as animal shampoo with Neem oil, often experience the frustration of trying to "hide" it within their concoction. Neem is likely to be helpful for yeast, fungus, and bacterial infections on the skin, and for insect repellant properties. However, many times we can substitute the use of other essential oils to replace these needs. While Neem oil is used in an array of animal products and sprays, it should be used with caution, knowledge, and respect. The true Neem oil is likely to be used at a concentration of 2-5% in actuality, and it is important to note that Neem oil may be toxic to fish and other aquatic animals. If you are using Neem, we must consider if a dog will be swimming in a fish pond, or other potential area that could transfer Neem in to the water.

The desire to use Neem oil could be replaced by the use of Neem Leaf Tea. Making a water-based tea of the plant, is a very safe alternative. Due to the wide array of unknowns about the source of Neem oil that most people obtain (diluted, pure, unknown concentrations) – if you wish to use Neem, you are better off to obtain a pure source, and dilute it yourself with known ingredients and concentrations.

Nigella – see Black Cumin

Oat Seed Oil (*Avena sativa*) – this oil contains some of the same properties as colloidal oatmeal, and may be beneficial for dry, irritated, and itchy skin conditions. It may be useful as an ingredient in some recipes, is edible, however is relatively new on the market, and is not commonly used with animals at this time.

Olive Oil (*Olea europaea*) – and easy oil that you are likely to have in your kitchen, it is often considered a good "emergency" carrier oil when dilution is needed for essential oil irritations. It has a long shelf life, and is readily available, edible, and often organic forms can be found. It is a wonderful oil when making herbal infusions, salves, or rectal or vaginal suppositories. It can be soothing and moisturizing to skin, however does not perform the best with animal fur and hair. Overall, while it can be used, it is not a favorite in terms of carrier oils when animals are concerned. In Traditional Chinese Medicine (TCM) Olive oil is noted as being good for nourishing the blood, so could be considered as a carrier oil for conditions with low platelets or blood cells (blood deficiencies/humoral).

Palm Fruit Oil (*Elaeis guineensis*) – this oil is often red or dark orange in color, due to beta-carotene. Lighter pale yellow versions of palm oil are more refined and less beneficial. An edible oil, it is an excellent source of Vitamin A and carotenoids. Many parrot owners supplement their birds' diet with Red Palm Fruit oil, however due to its intense color, it is rarely suited for topical uses as a carrier oil. However, as a carrier for ingestion of essential oils, this oil can certainly be considered. As there is an ecological impact with Palm Fruit oil production, it is important to source responsible suppliers of this oil, to avoid further destruction of wild habitats. In Traditional Chinese Medicine (TCM) Palm oil is considered ideal for Constitutional issues.

Palm Kernel Oil (*Elaeis guineensis*) – this oil is pale cream to white in color, and pressed from the kernels instead of the fruit. It is hard at room temperature, and is not recommended as a carrier oil for essential oils.

Papaya Seed Oil (*Carica papaya*) – this edible oil contains papain, the same enzyme within the fruit which is often fed to rabbits and other animals as an aid with digestion. While the fruit is most likely a more ideal source of papain, it is interesting to note. In humans, this oil is used for its enzyme action to reduce dark spots, rejuvenate, and exfoliate dead cells. It may have antibacterial and anti-inflammatory properties, and aid in the healing of wounds and skin-repair. Papaya Seed oil is not commonly used with animals at this time.

Passion Fruit Seed Oil (*Passiflora incarnata*) – this edible oil contains Vitamin C as well as calcium and phosphorus. Reported to have anti-inflammatory, anti-spasmodic, and sedative properties, it is not commonly used with animals at this time.

Peach Kernel Oil (*Prunus persica*) – this oil is mainly used externally in the human market, and while it may be considered edible, it is not widely used in this manner. This oil is not suggested as a carrier oil for animals at this time.

Pecan Oil (*Algooquian pacaan*) – this edible oil is primarily used for cooking, and has a similar consistency to almond oil. Due to the risk to humans and nut allergies, Pecan oil is not suggested for use as a carrier oil for animals.

Peanut Oil (*Arachis hypogeae*) – edible and low cost; due to potential human allergies, peanut oil is never recommended as a carrier oil for essential oils – for humans or animals.

Pequi Oil (*Caryocar braziliensis*) – native to Brazil, this oil is used for food preparations as well as external uses. Reported to be anti-inflammatory, anti-fungal, and anti-microbial, it is used for conditions such as eczema and psoriasis in humans. This oil is a bit thick and greasy, and is not widely used with animals at this time.

Perilla Seed Oil (*Perilla frutescens*) – an edible oil, it is quite unstable and tends to spoil quickly. It is not recommended for use as a carrier oil for essential oils.

Petroleum Jelly – also called Vaseline. Although some have fed this to cats for hairballs, it is indeed a petroleum product – and should never be used with animals in my opinion.

Pistachio Nut Oil (*Pistacia vera*) – a relatively stable and edible oil, it is non-greasy and readily absorbed by skin. While this may be used in some human applications, it is not recommended for use as a carrier oil for animals.

Plum Kernel Oil (*Prunus domestica*) – similar to peach, cherry, almond, and apricot oils; it is not suggested as a carrier oil for animals at this time.

Pomegranate Seed Oil (*Punica granatum*) – an edible oil, it is reported to have many potential health benefits. Punicic acid is a unique fatty acid within the oil, as well as many other beneficial phytonutrients. Research has shown promise with anti-cancer effects, and the oil is anti-inflammatory, regenerative, and healing. Pomegranate Seed oil is not widely used with animals at this time.

Poppy Seed Oil (*Papaver somniferum*) – an edible oil, it is also used in pharmaceutical and industrial settings. It is prone to oxidation, and should be refrigerated. It is not recommended for use as a carrier oil due to its unstable nature.

Pracaxi Oil (*Pentaclethera macroloba*) – solid at room temperature, this oil has native uses as an insect repellant and to minimize scarring and stretch marks. It has been used medicinally for snakebite and hemorrhage. This oil is not suggested as a carrier oil for animals at this time.

Pumpkin Seed Oil (*Cucurbita pepo*) – an edible oil, it is dark in color and thick. It is more used as a food oil than for topical use. It is not recommended as a carrier oil for essential oils.

Red Raspberry Seed Oil (*Rubus idaeus*) – caution should be used as some of these oils are hexane-extracted and would not be recommended for any type of use. With the increased popularity of CO_2 extracts, this oil is likely to be seen a bit more often. Claims to fame include possible UV-A and UV-B sun protection. This oil does have a long shelf life, however use with animals is not suggested at this time.

Rice Bran Oil (*Oryza sativa*) – an edible oil that is high in Vitamin E, it is often used with human massage, it is reported to protect cells against excess sun and suppress melanin generation in skin layers. While it can be used as a carrier oil with animals, it is not commonly used or recommended.

Rose Hip Seed Oil (*Rosa rubiginosa*) – this oil is high in GLA, and is valued for skin regeneration in humans. While it may be consumed, it is known to have laxative and diuretic effects, and may cause diarrhea, nausea, vomiting and abdominal discomfort. This oil has a very short shelf life and is not recommended for use as a carrier oil with animals.

Sacha Inchi Oil (*Plukenetia volubilis*) – this oil can also be called pracaxi but is a different oil than *Pentaclethara macroloba*. Native to Peru, it has been used for centuries internally and externally. It has a long shelf life, however it is not currently recommended for use as a carrier oil with animals.

Safflower Oil (*Carthamus tinctorius*) – this oil is edible, but oxidizes readily. While it could be used as an "emergency" carrier oil, it is not recommended for use with aromatherapy. In Traditional Chinese Medicine (TCM) Safflower oil is described as being indicated for use with vascular issues and blood stagnation, so it could be considered for use with vascular disease, with the caution of making sure it is always incredibly fresh.

Sea Buckthorn Oil (*Hippophae rhamnoides*) – this plant has a long history of use as food and medicine, and was supposedly fed to Greek horses to keep their coats shiny and healthy! CO_2 extracts have made this oil easier to find, instead of a macerated extract of the berries in other carriers. While it will not be a solo carrier oil, its addition into other recipes may impart some of its healing properties. It is reported to promote regeneration of skin cells, healing of wounds, reduce redness, aid with dermatitis, and reduce and aid in healing of gastric ulcers. In Traditional Chinese Medicine (TCM) this oil is used to treat problems associated with mucous membranes. The oil is orange in color, so staining must remain a consideration. This oil is not widely used with animals at this time.

Sesame Seed Oil (*Sesamum indicum*) – an edible oil that is readily available, it is a favorite oil for Ayurvedic medicinal preparations. Sesame oil is reported to be antibacterial, antifungal, anti-inflammatory, a potent antioxidant, and may even be helpful against cancer cells. Some have even used it to help eliminate lice, and it does provide some UV protection from the sun. There are toasted and unrefined versions of the oil, and the unrefined would be preferred for use. The toasted will have a strong odor. In general, this oil is not widely used with animals as a carrier oil at this time.

Shea Butter (*Butyrospermum parkii*) – this edible oil, softens and protects skin, and is likely a great addition to paw balms and other recipes. It is thick and creamy, and there are variations depending on the amount of refining that has occurred. It may help with circulation in skin capillaries, so consideration for use with conditions such as ear margin vasculitis, when creating a cream or salve recipe, may be a great idea. This oil is often used as a replacement for Cocoa Butter. Although not a direct carrier oil for essential oils, it is used quite often in many animal recipes and preparations.

Shea Oil (*Butyrospermum parkii*) – a more refined version of Shea, this oil remains liquid. It is still thick, and not ideal as a carrier oil; but may also be used within recipes. In general, the less refined Shea Butter would be preferred for healthful benefits. This oil is not as commonly used with animals at this time.

Shortening – also called Lard. This may be vegetable in nature, in which it is made from Soybean Oil. Other natural shortenings are derived from Palm Oil. These are thick and greasy, and not recommended for use with animals, except in extreme emergency conditions only.

Soybean Oil (*Soja hispida*) – although this is an edible oil, it is created greatly from a mass market, and heavily genetically modified crop. It is not recommended for use with animals as a carrier oil, unless it is the only option in an emergency.

Squalene – this is a fractionation of vegetable oils, especially olive oil, wheat germ oil, and rice bran. It may be used as a fixative in some perfumes. It is not recommended for use with animals.

Sunflower Oil (*Helianthus annus*) – an edible oil, it can oxidize easily. While this could be used for emergency situations, it is not suggested for use with animals at this time.

Tamanu Oil (*Caulophyllum inophyllum*) – also called foraha, and a variety of other names, it is reported to have many healing properties. However, the oil is very thick and dark green, with a pungent smell which often turns people off to its use. It is reported to be helpful for scarring, eczema, cracked and chapped skin, burns, infections, sciatica, rheumatism, and shingles. When this oil is refined to a more pleasant and liquid state, it is likely that most of the healing properties are lost. Large open wounds may benefit from the addition of this rather expensive oil to recipes. It is considered quite non-toxic, however it has not been used widely with animals at this time.

Tomato Seed Oil (*Solanum lycopersicum*) – as CO_2 extracts become more and more popular, oils such as this are entering the market. An edible oil, it is deep orange and color, and may provide some UV protection. It has not been used widely with animals at this time.

Vaseline – see Petroleum Jelly

Walnut Oil (*Juglans regia*) – also an edible oil, this oil is prone to going rancid quickly. It may have regenerative, moisturizing, antibacterial, anti-inflammatory, antiviral, and antiseptic properties, and has shown some ability is suppressing tumor growth. Due to rancidity concerns, Walnut Oil is not suggested as a carrier oil for use with animals at this time.

Watermelon Seed Oil (*Citrullus vulgaris*) – also called Ootanga, it is also becoming more available as CO_2 extracts enter the market. It is edible, and is reported to help dissolve excessive sebum in pores – so may be considered as an ingredient in sebum reducing washes and shampoos for affected animals. It may be anti-inflammatory and is reported to be very stable with a long shelf life, and has a light texture. It is often recommended as a replacement for mineral oil. This oil may show promise, however at this time it is not commonly used with animals.

Wheat Germ Oil (*Triticum vulgare*) – this ingestible oil is very thick and rich, and should not be used as a carrier oil for essential oils alone. Mixed into other recipes, it is high in Vitamin E so may extend the life of other blends. Use at approximately 10 percent of the carrier blend is recommended. Alone, this oil is not widely recommended as a carrier oil for use with animals.

Other Waxes and Ingredients

Beeswax – perfectly safe and ingestible for use in animal related products and recipes. Usually melted, then mixed with other carrier oils to create a workable substance; essential oils mix well within these recipes generally. One of the more common waxes used with animals, and often recommended first. Beeswax can act as an emulsifier in lotion and cream recipes.

Lanolin – this "wax" is derived from the fatty secretions of sheep into their wool. It is used for many purposes, especially water protection. It is safe for use with animals. Lanolin can act as an emulsifier in lotion and cream recipes.

Candelilla Wax (*Euphorbiea cerifera*) – this is a vegetable or plant-based wax, and is Generally Recognized As Safe by the FDA for use in foods. It is a nice alternative when animal-based waxes are not desired.

DMSO

DMSO or dimethyl sulfoxide, has been around for many years. It was first synthesized in the 1800's – and is actually an industrial solvent. It has been used in medicine as a vehicle for penetrating tissues, and bringing drugs into areas of poor circulation or for transdermal absorption enhancement.

DMSO has been used in the veterinary field in many ways. From use with horses topically and even intravenously, to nebulization with birds; DMSO has certainly made its rounds in a variety of applications. Although it is considered "natural" by some, or even organic – this description is based on organic chemistry more than anything natural. When I was first entering the veterinary field (even before vet school) it was quite commonplace to nebulize a parrot with a mixture of saline, DMSO, and antibiotics or antifungal medications in an effort to eliminate deep seated infections within the air sacs or sinuses. DMSO has the odd characteristic of being "garlicky" so even touching it or inhaling it – you would feel like you could repel vampires! I will never forget the smell or feeling of being exposed to DMSO.

Of late, DMSO has gained popularity in the naturopathic human world. Chiropractic and naturopathic colleges are actually promoting it as a natural medicine, which is really pretty far from the truth. And now that some of the naturopaths are also dabbling in essential oils – it was only a matter of time before they were mixing the two. Research articles have been written to show that essential oils penetrate cells, however this research included DMSO as a carrier to the essential oils. This is surely flawed science when an industrial solvent, known for carrying substances across membranes is included in your mixture.

Regardless of flawed experiments, DMSO is nothing to think lightly of. Although it appears to have a wide safety margin, I would not use it or recommend its use as a carrier for essential oils, or as a natural treatment for any condition.

Because of DMSO's amazing ability to draw items into the body, this also means that it will draw pollutants and other chemicals into a body as well. And most certainly, we do not wish to bring anything of detriment into our animals.

OIL COLLECTION METHODS

Essential oils are collected from plant materials in a variety of ways. Some are more appropriate for use with animals than others.

Steam Distillation

This method is where the collected and prepared plant materials are placed into a chamber, and steam is then passed through the matter to collect the volatiles. The steam is then re-condensed back into water and the essential oil fraction. The essential oil is removed off of the water (as essential oils and water do not mix) – and is used as the resultant essential oil. Some essential oils may require further actions, but in general this is the basic description of steam distillation. Each plant however, will have a variance of how the plant is grown, collected, handled after harvest, chipping or preparation of the plant for distillation, etc. There is a distinct art form to distillation, and I have certainly witnessed the quality fluctuations when new farm hands are thrown at the task without adequate training. Steam distillation remains the most appropriate collection method for use in Veterinary Aromatic Medicine.

Cold Pressing

The cold pressing of essential oils is most common within the citrus oils. Rinds of the fruit, are squeezed to release the essential oils. Some citrus oils can also be steam distilled, and result in a slightly different essential oil and essential oil profile. Cold pressed oils are also appropriate for use in Veterinary Aromatic Medicine, however only a limited number of oils are collected via the cold press process (Lemon, Lime, Orange…)

Hydro-Distillation

This process is often considered similar to steam distillation, but it is actually quite different. In this situation, all of the plant material is added to water, and then boiled. The steam is then collected and condensed. I relate this more similarly to boiled vegetables versus steamed (boiled is often over-cooked and mushy). Hydro-distillation does result in some deterioration of the constituents during the cooking process, and is considered less optimal for use with Veterinary Aromatic Medicine. Most who collect hydrosols for use, tend to use hydro-distillation within the process. I do feel that the hydrosols as well as the essential oil resulting from this process, are lesser in quality than I desire.

CO_2 Extraction

These extracts are discussed more fully in their own chapter. For Veterinary Aromatic Medicine, I do feel that CO_2 Extracts have a place, but just a more herbal, or topically related place. CO_2 Extracts contain more plant particles than essential oils, and will indeed carry more possible drug interactions and potential complications with their use, than with just traditional essential oils. Please see the chapter on CO_2 Extracts for more information.

Absolutes

Absolutes are obtained by chemical extraction. Hexane and other chemical residues may be present in the resultant "essential oil" which is not an essential oil at all. Absolutes are less expensive (Rose Absolute versus a steam distilled Rose Otto) – and so are often considered for use by those who do not strive for the utmost in safety or therapeutic effects. Often various flower extracts will be an absolute – and may not be specified in the ingredient listing. Items such as Honeysuckle, Jasmine, Violet – should spark concern immediately as to if they are solvent extracted absolutes. All absolutes should be avoided for use with animals in my opinion.

Hydrosols

Please see the next chapter on hydrosols. They are not essential oils, and often cannot replace what we desire to achieve with essential oil use. While they are "fine" to use – I do not find them as appropriate or to be a part of what I qualify as Veterinary Aromatic Medicine.

Flower Essences

Often confused with essential oils, flower and plant essences are completely different. Feline behaviorist Jackson Galaxy has a line of essences for animals, and I am over and over again asked about these as if they were essential oils. They are as different from essential oils as homeopathy is from amoxicillin. Please make sure to read and evaluate all products you purchase for use with your animals, to fully understand which modality they represent.

HYDROSOLS

Hydrosols are the by-product of steam or hydro-distillation. It is basically the water soluble portions of the plant within the water used to extract the essential oil. Also called hydrolats, floral waters, distillate waters, or hydrolates – they contain very small amounts of essential oil constituents. Hydrosols are extremely gentle, and can likely be thought of as a dilute tea when we consider herbal medicine. Not quite the herb, certainly not the essential oil, and likely not even a fully brewed "cuppa tea."

While hydrosols are often touted as being the more safe way to enjoy aromatherapy with animals, there are several flaws that we see in practice. Most notably, there are very few selections available on the market. While we can have access to over 300 essential oils, hydrosols often number in the 10's when you can find them. And they most certainly require special handling and considerations.

Hydrosols should be refrigerated, and often carry a shelf life of one year from the date that they were created. They can easily become contaminated or spoil with bacteria. In general, while their use may be lovely and gentle, it is a bit problematic in terms of convenience.

Most often, I just do not see enough response to the use of hydrosols, to warrant stocking them for the animals in my care. Although I obtained a very nice rose hydrosol as a face mist for myself, and can use it as a room spray or base for other items, when I want the aromatic effects of rose, I will still default to the use of a gorgeous steam distilled rose essential oil.

Hydrosols are not wrong (unless spoiled), they are just weak in nature, may not evoke enough of a response for veterinary aromatic medicine needs, and are a bit cumbersome to order, ship, store and use. For these reasons, I do not prefer their use.

INSTRUCTIONS FROM THE AUTHOR

As with the first edition of this book, it is important that you understand how to effectively use and read this book. There may be other books referenced to you at times, if you wish to learn more about chemistry or individual chemical constituents or distillation. This book will focus more on Veterinary Aromatic Medicine, and not on the essential oil industry as a whole – except for the parts that are more critical to understand in regards to animals.

Do not be afraid of the phrase Veterinary Aromatic Medicine. It is the same as animal aromatherapy, or the use of essential oils with animals whether you are a veterinarian or not. All people can use veterinary aromatic medicine, however I believe we need to invoke a name that demands the respect deserving of the modality. So this is the one I have selected.

As there are so many species of animals, it becomes difficult to cross reference each essential oil differently for a horse versus a bird versus a cat or dog. You will find a section for each species, listing some of the most common veterinary conditions for that species. Then, you will find the essential oils that I find most helpful for that condition listed. You may even find some frequency recommendations within the "CONDITIONS" listing. However, if you are then interested in using Copaiba for a concern, you will need to go to the individual essential oil listings (SINGLES), and then read about how you would use Copaiba for the species you are interested in. This way, I am not repeating over and over again how to use a certain essential oil.

Find the essential oil you are interested in using within the condition, then read more about how to use that essential oil for the species you are interested in. It may seem confusing at first, but you'll get used to it!

The recommendations in this book are in no means the only protocols that will work or that can be used for various conditions. However, I will recommend those items that are the most friendly to that particular species, as well as have good results. If you encounter a condition that is not responding to the initial recommendations, it is important to use something different. However, it may be best to consult with an experienced animal aromatherapist or veterinary aromatherapist if you are "breaking new ground" in treatment philosophies or oil usage.

As much as possible, I encourage people to start with protocols that have been used in a particular animal species before. Veterinary aromatic medicine is relatively new to our society, even though animals have used aromatherapy throughout the ages, through natural exposures. Be sure to learn the most common ways oils are used in your individual species of interest, and if you are faced with a condition that is not yet listed in the ADR, or need to modify your oil usage, continue to use the oils in "species friendly manners."

Species friendly use, also means considering which methods the animal may "like" more than others. There are oil selections and oil techniques that may be more appropriate for a cat than for others. It is important that you also read the chapters regarding use of essential oils in the litterbox, or in drinking water whenever you plan to expose an animal to a method of use. Learn as much as possible about each specific METHOD OF APPLICATION as well as you learn about the condition or the essential oil recommended for it.

Some of the sections and concepts described in this book may start to sound like a "broken record". Repetition of important concepts and fundamental skills may be noted throughout this book. I find that most people learn better by encountering the same concepts several times. So if you feel like you have "read this before" – you may have – and take it to heart that you will absorb the concept more fully!

How To Use This Book:
I would like to describe to you how I best see you utilizing this book. I would like to encourage you to read the entire book, each section, even those for animals that you do not have or do not wish to ever have contact with! It is not about which animal you will see, but often more about the knowledge to be flexible for individuals. If you can gain a clear understanding of how we modify the use of essential oils for animals such as birds, you will easily be able to modify your use of oils for a particularly sensitive dog or horse. Each animal is an individual, and you will encounter a dog someday, that needs to be treated more like a cat! For those of you who are squirming thinking of a snake or lizard right now, have no fear! The descriptions of the use for exotic species are not explicit, and you should not be plagued by nightmares upon reading it!

There are several different sections to this book that you may find helpful. Reading basic instructions will give you a foundation for how we use oils in animals. Reading about each and every single essential oil will give you valuable information and qualities for each individual oil. Then, the conditions listings for each species, will recommend items that are indicated for each condition. If you find a condition listed for one species of animal, but not for another – you can rest assured that the same recommendations will apply for your species. So as Vestibular Disease is not listed in the Feline Conditions, but it is in the Canine Conditions – you can easily refer to the oils recommended and learn how to best use them for a cat instead of a dog.

As you navigate through the conditions listings, you will also want to reference basic instructions as well as species specific instructions and comments. For example, if using certain essential oils in a litter box is suggested for a cat, you will want to read the basic information on THE LITTER BOX and also any other feline specific recommendations listed for the individual essential oil. Feline specific instructions will be found at the beginning of the Feline Conditions listings.

Single oils will be recommended in each condition listing. Within the SINGLES essential oils section, the oils will be listed in alphabetical order by common name, followed by the scientific name. While there are many flaws to listing items by common name (there are a few that still get listed by their Latin name), it remains how most people learn their essential oils, or recognize them. So for the most efficient and easy referencing, I have still selected to mainly list in this way.

FIRST LINE RECOMMENDATIONS:
There will be First Line Recommendations made for each individual condition. These are the methods that I will generally select first for a specific condition and for a specific species. These recommendations are made based on what is widely accepted and tolerated by my patients, as well as have good results. In some conditions, you may only see these First Line Recommendations listed, as I felt it was more important to give you a start to what you could use, than to exclude a subject from the conditions listings if I was unable to include the full information on the listing at this time.

In this current edition, you will see a listing of single essential oils that may be beneficial to the condition listed.

INSTRUCTIONS

It is greatly important to recognize that not every single essential oil should be used for the condition. However, the FIRST LINE RECOMMENDATIONS can often be layered and used together to create more effects for an animal. When we can expose a cat to diffusion, litterbox use, and appropriate topical applications, we can affect the condition with even greater support. This has changed for me over the years, as I have learned more and more appropriate ways to use oils for animals. Many light layers are far more effective, and easier on an animal than administering one large "hit" or a more aggressive concentration. The body truly loves exposure to small amounts, more frequently in its use pattern. And by using diluted exposures more often, versus a very strong essential oil once, we will see the body respond far better. Certainly starting with just one method in more sensitive animals, then building in exposure as necessary is just fine. And in more critical situations we can use more suggestions all at once. With previous more aggressive recommendations, if we used too many at once, an animal could feel worse rather than better. A situation that is best avoided, and completely unnecessary for results to be seen.

Single Oils:

These will be listed in the conditions listing in alphabetical order. It is important that you go to the description for each individual oil that you choose to utilize, and read more about its use in your species. For example, for a feather picking bird, an oil may be recommended for diffusion, that would not be appropriate for topical application. By reading the description and methods of use for that single oil, and for that specific species, you will gain more knowledge on how to appropriately use the qualities of a given oil, in a safe and effective manner for each species.

Once you have determined which oils you will be using, and have read the methods of how to use them for your species, you can gather more detailed information in the specific chapters at the beginning of this book. So, if you have determined that you would be adding Copaiba to the food of a bird, please read the chapter "Mixing Oils into Food", to gain a wider understanding of how we use this method.

THE SAFE USE OF OILS

The great controversy encircling the use of essential oils in animals has always intrigued me. I was never willing to just accept what others reported to me, I wanted to evaluate a case fully, and know more. In the case of essential oils, you will find so many reports of how you cannot use them for cats or ferrets, or how they are toxic to animals. One simple search in the internet, has lead people to email me in a frantic state, worried that they have somehow harmed their animals.

Thankfully, the truth is that even with most poor quality oils, the adverse reaction rates and toxic effects are actually quite low. Safety of essential oils is actually quite good. There are thousands of products containing essential oils in our everyday lives, and most people would be shocked to learn just how wide spread it is. Almost all of the cola you drink, ice cream you eat, or dishwashing soap you use, now contain essential oils or parts of them. And this industry is huge. Food and fragrance is the largest sector of the essential oil market, so most of the essential oils available are obtained with this market in mind. This means that these purchasers would like essential oils that are very consistent and offer a special flavor or specific fragrance to their product. These essential oils will not always be something that is particularly medically beneficial. But as the market grows and grows in terms of consumers of essential oils, you can be assured that much of the "therapeutic" essential oils placed within the market base, will start to come from this vast pool of available oils.

In my research on how and if essential oils present a toxicity concern in animals, I find a few things to be quite consistent. In almost all reports of deaths or illness, the essential oil used is almost always of a questionable quality. In one feline case, a lavender essential oil was used which was obtained online as supposedly high and therapeutic grade. However, when 4 ounces of such an oil is available at the going rate of $14.95, I can guarantee you that this is nowhere near a lavender essential oil that should be used for neither man nor beast. Combine that with the fact that it is sold and housed in a bottle with a rubber dropper, and we have an even more worrisome combination. I have witnessed many essential oils degrade and "explode" the rubber bulbs at the top of the bottle. Any company selling essential oils with this set up, is clearly not within good industry guidelines.

I truly do seek out reports and issues with essential oils. It is not uncommon for other veterinarians to seek me out if they feel they have a case of concern. And quite honestly, I enjoy the challenge of gathering important data. It is sort of like a mystery novel that I want to get to the end of. Where is the important information? Where is the smoking gun? And out of hundreds of cases evaluated, I can still say, that I usually find an error in the evaluation of the case.

Another case was of a cat that had Myrrh essential oil (of unknown quality or source), applied to the back of its head. The cat proceeded to be unhappy, and ran away from home. It was missing for two days, then returned in a sick state. It was automatically assumed that this cat's illness was due to the essential oil application, but not to the fact that while missing for 2 days, anything could have occurred, including drinking antifreeze. While I will not eliminate the potential problems that the cat may have experienced from the Myrrh application, all of the case facts pointed to symptoms that we are less likely to see with just a topical application of essential oil, and the subsequent issues therein. However, reports like these fuel the aromatherapy industry, to continue their safety concerns and talk about essential oil toxicity, especially in cats.

When we consider these passionate warnings to avoid the use of essential oils in certain ways, and in certain species, we need to remember a few things. The people conveying this information truly have the best interest of the animal at heart. But unfortunately, most are only regurgitating information that was taught to them decades ago – and evaluated by non-veterinary professionals, with no training in animal physiology, medicine, or pharmacokinetics and pharmacology. Yes, the information to remain "super safe" is not wrong, and it certainly will protect animals from unsafe use. However, I find more often that I and others are attacked when they offer that they have used oils in all of the ways that are "dangerous". The ability for some of the industry to accept something new, seems largely closed.

This is why I would like to change the wording of animal aromatherapy or veterinary medical aromatherapy to exclude "aromatherapy" in our verbiage. Aromatherapy is often misconstrued as to what it truly means. It is not just candles and scents to make you happy. True aromatherapy has real physical and emotional benefits. These benefits should demand respect, similarly to any other veterinary modality or drug I use. Anesthesia is certainly life-saving in many situations. But I think all would agree that it has to be calculated carefully, and used by trained and skilled personnel. I would never want my veterinary client to go online and select which anesthetic I would use for their animal. They are not trained properly to do so. Nor would I want them to source their own injectable antibiotics to use on their flock. I have experienced firsthand, someone who was purchasing liquid enrofloxacin online to use with her birds. As a veterinarian, I recognize that this drug has quite a distinct smell to it. When her source didn't seem to be working, I hated to inform her that because it had absolutely no smell, she was likely not even purchasing enrofloxacin, and who knows what she had actually been administering to her precious birds!

Veterinary Aromatic Medicine is not just for veterinarians. Just as a veterinary supplement or a veterinary recommended diet isn't only for a veterinarian to use or have knowledge of. However, I feel that the wording helps to impart the respect and ability we have with plant based medicine. Plant based medicine is evolving greatly in the veterinary field. Essential oils remain a huge addition that will continue to advance in the years to come.

To me, I consider essential oils to be quite similar to the use of Morphine in cats. When I was in veterinary school, we were taught that cats could simply not have Morphine. They would become dysphoric, and it was just a horrible thing, and could not, and should not be done. Then a few years later, someone gave a lecture on using Morphine properly in felines, and how wonderful it could be. Others started to dabble in it, and although I must admit, there was a bit of a learning curve, it became more and more widespread in its use, and painful felines everywhere, started to benefit from this drug. As long as it was used in the specific ways that cats needed it to be used.

It took quite a few years to change that dogma. And almost 20 years later, I am pleased to have blank stares of current veterinary students, who have never even heard that Morphine could not be used in cats. They are just automatically taught the proper use of the drug. This, seems to be the fate of essential oil information in my opinion. It may take a while, and a bit of convincing to a non-medical and non-scientific community (which can be harder), but eventually, we will recognize the full spectrum in which essential oils can be used with all species, as long as we do it safely, and with respect to their individual species needs.

You can read more in the cat specific chapters on their individual nuances, and the information that backs up what true veterinary medicine knows about their physiology. Information is nowhere near complete, and even I am greatly behind on my potential for publishing data. However, we must start to look at current data instead of decades old "urban legends".

I'll quickly comment here on the subject of Detoxification, and if a "reaction" to essential oil use is normal, to be expected, or a beneficial event. It is common for some people using essential oils to teach that this is a great thing. And that the body must be mounting a beneficial response to the use of oils. However, in clinical practice I do not feel that a healing crisis is necessary, nor beneficial. They can happen, but more often than not, I can get all of the benefits, without any of the woe when essential oils are used more appropriately. Any response that is not beneficial to your animal, or uncomfortable in any manner, needs to be re-evaluated and adjusted.

This may not include the overall dislike of being touched, applied to, or being "messed with" in general. There are many dogs who do not like water or rain on them, and will rub furiously along carpets and couches to get the offending rain drops off of them! However, any red skin, a worsening of conditions, diarrhea, etc…is something to avoid. As a veterinarian, I am not opposed to "forcing" a little bit of something on an animal to gain beneficial effects. Just like with oral medications in cats, they often do not volunteer at the chance to have a finger shoved down their throat. But Western Medicine is not the enemy – and we have to have an integrative approach. When something in my traditional tool kit is indicated, and needs to be used, I will still use it; whether the animal enjoys it or not. We certainly strive to make all things better, such as warming subcutaneous fluids, using a nice new and sharp needle, etc…but when push comes to shove, an animal doesn't always like everything that is necessary for their health.

The information provided within this book, should give you a great starting point for what is realistic for animals to use, and in safe methods and manners. Every animal is an individual, and some have more intricate health concerns than others. I will discuss the foundation of use for all animals in future chapters, but whenever there is concern, starting with a very light regimen and working your way up to more concentrated or aggressive use only as needed is the best advice.

The guidelines in this book will often give the average amounts or "end point" amounts that I often consider for an animal. This by no means, assures that this is the proper amount for every animal. Some animals may need more, and some animals may need less.

OIL SELECTION

It is possible for you to learn how to select oils, and how to evaluate their quality. The fact is, it takes a dedication, and a certain level of investment to do so. Here I will answer the most common questions I get on oil quality, and sources. And explain a bit of what proper selection can entail.

A common question is to wonder if you have to use organic or organically certified oils all the time. The easy answer to this is no. I often find that non-certified oils may have actually better quality and chemical parameters for my purposes in Veterinary Aromatic Medicine. In some cases, farms that have undergone certification, do so at the detriment of the actual plant. There are just some oils that are better when wild harvested, and allowed to grow in their native environment. When possible, we always opt for "certified" organic sources, but by knowing your suppliers and evaluating all oils regardless of various certifications, you are likely to encounter some gorgeous oils that should not be excluded from use.

For some farmers and distillers, their operation is small and more to what I would classify as artisan. It would not make financial sense for these farmers to certify their crops as organic, however, they still would technically qualify in standards. Artisan oils give us a great opportunity for wonderful and medically beneficial heritage plants to be harvested and distilled.

In sourcing, people have varying considerations of what a supplier is. Often times, people are considering only brand names. Many of these "brands" will be sourcing their oil supplies from the very same supplier in fact. There are companies that only supply large volumes of oils, companies that supply to the general public as well as some bulk purchasing options, and all shades in between. For the most part, an end consumer will be using a particular "brand" of essential oil most commonly. Many of the larger companies that supply oils to these retailers, are not readily advertised online or to the public. There is a bit of an "old boys club" in some aspects of sourcing oils, and it sometimes comes down to who you know, as to if you are alerted to some excellent oil availability.

Sources are often tightly guarded in the industry. It is a bit of a fallacy that you should be able to ask where the oils are coming from for any given retailer, and get a full answer. I have personally spent tens of thousands of dollars on evaluating my sources and suppliers, and so this is not information that I readily give out. There are definitely industry friends that I have, and we talk about our similar mutual suppliers, however, resources are not unlimited, so when I find an oil that I think is spectacular, I am not generally going to publicize it all over social media!

Certain essential oils may only be harvested once a year, and have very limited yield during distillation. For example, Melissa essential oil is one of my most precious oils. Not only is it only available in limited quantity, but I have only found one source that I truly adore. There are times when I am limited by my supplier (the person who imports this oil into the United States) on how much I can purchase at one time, or even on a monthly basis. To say I covet this oil is an understatement. Being without this oil, is not an option for me, and I would say it is a closely guarded secret as to where I find my preferred oil.

This is just standard for the industry as a whole, and many other industries as well. A pet food manufacturer is unlikely to tell you the sources of all of their ingredients, unless they have some exclusive relationship with that particular farm or supplier, and then the promotion of that information becomes valuable and logical for them. So, use common sense, when companies freely share trade secrets, it usually is a marketing strategy.

Another common misconception is the fact that any company could provide sometimes hundreds of different single essential oils, and truly farm, harvest, and distill all of these oils for themselves. While they may know their farmer or supplier, it would an astronomical impossibility for any one company to actually own and operate all aspects of this industry. And likely, you would not want them to. There are such intricacies to each individual crop and distillation process, that I feel we are in better hands allowing someone who understands lavender farming, harvest, and distillation backwards and forwards in their sleep, to work with their preferred plant in their own area of specialty. This is another area that parallels veterinary medicine. Just because a veterinarian will "see" your parrot in practice, does not make them a qualified avian vet. I think areas of specialty and focus, improve what we obtain in the final outcome.

What do you do if you want to start sourcing oils for yourself then? The answer is simple. You have to dive in, and start experiencing all parts and sources of oils for yourself. You will need to search on the internet for suppliers, and invest in the purchase of many essential oil "samples" to evaluate. The more you evaluate side by side, the more you can appreciate subtle differences in the country of origin, person who distilled the oil, and even in the year of harvest. Most people who guarantee that their oil is the best, or who feel certain that they need no other essential oil source, have never experienced multiple supply sources. If someone is encouraging you to believe that their oil is superior, make sure they have evaluated at least 10 different suppliers or brands of that same species, and that they can fully explain all of the subtle differences and reasons why they then handpicked their selection. When I speak to a potential new supplier, I can tell very quickly if they truly understand their product, and the processes of essential oil use, or if they are merely a sales person. The vast majority will be sales people.

While evaluating most essential oil samples, we will be using what is termed organoleptics. This is the basic smelling, experiencing, and sometimes tasting of the essential oil. It is truly important, and actually often more sensitive and accurate than computerized testing. While Gas Chromatography (GC) and Mass Spectrometry (MS) tests are also evaluated, these tests can be some of the more difficult areas to understand unless you train with a chemist, or have vast experience in what each individual oil should carry for constituents. Most people should rely on the experience of chemists whose job it is to evaluate essential oils on a daily basis for chemical analysis of oils. And in the reference section of the book – are several companies who provide well respected and independent analysis of essential oils.

After you have found your source of essential oil, to me it is a critical next step to actually use them. This may sound like a bit of a "no-brainer" – but I was amazed at the prevalence of products being added to the marketplace by companies, whether for animals or for humans, that had absolutely no prior use in the public or in clinical cases what-so-ever. A new animal blend could be whipped up, and on the shelves in a matter of months. All the while, the product had never actually been utilized with animals. Again, it is a buyer beware situation. Ask for some clinical cases or experiences, instead of only testimonials. Although I do believe that testimonials are important in how we learn more about what essential oils can do, I always hope for a little more data from any company who may be marketing a product specifically for an animal related need.

While this book is not to promote any one brand, it is good to note that there are single essential oils available to you that are specifically screened and evaluated for the use with animals. If you are unsure in any way that you may be hearing more marketing than truth, or if you are not confident in your ability to select essential oils to use, I suggest that you utilize only essential oils that have been selected for Veterinary Aromatic Medicine in the resource section.

If you are lucky enough to have a veterinarian who is recommending essential oil use with animals, here is a quick guideline to determine where your level of trust should lie. While a veterinarian may recommend a brand to you, and ensure that as long as you "order these" you will be safe – we need to carefully consider this statement. My preference would be that if a veterinarian recommends "xyz" brand that is not typically screened or created for use specifically with animals – that they personally evaluate each bottle you would purchase. Consistency of quality may fluctuate, regardless of company or source. And having an experienced person evaluate each and every bottle that you will use with your animals, is worth its weight in gold.

ORGANOLEPTICS

A fun and fancy word, it means the evaluation of an item through the senses of sight, touch, smell, and taste. Sight might include the color or turbidity of an essential oil. If it is clear, cloudy, yellow, green, containing debris, etc. Touch is likely less descriptive for essential oils, but I would include using the essential oil as intended, as part of this category. After all, we may have experienced the burning "touch" or sensation of a "hot" essential oil, or the cooling feeling of Peppermint. All of these factors are traits of an individual essential oil, and so can be valuable in its overall evaluation.

Smell is obviously one of the first characteristics we consider when evaluating essential oils. Watch anyone with a new oil, and the first thing they will do is to smell it. How they smell it can be a telling adventure. Most just grab a bottle, open and sniff. But you will find more experienced evaluators to request or use a paper strip that the oil has been applied to. While I still smell the bottle initially, there is much value to removing the oil from the bottle, and evaluating it away from oxidized oils that may be present on the bottle threads, or without the "headspace" that would be present above the essential oil within the bottle itself. Headspace is the unfilled space present above the essential oil, within a bottle. Depending on how much of the essential oil is missing from the bottle, there can be more or less air or oxygen in contact with the essential oil. Different volatile components may be present within that headspace than what are present in the whole oil. Upon first "whiff" of the bottle, different things may be detected than from a scent strip. There are certain oils in which I find this "headspace whiff" to be an important organoleptic, such as when evaluating for spoilage or oxidation, but we should always include proper smell evaluation in our organoleptic procedures. Some may select to smell the cap of a bottle, however, one must be careful with this practice as well, as there may be presence of more oxidized or evaporated oil within the threads of the cap.

Smelling with one nostril, and then another is also a technique of experienced aromatherapists. You will smell an item differently with your right nostril versus your left. These variances are important once you train your body to how different essential oils smell or should smell. For those who are inexperienced, they need to be mindful of smelling through one nostril or another, as they may assume the essential oil is noticeably different just from accidentally smelling on the right versus the left.

Another aspect of smell, which can be related to the sense of touch, is how the essential oil makes you feel while you inhale it. It is important to note how an essential oil makes you feel. Does it expand your sinuses? Do you get a feeling of dilation? Is there any ache or pressure that you feel within your nose, nostrils, or sinuses? Do you get an ache, sharp feeling, or pressure in any part of your head, or behind a specific eye? These things may sound unusual, but once trained, there are specific extenders, synthetics, or chemical presences that you can detect from the "feel" of the inhalation. Often it may be only to alert yourself that something is "off" – and you may not be able to pinpoint a direct issue. But I find more often than not, by being in tune to my body, I recognize a problem with an essential oil, before testing has ever revealed it.

When you trust your instincts, you will find that the human "computer" is actually quite sensitive. I once evaluated a sample from a well-respected supplier, and was quite surprised actually that I did not like the oil. There was just something about it that made me feel it was not the oil for me. The sample was filed within my essential oil library, and later that year I was informed that the product was actually an extract, and not a true essential oil. I then knew why I did not like that particular sample. Even if all of the specs and reputation is there, we are still wise to do our own personal evaluations, and to trust our interpretations.

The sense of taste for me is closely associated with smell. Many times, after inhaling an essential oil, I will detect varying tastes within my mouth. It has always been true that these senses are closely related, and I find that certain chemical constituents, extenders, or synthetics will literally leave a bad taste in my mouth. There may be some evaluators who truly taste their essential oils and can detect many things in this way, but for me the simple fact of being aware of this sense during inhalation is often enough.

GRAS STATUS

You'll hear this term bumped around a lot. Like it is some magic term that makes all essential oils perfectly harmless and okay to use. GRAS means "Generally Recognized As Safe". This is a list generated by the EPA (Environmental Protection Agency) of which substances are considered safe for use in foods. Unfortunately, this means that they have been evaluated for use with levels generally used in flavoring, and not in therapeutic levels that we use in aromatherapy.

While still helpful, as items that go into our foods have usually been researched a bit more heavily in toxicity studies, it still should not be used as the magic bullet to claim an oil to be harmless. It still is "all about the dose". However, for the veterinary world, most of the research on safety of essential oils starts with animal based studies. So in reality, Veterinary Aromatic Medicine is likely to hold more truth and answers when we evaluate available research, than actual human data would.

The FDA includes on the GRAS list these "Essential oils, oleoresins (solvent-free), and natural extractives (including distillates) that are generally recognized as safe for their intended use":

Allspice (Pimenta officinalis)
Almond, bitter (free from prussic acid)
Angelica (Angelica archangelica)
Anise (Pimpinella anisum)
Basil (Ocimum basilicum)
Bergamot (Citrus bergamia)
Black Pepper (Piper nigrum)
Cananga (Cananga odorata)
Caraway (Carum carvi)
Cardamom (Elettaria cardamomum)
Carrot (Daucus carota)
Cassia (Cinnamomum cassia)
Celery Seed (Apium graveolens)
Cilantro (Coriandrum sativum)
Cinnamon, Bark/Leaf (Cinnamomum zeylanicum)
Citronella (Cymbopogon nardus)

Clary Sage (Salvia sclarea)
Clove (Eugenia caryophyllata)
Coriander (Coriandrum sativum)
Cumin (Cuminum cyminum)
Fennel, Sweet (Foeniculum vulgare)
Galanga (Alpinia officinarum)
Geranium (Pelargonium graveolens)
German Chamomile (Matricaria chamomilla)
Ginger (Zingiber officinale)
Grapefruit (Citrus paradisi)
Helichrysum (Helichrysum angustifolium)
Hops (Humulus lupulus)
Hyssop (Hyssopus officinalis)
Juniper Berry (Juniperus communis)
Laurus nobilis
Lavender (Lavandula officinalis)
Lavender, Spike (Lavandula latifolia)
Lavandin
Lemon (Citrus limon)
Lemongrass (Cymbopogon flexuosus)
Lime (Citrus aurantifolia)
Mandarin (Citrus reticulata)
Marjoram (Origanum majorana)
Melissa (Melissa officinalis)
Mustard (Brassica spp.)
Neroli (Citrus aurantium)
Nutmeg (Myristica fragrans)
Onion (Allium cepa)
Orange (Citrus aurantium)
Oregano (Origanum vulgare)
Palmarosa   (Cymbopogon martini)
Paprika (Capsicum annuum)
Pepper, Black (Piper nigrum)
Peppermint (Mentha piperita)
Petitgrain (Citrus aurantium)
Pimenta (Pimenta officinalis)
Roman Chamomile (Anthemis nobilis)
Rose (Rosa damascena)
Rose Geranium (Pelargonium graveolens)
Rosemary (Rosmarinus officinalis)
Rosewood (Aniba rosaeodora)
Sage (Salvia officinalis)

Savory, Summer (Satureia hortensis)
Savory, Winter (Satureia montana)
Spearmint (Mentha spicata)
Tangerine (Citrus reticulate)
Tarragon (Artemisia dracunculus)
Thyme (Thymus vulgaris)
Turmeric (Curcuma longa)
Vanilla (Vanilla planifolia)
Wild Orange (Citrus sinensis)
Ylang Ylang (Cananga odorata)

GAS CHROMATOGRAPHY & MASS SPECTROMETRY

Commonly referred to as GC/MS or even simply GC analysis, these tests are often considered the hallmark of how to evaluate an essential oil. Unfortunately, they are difficult tests to evaluate for most people, and many would not even know where to begin in reading one or what to look for. Sadly however, you will hear lay persons demanding to see the GC report quite often, and it has become a bit of a falsehood that the quality of the essential oil depends on if the company is forth giving of these reports.

With many essential oil companies now posting their GC reports online, we have entered into the age of falsification. Unscrupulous companies wishing to cash in on the essential oil band wagon have been caught selling essential oils that are not even of the species that is reportedly being sold. I have no doubt that there are many falsified documents floating around within the retail world, and this too becomes a buyer beware situation. Not many people can afford to have their recreational essential oils tested by well-known laboratories and chemists. Knowing and trusting who you obtain your essential oils from, and who has done any existing testing and evaluation of them is still key to using this evaluation.

A Gas Chromatograph is a way to analyze the components of an essential oil. This technique is used in other areas of medicine and laboratory research as well. Even the spice industry uses GC to evaluate their spices for accuracy, identity, and purity. Each GC machine, however, needs to be specifically set up for the type of material you wish to run on it. And in the case of essential oils, often times the Gas Chromatography technician will need a bit of additional training to understand and work with the nuances of evaluation of essential oils. Not just anyone with a GC will be capable of properly evaluating an essential oil.

With a GC analysis, a sample of the essential oil is often heated in the presence of a carrier gas such as helium. Essential oils are volatile substances, and each individual chemical constituent will carry a different molecular weight. This fact means that each constituent will leave the body of the essential oil at a different time. Sort of think of it like people jumping off of a sinking ship. Some people may jump first, while others hang around for a while. With essential oils, the more volatile essential oil components will "jump" away from the whole essential oil and down the tube of the machine first. A simplistic view, but pretty accurate. The computer and advanced laboratory detection units, will record who jumped first, at what time, and how much of a splash they made (basically how much they weighed!) Each constituent is often identified by its own characteristic trait of when it jumps. Then, the percent of the individual constituents found within the essential oil is reported on the end document.

Mass Spectrometry (MS) measures the mass of each particular chemical within a sample. By calculating the weight and percentage of each chemical constituent within a sample, in theory it should add up to 100% of the sample detected on the GC. If all of the chemicals detected on the GC only added up to 90% of the sample's mass – then 10% of that sample is something else that the GC did not even detect. In this way, we can use this tool to find other items which may be included within an essential oil sample that are not truly volatile, were not dectected on GC, or are not supposed to be there.

ESSENTIAL OIL DILUTION RATES

In general, there are a few guidelines that we can start with in terms of how dilute we should be using essential oils with animals. Because of the wide range of species we can be dealing with, it is not only important to consider if you are working with a cat, dog, or bird – but to also fully understand that for example – applying a greasy carrier oil solution to a birds feathers would be wholly inappropriate. So there are other considerations than just basic concentration of the essential oil presented in every situation.

Concentration and dilution of the essential oil, are related words discussing much of the same idea. In technical terms the concentration should refer to how much essential oil is present within a carrier oil for instance, unless specified differently. If I made a Lavender solution at a 5% concentration – this should mean that there is 5% of the Lavender present and the remaining 95% is the carrier substance. However, some people will change up this statement describing the mixture as 5% diluted. This is technically inaccurate.

A 5% dilution would really mean that you diluted the Lavender by 5%. All in all, we just need to be careful with how we speak, and how we relate accurate recipes to others. Years back, I polled a Facebook group to ask what people thought a 5% dilution or concentration was. Even among certified aromatherapists, there were conflicts about which term to use, what it exactly meant, what recipe would result in said concentrations, and many, many people (aromatherapists included) had the wrong answers in terms of actual concentration results.

For me, I like to keep things as simple as possible. Most often, this may mean relating recipes in the easiest terms for most people to work with. Often drops and a common volume of carrier to be used. However, although widely understood and easy to work with – drops are not the most accurate way to prescribe, measure, or record essential oil use.

We'll cover drops and milligrams contained in essential oils in the next chapter, but for now back to general dilution concepts. When using essential oils clinically, we can consider their dilution to occur in several ways. First, a stronger essential oil may be functionally diluted within a more mild essential oil. Although the total concentration of essential oils still would be a "neat" or undiluted mixture, we can understand that a drop of straight Cinnamon oil would be far more intense than one drop of Cinnamon oil mixed into 10mL of Tangerine essential oil.

Also, although I might put an undiluted essential oil within water – it is in effect diluted in the way it is presented. This is a harder concept to wrap your head around, so I'll explain it in terms which most people get confused about. If I add 4 drops of Lavender to 4oz (120mL) of water; it is true, the essential oil is not going to be fully dispersed within the water. However, when I shake up the water, all of the little neat (undiluted) droplets of Lavender will be spread apart. Think of it as a crowd of people. If you are all crammed into a box car on a subway train, your concentration is really dense (neat oil). If we put one person in each box car, you are spread out, and much less likely to be encountered, stepped on, or annoying to others. So, by placing an essential oil within water, we use the water to not truly "dilute" the essential oil, but to obtain a method of distributing it far and wide, and in teeny tiny amounts over a larger area.

When I shake up a water mist with essential oils in it – I can spread one drop of essential oil over an area of a square foot, instead of one drop hitting the skin directly and intensely. While we still have to consider which essential oils we perform "water-misting" or "spritzing" with – this can be a very effective way to have very small amounts of essential oils applied. I often prefer a water mist for application situations for which greasy or fatty carrier oils will not be idea. Such as for misting birds, or for a wound that is moist and added moisture would not be desired. If a wound or infection would most likely benefit from being "dried out" – then a water mist is an excellent way to apply a very tiny bit of essential oil, especially over a larger surface area.

Situations where water-misting is ideal – over incision areas, onto feathered creatures, onto hot spots and other moist wounds or infections. Of course, the essential oil to be misted has to be considered. While we may be able to do a light mist of even a hot oil like Oregano to a horse for a case of Scratches (Greasy Heel), it would of course be totally inappropriate to mist a bird with an Oregano water mist.

Depending on the essential oil to be water-misted, we can vary our concentration within the water to the effect we need. For very conservative cases, with highly sensitive animals, we may add only 1 drop of essential oil to 1oz (30mL) of water. However, with more mild essential oils, or for more effect needed, we may even use 15 drops per 1oz (30mL) of water. You can read more about water-misting in the chapter Topical Applications, or in the animal specific recommendations for each species.

Another form of dilution of essential oils is when we add them to carrier oils. These in general are fatty or greasy oils such as Fractionated Coconut Oil or other seed or vegetable oils. See the chapter on Carrier Oils for more specifics on the differences in these items. Of all of the carrier oil options available, Fractionated Coconut Oil remains the most suitable for most animal needs. It handles well with fur, absorbs nicely into skin, has very little if any allergen concerns for human or animal, and does not tend to stain materials or fabric that the animal may come in contact with.

When considering the dilution of essential oils for use with animals, we should usually consider the species first. Below is a quick reference for each species, and the approximate percentage in which we use essential oils when mixed into a carrier oil. Certainly variations may be needed – certain essential oils may be more appropriate at higher or lower percentages of use, or certain animals may require higher or lower percentages.

Avian, Birds, Parrots, Finches – often do not use fatty carrier oils. 1-5% of total essential oil concentration is suggested.
Chickens, Fowl, Duck – these birds can often tolerate higher concentrations of essential oils, mainly applied to feet. 5-30% total essential oil concentrations have been used.
Lizards, Reptiles, Turtles – often do not use fatty carrier oils. When indicated 1-5% total essential oil concentrations are generally suggested.
Chinchillas – often do not use fatty carrier oils due to hair coat. When applying to hairless regions, 1-3% total essential oil concentration.
Rabbits – 1-5% total essential oil concentration.
Guinea Pigs, Rats, Rodents – 3-5% total essential oil concentration.
Ferrets – 3-7% total essential oil concentration.
Cats – 3-7% total essential oil concentration.
Dogs – 5-50% total essential oil concentration can be used.
Horses – 10-50% total essential oil concentrations are suggested.
Sheep, Goats, Llama, Other Livestock – 10-50% total essential oil concentrations are suggested.

Concentrations and Percentages of Essential Oils
It is the most important thing for you to understand what a 1% essential oil solution will be, and how to create it.

To calculate out the percentage of essential oils within a solution you create, you must do a bit of math. Say you add 24 drops into 30mL (1oz) of a carrier oil. First, the size of the drop will matter with the actual volume of essential oil that is added to your creation. Since a drop may be anywhere between 0.02mL to 0.04mL (and really could still vary depending on the dropper or pipette you selected) – if we average a drop to be 0.03mL – we can say we added 0.72mL to 30mL of carrier oil.

In math – to find the percentage of the essential oil concentration – we will divide the essential oil volume, by the volume of the TOTAL solution (and these must be in a common measurement type so drops to drops, mL to mL, etc…). So the inaccurate math would be 0.72 ÷ 30 = WRONG. This calculation yields 0.02 which is 2%. The correct calculation would be 0.72 ÷ 30.72 = CORRECT. This instance still yields a 2% concentration value, however as volumes get larger and larger, this becomes a greater issue.

If you used the same size drops – then 24 drops in 1000 drops of carrier oil – would yield a 2% solution, or concentration of essential oil within a carrier oil. However, not many people really want to count 1000 drops! So we usually default to using volume, with milliliter (mL) being the most common volumetric used with essential oil work.

For a larger batch of essential oils – let's consider a more bulk situation to see how the calculation can become faulty. I add 200mL of essential oils to 900mL of a carrier oil. If I divide 200 ÷ 900 = my answer is 0.22 or 22%. This is WRONG. Your actual concentration of the essential oil is 200mL within the TOTAL volume of 1100mL (900+200). The correct calculation is 200 ÷ 1100 = 0.18 or 18%. That is a 4% calculation error – and with small animals this may be a potentially harmful calculation error.

Another example may be if I am adding 2mL of essential oil to 8oz of shampoo. Now, math can become more difficult. We need to convert each measurement of volume, to the same type of measure. So mL to mL, or oz to oz. Let's convert the 8oz into mL. There are 30mL in 1oz. So 30mL x 8oz = 240mL in 8 ounces of shampoo. To figure out the concentration now of the essential oil within the shampoo – 2mL essential oil ÷ the TOTAL solution volume of 242mL = 0.01 or 1% concentration of essential oil within the shampoo we created.

If you are one that does not thrive on calculations and math – it is best if you follow specific recipes that give you distinct and easy to follow measurements.

DILUTION RATES

Another few chemistry points for those who are really particular...The volume of two solutions added together, does not always equal a truly additive result. What does this mean? Well if we add 2mL of something to 30mL of something else – we do not ALWAYS end up with 32mL of liquid. Certain chemical reactions can occur, and so it "could" be possible that we end up with less total volume. This does not appear to be a common occurrence with essential oils, thank goodness, and when we add a certain number of mL to a certain amount of carrier oil, true additive properties seem to hold true. But, if any student needs a research project, I am pretty sure they could add volumes together all day long, with different oil types, and different carrier oils to see if they could find a difference. Sounds exciting! I won't be getting right on that!

Let's give you a few measurement conversions that are often needed in Veterinary Aromatic Medicine.

1 teaspoon (tsp) = 4.93mL (5mL)
1 Tablespoon (Tbsp) = 14.79mL (15mL) = ½ oz
1 ounce (oz) = 30mL
½ ounce (oz) = 15mL = 1 Tbsp
1 drop = 0.02 to 0.04mL
1mL contains approximately 20-40 drops (30 average)

Therefore in an essential oil bottle:
5mL contains approximately 150 drops (range 100-200)
10mL contains approximately 300 drops (range 200-400)
15mL contains approximately 450 drops (range 300-600)
30mL contains approximately 900 drops (range 600-1200)

mL = milliliter. A "cc" is the same as a mL – just in a different unit of measure (cubic centimeter). There are 1000mL in one Liter (L).

Let's give you a cheat sheet of various concentrations used with animals. All calculations are based on an average 0.03mL per drop. While it will remain more accurate to measure your volumes while diluting, even the variations within drop size will generally result in recipes which are still safe in concentration. It is important to recognize, that measurement by kitchen teaspoon or Tablespoon, is far less accurate than a graduated cylinder or syringe.

How to Obtain Percentages

1% Concentration:

Essential Oil	Carrier
2 drops	5mL (1 tsp)
3 drops	10mL (2 tsp)
4 drops	15mL (½ oz)
9 drops	30mL (1 oz)

2% Concentration:

Essential Oil	Carrier
3 drops	5mL (1 tsp)
6 drops	10mL (2 tsp)
9 drops	15mL (½ oz)
18 drops	30mL (1 oz)

3% Concentration:

Essential Oil	Carrier
5 drops	5mL (1 tsp)
9 drops	10mL (2 tsp)
13 drops	15mL (½ oz)
27 drops	30mL (1 oz)

4% Concentration:

Essential Oil	Carrier
7 drops	5mL (1 tsp)
13 drops	10mL (2 tsp)
19 drops	15mL (½ oz)
37 drops	30mL (1 oz)

5% Concentration:

Essential Oil	Carrier
8 drops	5mL (1 tsp)
16 drops	10mL (2 tsp)
24 drops	15mL (½ oz)
48 drops	30mL (1 oz)

You'll notice now that if you want a 6% concentration – you can NOT simply double your drops added, from the 3% essential oil amount. This is because total drops do not equate to a set volume to percentage conversion, and so as our drop numbers increase, we may not get a match for match on the resulting concentration. Individual calculations for each solution is recommended when strict requirements of dilution may be needed.

We'll calculate out a few more of the common dilution rates recommended, especially for the cases of work with smaller animals – so that you will have an easy and quick reference.

6% Concentration:

Essential Oil	Carrier
10 drops	5mL (1 tsp)
20 drops	10mL (2 tsp)
30 drops	15mL (½ oz)
59 drops	30mL (1 oz)

7% Concentration:

Essential Oil	Carrier
12 drops	5mL (1 tsp)
24 drops	10mL (2 tsp)
35 drops	15mL (½ oz)
70 drops	30mL (1 oz)

10% Concentration:

Essential Oil	Carrier
18 drops	5mL (1 tsp)
35 drops	10mL (2 tsp)
53 drops	15mL (½ oz)
105 drops	30mL (1 oz)

As we move into higher concentrations – it is best if larger total batches are measured with glass graduated cylinders. Always measure "to the bottom of the meniscus" (you can google this if you are not aware how to accurately measure liquids with a graduated cylinder) – and you will be much happier than counting upwards of 100 drops!

Another consideration that makes "real sense" is that fact that we cannot add 5mL into 30mL of carrier oil, within a bottle designed to carry 30mL. While we can often fit a certain number of drops within a 1oz bottle (30mL) beyond that actual 30mL amount (consider that most essential oil bottles are not full to the top when you purchase them) – there does become a limit. So you will note in the following concentrations – amounts to derive a total bottle volume, more so than how much to add to a standard volume. Because let's face it – this is the *real world*. And I want to use real bottles! *Real world* recipes will be in *italics*.

Then, you will also note that there is a part to part designation now behind the concentration. So 1 part: 6 parts. This allows for a bit easier dilution "on the fly" or the ability to customize to any volume you want. The part can be a drop, it can be 2 drops, 10 drops, 1mL or any measure you select. The part to part conversion is not always 100% accurate. For example the 15% Concentration – 1 part to 6 parts truly equals a bit over 14%. You get this percentage by dividing 1 by the TOTAL amount of parts – so $1 \div 7 = 0.1429$ or 14%. Basically, you'll still be quite safe and effective, but when crunched for time, you can quickly dilute even in your hand – by adding 1 drop essential oil, and 6 drops carrier oil.

Note: while syringes may work wonderfully to measure carrier oils, they do not work well for essential oils. Essential oils tend to cause degradation of the plunger, and risk of plastics dissolving into your essential oil is high. Even with syringes that appear to be "made" for essential oil use. I advise against the use of plastic syringes.

15% Concentration (~1 part: 6 parts)

Essential Oil	Carrier
29 drops	5mL (1 tsp)
57 drops	10 mL (2 tsp)
85 drops	15mL (½ oz)
(73 drops)	*(13mL)*
5.1mL	30mL
(4.25mL)	*(25mL)*

20% Concentration (1 part: 4 parts)

Essential Oil	Carrier
42 drops	5mL (1 tsp)
(34 drops)	*(4mL)*
84 drops	10mL (2 tsp)
(67 drops)	*(8mL)*
(3mL)	*(12mL)*
(6mL)	*(24mL)*

25% Concentration (1 part: 3 parts)

Essential Oil	Carrier
1mL	3mL
2mL	6mL
3mL	9mL
7mL	21mL

30% Concentration (~1 part: 2 parts)

Essential Oil	Carrier
1mL	2.3mL
1.3mL	3mL
3mL	**7mL** – easiest way to create TRUE 30%
4.5mL	10.5mL
9mL	21mL

35% Concentration (~1 part: 2 parts)

Essential Oil	Carrier
1mL	1.8mL
1.6mL	3mL
4mL	**7.5mL** – easiest way to create TRUE 35%
8mL	**15mL**
9mL	17mL

40% Concentration (1 part: 1.5 parts)

Essential Oil	Carrier
1mL	1.5mL
2mL	**3mL** – easiest way to create TRUE 40%
4mL	**6mL**
5mL	7.5mL
10mL	15mL

45% Concentration (~1 part: 1.25 parts)

Essential Oil	Carrier
1mL	1.2mL
2mL	*2.4mL*
6mL	7.5mL
13.5mL	**16.5mL** – easiest way to create TRUE 45%

50% Concentration (1 part: 1 part) (50:50) (1:1)

Essential Oil	Carrier
2.5mL	2.5mL
5mL	5mL
7.5mL	7.5mL
15mL	15mL

At the higher concentrations, you notice that I go up by 5% increments. While you may certainly calculate out each increase in concentration by 1% at a time, when moving to a higher concentration, especially if I have already been at a 20% concentration or higher, I find that the increase by 5% is overall a decent decision. However, for those in the 10% and under range, much more sensitive adjustments to total concentration should be observed.

USE OF NEAT OIL

Some subjects just bear repeating, and a whole chapter unto themselves. In the past, we did use some "neat" or undiluted essential oil application techniques. And for the most part, we still can to some degree. However, the thing to consider now, is how much have we learned since 2011 (yes my first edition book was written in 2011, and published in 2012)... Quite a bit really. And while larger companies will still like for you to use neat oils (it does use them up a bit faster so you have to buy more) – their recommendations are not based on what is best for an animal (or human) – but out of what is convenient to lazy humans, and best for their resales. Doing the work and recognition of what actually works better, and being willing to admit that change is good – is not in the wheelhouse of most larger companies.

Let's go through some of the reasons why we will use neat oils. Certainly with diffusion is one of the primary reasons for using neat oils. The fact that a carrier oil may be within a blend or used to dilute a single oil, will not be the best thing for your diffuser. Both water-based or air-style diffusers should not be used with carrier oils. Now, if you have already accidentally done this – do not worry. If your diffuser did not break, and is still running. Just stop this practice. And no, you did not do any harm to yourself or your animals. We have nasal hairs, and a respiratory system in place, that filters out harmful things in the air that we are not meant to breathe. So any fatty droplets that "might" have made it into the air (they are less likely to do so because of their weight and lack of volatility) – likely got trapped and excreted in nasal hairs, and cells lined with mucus and cilia to remove the offending foreign material.

There are other situations in which we use neat oils as well. Within water-mists for example. Although water-mists "can" be created with an essential oil or blend that has been diluted in a carrier as well. For certain lesions, wounds, lumps, or bumps we may find that neat application is more indicated. Such as for skin tags. It won't do any harm that we start with diluted oils first, unless the lesion is already super moist or greasy, and our goal is to have drying effects. But, for discrete lesions, occasionally we will note that a very small amount of a neat oil applied directly to it, is far superior.

When adding essential oils to other carriers, such as shampoo – then also a neat oil is more indicated. Although we can also certainly add essential oils within a carrier oil to a shampoo – it becomes a bit harder to obtain a therapeutic concentration of essential oils, depending on how diluted that blend may be.

And of course, if there is a lot of carrier oil added to a shampoo, it will start to degrade the oil cleansing actions of the shampoo, and create too greasy of a situation.

Likely the most confusion I hear, is about how a water-mist made with neat oils and misted on an animal is different from a "neat application". My best advice is also to try it on yourself. Have you dripped neat oil onto your skin? There is a small dot of a very intense item, right at that location. Now add that drop into water, shake the bottle, and mist it over your entire arm. Is it different? It sure is! So, while you are still technically having a neat oil misted onto you, the tiny droplets of it are so small, and so wide spread (dispersal), we really see it more as a "diluted" application, and one that a body and skin can handle far better. Water is technically a dispersant in this situation. Remember, an essential oil within a carrier oil, is also just spread out in the carrier vehicle. While some carriers may bind a bit to the oil, you are still just creating the situation where the "total amount of essential oil" becomes spread out over the body. So in this way, we will view them as quite similar.

What did we see clinically that made us start to deviate from neat oil use? First, and possibly most importantly, it just showed itself as being completely unnecessary. When I encountered a horse who had an application of 30% concentrated oils within a carrier, versus a horse who had neat oils applied – they both saw results. However, the horse with diluted oils had the effects last longer! That was where my veterinary brain started to pay attention. If we could do daily applications with diluted oils, instead of three times a day with neat oils – why was this occurring?

Here are the reasons why a neat application may work differently. First, we have a hair coat on most animals. So the oil is destined to contact there first, even with a petting technique. Neat oils evaporate much more readily, so by the time the oil contacts the animal, or is absorbed through the hairs, a large majority of the oil has already evaporated away. When an essential oil is mixed into a carrier oil, the fatty substance protects the essential oil from immediate evaporation, allowing it to stay in contact with the animal longer. We saw this distinctly with fly sprays for horses. If we applied a water mist with an essential oil, we saw that it might work well, but as soon as it was dry it had evaporated away – and there was not as much benefit. So we started to make our bug spray solutions within Fractionated Coconut Oil for my horses and cow. And it lasted a lot longer! It was far more economical for large animals, definitely made more sense!

This holds true for other topical applications. While some may think that a neat application is more powerful, it is, but in a different way, and for a different length of time. I often say a neat application is like being punched, while a diluted application is like a massage. They may both get blood moving to your muscles, but one is likely to take longer, be less damaging, but also be more rewarding in the long run! A neat application will have a shorter time to absorption. So any neat oil applied is absorbed faster – but this also means it will often be metabolized and eliminated faster as well. A diluted application will have a slower onset of actions generally, but will continue to deliver its benefits far longer as it continues to be absorbed.

With petting applications, this is likely where most people are destined to continue to use neat oils. And this is still fine, you are still "diluting" your exposure to the neat oil by distributing it throughout your hands, and because there will be a lot of absorption and evaporation into your hands as well, and less reaching the animal as the final result. However, petting with a diluted oil is likely to achieve a little bit longer acting time as well.

The other thing that was distinctly different with neat applications versus diluted, was the issue with horses and what we used to term "Raindrop Welts". You can read more about this in other chapters, but the basic facts are – we saw these with neat application of oils, we did not have to see these welts for a treatment to be effective, and indeed applications of diluted oils did not cause welts or discomfort, and still were just as effective, if not more. We do not have to irritate a body to make a treatment effective.

The simple fact is that while we "can" apply neat oils to some animals, we just don't always need to. And in fact, we can see distinct benefits in NOT applying neat oils versus diluted oils as well. And that is good enough for me.

FORMS OF DILUTION

This is likely a good time for some clarification of a few terms. Things like dilution are often used to describe a variety of actual processes. However, for animals, we will remain a bit more limited than the human world on what is appropriate to put into a spray or use around an animal.

First, surfactants. These are mainly chemicals used to reduce the surface tension between liquids. If you have heard some popular quotes "they make water wetter"...but in reality surfactants help to combine materials that would otherwise not mix together. So, when we use a shampoo with a surfactant, dirt or oil is more readily mixed into the soapy water, to be washed away.

Surfactants are used in a variety of industries, and most commonly you'll see them in soaps and shampoos. While there are some "more natural" surfactants in this world (derived from seeds or plants) – they remain a bit on the "aggressive" side for what we want to expose animals to directly. So for any formulation that will involve adding essential oils into water for use on animals – I will recommend leaving the addition of surfactants out. If you are adding essential oils to a cleaning recipe, that contains natural surfactants – this is fine. Likewise, if you are adding essential oils to a natural shampoo that contains natural surfactants, this is also fine. The main goal is that you will not be creating a water mist, intended to be misted onto an animal while adding a surfactant to it. Basically, avoid the addition of surfactants into direct animal intended blends or sprays.

Dilution. This word is likely least understood in the technical sense. And even I will call a "dispersment" a dilution of sorts – although technically wrong. Dilution is when a substance is reduced in concentration, generally by another like substance. When essential oils are mixed into fractionated coconut oil, they become joined together in the dilution. Rarely do we see the essential oil separate from the fatty carrier oil again, and sit on the top. However, if we add the essential oil into water, after a while it will separate and float on top. Sort of like oil and vinegar – while you can shake it and mix it temporarily, it will separate eventually. Oil and vinegar are not a dilution. But essential oils within fatty carriers are a dilution. Another dilution would be when you add water to a juice concentrate (can of frozen orange juice). Once mixed together, your juice remains "juice" and does not separate out again. A dilution is a more permanent way to achieve a lesser concentration of an essential oil single or blend.

Dispersment. This situation most accurately described when we add an essential oil blend or single to water, then shake it really well. This will break up the essential oil particles into tiny bits, and scatter them throughout the water. Dispersing them. Then, if we use this water to "mist" or spritz out of a spray bottle, we are further dispersing the droplets of essential oil far and wide. If we let the shaken mixture sit long enough, eventually the essential oil (if lighter than water) will separate out and float on the top. There can be essential oils and blends which are heavier than water, and could sink.

Emulsions and emulsifiers. An easy emulsion to think of is lotion or mayonnaise. These are created by "whipping" the items quickly to change the molecular bonding, so they want to stay together. With lotion, a water and a fat are whipped quickly, and may include some sort of chemical emulsifier to help accomplish stability. Chemical emulsifiers are less appropriate to use with animals, and may be toxic. However, natural DIY lotions and recipes are fine to use when appropriate for the condition, and essential oils generally mix well into an emulsion. However, it is not necessary to use an emulsion when we are considering the dilution of essential oils for use.

Solvents. This is something that dissolves the essential oil, and essentially makes it easier to incorporate into another item. The most common situation for this is the addition of essential oils into an alcohol, such as ethanol (or grain alcohol, vodka, or Everclear), and then adding this mixture into water. As you can imagine, the use of alcohol, even if consumable by humans, for animal products is less than ideal. Misting a bird with a bit of a vodka mixed tonic, would not be appropriate in the least. However, for a few select situations, such as an ear spray recipe – we can see benefits to adding alcohol. Not only will it act to solubilize the essential oil, and make it easier to carry within water, but the alcohol itself can carry some beneficial drying properties. For the most part, any solvent that is not edible should not be considered for animal use. However, even with edible (or drinkable as it were) solvents such as vodka – extreme caution and common sense should be used. Great consideration of the location of treatment, any licking that may occur, and total exposure to the alcohol has to be carefully weighed. Alcohol can also be an item that will sting on open or broken skin – so caution should be used. Everclear remains the most recommended form of alcohol used when a solvent is considered for animal use.

Take home message – when reducing the concentration of essential oils that an animal will be exposed with there are a few common factors to be considered. All ingredients should be consumable; that is, perfectly safe for ingestion. Artificial chemicals should be avoided as much as possible, however when surfactants are already present in natural shampoos and similar animal safe items, this remains fine to use. Most dilutions should be performed with fatty carrier oils – and Fractionated Coconut Oil remains the favorite choice (see chapter on Carrier Oils). Dispersment is an effective form of the reduction of exposure to essential oils with animals – and a plain water addition (generally distilled water) is recommended and suggested.

DROPS & MEASUREMENTS

A drop is not a drop, is not a drop, is not a drop. As you were exposed in previous chapters, in the world of essential oils, we tend to discuss everything in drops. Each essential oil bottle, each essential oil dropper insert, each essential oil, each pipette...all have their own calibration in terms of what a drop contains. And this information bears repeating in its own chapter.

In general we widely accept that most drops are about 0.03mL or cc. This is a volume measurement of liquid. For most veterinarians we are very comfortable with milliliter measurements from syringes. Essential oils and syringes do not mix however, and attempts to draw and measure with syringes are often met with stuck plungers and destroyed and non-functional materials.

There have actually been scientific investigations on the size of a drop of essential oil. The number of drops per mL of essential oil, was recorded from different dropper styles and for different essential oils. On average, 20-40 drops were contained per mL. This is a pretty wide range actually, however thankfully the differences are unlikely to greatly affect an essential oil recipe you may be using.

As a veterinarian, my medical brain craves a more accurate solution. I wanted to know the direct milligrams per milliliter of an essential oil – just like I would with an injectable medication. All of our drugs are calculated in milligrams (mg) and so a pill has a known milligram amount within it, and an injectable has a known milligram amount per milliliter. Then we can carefully and exactly calculate how many milligrams we want to administer based on the weight of a patient.

But for essential oils, this information seems to be widely ignored. In actuality, it is a pretty simple thing to calculate out the milligrams within the essential oil drop, or within a milliliter. You weigh the essential oil! I was actually sort of disappointed when I figured this out. It is a straight weight measurement. I expected that I would have to do some back flips, while crunching numbers based on the molecular weight of the essential oil, while considering the room temperature in which I did those calculations. But nope, just weigh it. Simple as that. So if my goal is to give 50mg of an essential oil – just weigh out 50mg of the essential oil. Of course, each essential oil will have a different milligram amount present within a drop or within 1mL. This variation is due to its own molecular weight.

A milligram scale can generally be found fairly affordably online these days, and if you desire to measure in "super nerd-dom" – then weighing is for you!

One drop is generally accepted to be between 20-35 milligrams (mg) of essential oil. Many aromatherapists today utilize 35mg as the average drop, maybe erring on the side of safety, while old school sources may assume 25mg per drop. We will simply assume 35mg per drop for our purposes within this book – but remember, your truly accurate way to measure an essential oil is by weighing it.

Naturally, we can transfer these milligram measurements to assume that if there are approximately 30 drops in a mL, then there are likely 900mg per mL. But again, this is not highly accurate, especially as we get into higher and higher numbers of drops. Weighing should still remain the most accurate way to know a true dose of an essential oil.

You can also blend via weight. If you had a blend that contained 1mL of Peppermint, and 2mL of Ginger, and so forth; you could instead measure the weight of the 1mL of Peppermint, and the weight of 2mL of Ginger. Then, as with most chemical scales, we can actually tare (or zero out) the scale between each addition. Even before blending begins, we can tare the scale to "ignore" the weight of the container we are blending into.

Just another way to add accuracy to our activities. So a blend may now go together in this way. Place your bottle onto the milligram (or even gram scale in larger batches) – and tare the scale (setting it to zero to eliminate the weight of the bottle). Then, your recipe for oils to add into your blend, will then be based on weight. So 30mg of Peppermint, 60mg of Ginger, etc. You could tare the scale between each addition, or write your recipe in terms of totals. Whatever is better for your brain. In terms of totals – your recipe may start with the tared scale and bottle, then "add Peppermint to 30mg" then "add Ginger to 90mg", etc...

Basically, blending is an art form. And no two artists do it the same way – nor should they. Independent creative juices add character and love to our end result. I personally currently blend by measuring each essential oil in a glass graduated cylinder. Usually one at a time. For a few blends, I may add three of my essential oils into a larger cylinder, then pour them all at once into my blend bottle. However, this can take a bit of care in addition and tracking of "ingredients". Making a recipe sheet is a wise idea, and creating it however you feel your blending ritual calls to you – is the best route.

See the chapter on blending, to see a sample of a blending chart.

OILS & REPRODUCTION

I am commonly asked if essential oils can be used for breeding animals, during pregnancy, and during lactation. I have found that not only can oils be used during these times, but are indeed helpful instead of harmful. We have used essential oils in many reproductive situations. Birds and eggs have been exposed to water-based diffusion of many types of oils, laying hens have ingested essential oils consistently in their drinking water, and drops of essential oils have been placed into the nest boxes of chickens. Pregnant and nursing cats (as well as babies) have received the Body Supporting recipes, used essential oils in their litterbox, and have also been exposed to water-based diffusion of almost every essential oil, and at quite high concentrations (sometimes higher than we recommend). The oils have always been well accepted and never appear to influence milk flavor, nursing drive, or cause harm to the fetus or neonate in any manner when essential oils are used in the proper methods and with the proper ratios and dilutions.

Certainly, we need to use common sense and avoid hot and potentially irritating oils directly in the areas of the nipples. However, full dog Drip & Rub Techniques have been administered to nursing moms, and the puppies just seem to reap the benefits of having a "diffuser mom" or by coming into contact with the residual oils on the mother's back.

Horses, Cows, Goats, and many other animals have received regular topical applications of essential oils, and even oral essential oils throughout their entire reproductive period. I have never been concerned about the use of essential oils for mother, father, or offspring.

In the case of rabbits and other exotics, water diffusion of almost every form of essential oil has been used. Tiny newborn rabbit babies were noted to be far healthier when the owner started to disinfect her hands with a drop or two of essential oils prior to handling the still wet babies. Although the essential oil was completely absorbed into her hands, the residual benefits were absorbed by the baby rabbits. Even such a light exposure to essential oils can be extremely powerful and beneficial.

OILS & REPRODUCTION

There is always concern if certain products can be used during pregnancy. Certainly, essential oil use should be carefully considered and discussed with your veterinarian if you have any concerns. What I have personally noted in my work with pregnant or reproductively active animals - is that the proper essential oil use has been safe, effective, and even beneficial to conception, pregnancy, and birth. There are cautionary statements on almost every essential oil, and for almost every situation known - whether it is based in full truth or not. We often prefer to err on the side of being overly cautious, than to ever hurt a living being - especially a baby. For the most current safety information on essential oils - I do suggest the book by Robert Tisserand and Rodney Young - *Essential Oil Safety*, Second Edition. This book compiles data regarding each essential oil, and presents known safety information about them. It is a respected reference, and in general - I am very happy with the realistic comments made by the authors at the end of the presented information.

Let's review an oil which is listed in the "should be avoided by any route throughout pregnancy and lactation" table in the Tisserand *Essential Oil Safety* book. There are many in this table including these more commonly used oils of Anise, Carrot Seed, Cassia, Chaste Tree (Vitex), Cinnamon Bark, Blue Cypress, Dill Seed, Fennel, Hyssop, Lavender (Spanish), Myrrh, Aniseed Myrtle, Oregano, and Rue.

Rue is "nicely controversial" at times - so we will discuss it here. So many essential oils get a "bad rap". It is almost becoming humorous to me, when I hear of an essential oil that is clearly in the "super safe" category - being described as dangerous and to be avoided. No matter what the oil - if you want to find somebody who will tell you it is bad for something - rest assured, you can find it! The problem is that hearsay is clearly becoming the truth of the rumor, instead of good hard evidence.

So in the case of Rue oil - it has been reported to have effects on the uterus and pregnancies. However, most of the information is based on "research" that is so incredibly and massively strange - it would be like saying that Chevrolet Trucks cause pregnancy loss in dogs and so no dog should go near a Chevy while pregnant. What that statement doesn't tell you, is that the Chevrolet Truck ran over the dog...causing the pregnancy loss. As ridiculous and disgusting as that scenario sounds - that is literally what most of the research is like. Even in the Tisserand book - this quote describes Rue essential oil and pregnancy - "Used in massive amounts on pregnant rabbits (12 mL/kg) and guinea pigs (50 mL/kg) rue oil, not surprisingly, was toxic to both mother and fetus, causing widespread tissue damage and some fatalities (Patoir et al 1938a, 1938b). These dose levels are equivalent to human ingestion of approximately 800 mL and 3.2 L. Two pregnant guinea pigs, each fed 12 drops of rue oil, aborted; rue oil was found in the fetal tissue, and was considered toxic to it (Anon 1974). This is still a very high dose, around 3 mL/kg, and equivalent to human ingestion of some 200 mL. In teratology studies on rats and mice, at doses of rue oil up to 820 and 970 mg/kg, respectively, no significant maternotoxic, embryotoxic or teratogenic effects were observed (cited in Committee for Veterinary Medicinal Products 1999)."

However, Rue oil will remain in the listing of contraindicated essential oils for pregnancy - because NO ONE wants to be the person who says Rue Essential Oil is "okay to use" during pregnancy; and maybe, just maybe - be on the wrong end of that answer. I also won't be the person who says 100% yes, you can use these things during pregnancy, breeding, or lactation. I personally do not thing that there is ANYTHING that is 100% safe for pregnancy or "life" for that matter. Heck, just drinking city water is detrimental to health in my opinion. It may not be an immediate revelation, but how many of us know 100% if a fading kitten or a mother who needed a C-section for delivery of her pups - was not affected by the hairspray or perfume that the owner wears daily? With essential oils, there is so much concern - that is sometimes only based on horrendously irresponsible research - that I think we start to become freakishly neurotic with worry.

I have often stated myself in this way - "I am a response-oriented veterinarian"... What the heck does that mean? Well, if I see something work, and work really well - I am REALLY happy with it! Like changing animals from city water to bottled spring water. Is there scientific proof that tap water is bad for you? Likely not anything that the government would let you see! It might even sound a bit crazy to some of my clients - but what harm is there in providing a different water source for a few months? Maybe a few bucks, and gas money to go to the store...but let's try it out. More often than not - and certainly with a frequency that makes me recommend it for ALL of my clients - spring water drastically improved the health of my patients.

And so this is the case with essential oils. What I can tell you of the use of essential oils with pregnancy, breeding, lactation, and neonates - is that when used PROPERLY - essential oils appear to be incredibly helpful and not harmful. Through our veterinary clinic, and through the communications with thousands of people using essential oils EVERY DAY with animals - I have accumulated personal experience and knowledge that would be difficult to publish or share as a whole - but it is there.

Oregano is included on the list of oils that should not be used during pregnancy and lactation. But, as an ingredient within the body supporting blends, and as an oil that is often used the animal aromatherapy world - I can attest to the fact that thousands of animals have used Oregano essential oil during conception, pregnancy, throughout lactation, and even on neonates without concern. And, if someone "does something wrong" - I tend to be contacted with questions. In this way - I suppose it is an excellent learning opportunity for me. I get to see cases that have been "messed up" - and at least get to harvest the knowledge of that event. If someone mixes up their own homemade blend of essential oils, applies it to their cat for the last month, but then reads or is told online that they could "kill their cat with that"... it seems that I am the person to contact!

I do collect the information on which essential oils were used, at what concentrations, and how often - along with health information whenever available. Occasionally, I'll even pay for additional lab work to be performed on the animal for my own curiosity. I can truthfully say, that when high quality essential oils are used in less than ideal ways, I am usually impressed at the actual range of safe dosages that can be used.

Some oils may provide a cautionary statement in references, regarding using caution during pregnancy and with children under 18 months of age. With any pregnant animal, it is a good recommendation to use oils without any warning statements regarding its use during pregnancy. However, in practice, we have not noted any ill effects in any pregnant animal from the use of essential oils at this time. As for the use of oils with this recommendation in young animals, there are often other oil selections that can be made. Since animals have different age relationships than humans – I would suggest that this recommendation would apply to animals 6 months of age and less.

SENSITIVITY TO OILS

It is important to recognize that an animal's sense of smell is incredibly more sensitive than humans. This does not mean that they cannot be exposed to intense smells, it merely means that anything that may smell strongly to us, smells infinitely stronger to them. For example, a search and rescue dog sniffing from the bow of a boat, can actually smell and detect a dead body underneath the water! A bloodhound can smell traces of your body cells that exfoliate and fall off of you as you walk!

It is no wonder that many people interpret an animal's response to an essential oil as "dislike." What I find in my work with hundreds of cases, is that animals that project a dislike of essential oils, have usually been introduced to them in an overly aggressive way. Holding a bottle out for an animal to sniff, may well be like shoving your head into a rotten smelling garbage can. Surely you could smell the rotten garbage from across the room. But, burying your head inside the garbage can is a whole new level of intensity. And, likely if anyone came at you with a garbage can in the future, you would have an aversion to ever smelling it again. It didn't hurt you, but it was an episode you soon won't forget.

We also need to remember that studies have shown that hair follicles enhance the transdermal absorption of most chemicals (essential oils). As animals are covered in hair follicles, this makes complete sense why some would appear more sensitive to oils than humans or even other animals. A cat has more hair follicles per square inch of skin, and a finer coat than a dog or a horse. And with an animal such as a chinchilla, with the densest amount of hair follicles of any land animal, one can see why exotic pets may be perceived as much more delicate. I have seen strong and clear responses to mere diffusion alone, convincing me that the hair follicles aid in the absorption of air borne essential oils.

It is likely that species such as chinchillas and rabbits can absorb therapeutic and systemic levels of essential oils, purely via diffusion.

This scenario also raises incredible insight into the dangers of exposure to household chemicals and toxins in an animal's life. The cleaning chemicals on our floors, fabric softener on our sheets and blankets, odor eliminating sprays on our couches, and air fresheners in our homes; may also be exponentially absorbed by the hair follicles of our furry companions.

Many people have expressed to me the concern that to apply essential oils effectively, we would have to part the fur and ensure that the oils come in direct contact with the skin of an animal. In practice, this theory has been shown to be untrue. I find that a broader "petting" application of an essential oil over a large area of fur or hair, is actually more effective, and certainly less potentially irritating, than one drop applied directly onto the skin.

If you would encounter a situation where the skin, paws, or animal became irritated from an essential oil application, it is important to apply a diluting oil, or carrier oil, to the site. Do not use water or attempt to wash off offending essential oils with water-based soaps or shampoos, as this can act to drive or spread the essential oil only further into and onto tissues. Fractionated Coconut Oil is my first recommendation as a carrier oil, but in a "pinch" any sort of fatty vegetable oil or substance containing fats can be used. It is wise to plan ahead, and to always have a carrier oil with you if you intend to be using oils. However, as I have found with my children, they sometimes need dilution of oils when you least expect it. In cases of urgent need – items like whole fat milk, creamers from restaurants, and butter can be used to calm down a "hot" response to an essential oil or an accidental contact with sensitive tissues (especially in or around eyes.)

The act of diluting an essential oil application basically involves applying the carrier oil to the site of irritation. For skin irritations it is tempting to apply another essential oil, which may be known for soothing effects, to a site. I never recommend "fixing an oil problem, with another oil." Since the majority of issues seem to occur from too aggressive of use at the site of application; the act of applying additional essential oils may only serve to increase the amount of discomfort at the site.

A common issue that is brought up to me is the fact that there are many oils that are listed to be avoided for use around small children. Eucalyptus oils, and oils rich in 1,8-cineole are often implicated (Rosemary). Most of these precautions are related to the fact that breathing issues have been noted when children are exposed to intense odors. Unfortunately, most of the respiratory distresses when researched, were clear cases of actual poisoning or aspiration of the oil into the airway. With normal and proper use of oils high in 1,8-cineole, we should not see such aggressive reactions in response to the essential oil. In clinical work, we quite see the opposite. These oils are highly beneficial for respiratory concerns, and yes even asthma.

Even our basic friend Lavender, has been implicated as "use with caution with asthma" – however I will beg to qualify that most of these relationships may relate to how the oil was used, and the presence of adulterants and synthetics.

When I was young, strong odors greatly affected me. Even walking into a store with a popcorn popper, would result in a form of apnea (or restricted and stopped breathing). It was quite a stressful situation, and even smells such as corn chips being opened too close to me would result in a similar action. I couldn't breathe. This is similar to what is reported in some children who smell very strong oils such as Eucalyptus or Peppermint. And in speaking with many other people over the years, apnea in relationship to strong odors is certainly not uncommon, nor restricted to only essential oils.

Peppermint (Menthol) and Eucalyptus (1,8-cineole) – are often implicated in this relation of essential oils to respiratory distress. But when you look at the actual cases which are used to document these concerns, there is such gross mis-use of the oils, it bears some evaluation of its own. In most situations, the essential oils were instilled into the nose, certainly something we should avoid doing.

The National Association of Holistic Aromatherapy (NAHA) does not recommend the use of Peppermint for children under approximately three years of age, due to the fact that basically the nasal mucosa can act as an autonomic reflexogen organ, which may lead to sudden apnea and glottal constriction.

As someone who has experienced this condition first hand, I would say it does not matter what the essential oil is, but if it is strong and intense in odor – you should use caution around any small child if you are using the oil incorrectly. In the ways we suggest in terms of water-based diffusion, diluted topical applications, and use within blends – there should be no reason to have untoward worry in regards to use of these oils. So if you are applying the Canine Supportive Blend to your dog, who then sleeps with your child; there is such a low concentration of Peppermint within the blend, that it should be of no concern to the child.

Even in Essential Oil Safety by Tisserand & Young (2nd Edition), there are only cautions made in regards to Peppermint – to not apply near the face of infants or children. However, it would appear that when truly diluted, diffused from a water-based diffuser, or within a blend – smelling an animal or diffusion recipe containing Peppermint, is no more likely to be any more intense than smelling someone's chewing gum.

PHOTOSENSITIVITY

Animals are a bit unique in this sense. While we greatly respect and mention when an essential oil may carry photosensitive properties with it, it is mainly for human consideration. Unless you have a fully hairless breed, it has not been documented that animals show concern in regards to photosensitivity.

This is not to say that it cannot or will not happen. Nor is it to say that "hot" or even very "cool" oils such a peppermint, cannot cause uncomfortable feelings to the skin of a horse if left to stand in the sun. But, in general, we have not noticed the same odd skin photo-reactions that we can with humans.

It is wise to use additional caution for birds with bald face patches, or lack of feathers, when using Feathered Spray. Do not leave animals outside under intense sun, or even intense cold or heat after essential oil applications. If you have a hairless animal, be especially aware of any photosensitizing oils you may use. And finally – as a human – use caution for yourself if you apply oils to your animal that contain photosensitizing oils within them, exposing your skin to these items.

It is good to note – that due to the fact that most essential oils used for animals will be diluted, we are already eliminating some need for concern. Many oils can be used at appropriate dilution rates, to eliminate the concern for photosensitivity reactions (darkening of the skin, discoloring, blistering…). And due to the use of blends, we are often further "diluting" the total amount of the photosensitizing agent as well.

ESSENTIAL OIL AVERSIONS

By far one of the most common concerns I hear is that an animal or pet does not like oils. What I usually find in these circumstances is that there has been some sort of event in the animal's history of using essential oils too aggressively for that individual. For example, actions such as dripping peppermint onto the hips of a cat, dropping oils directly into the mouth, tipping the ears with oils, applying oils to the feet or foot pads, or applying oils near the face or nose of an animal, have resulted in certain aversions.

Although these applications can be well tolerated by many, sensitive animals seem to hold a grudge to certain experiences. This is very similar to traditional veterinary medicine where a cat will hide under the bed and not come near you after a few "pilling" episodes.

It is worthwhile when exploring routine and non-critical use of essential oils for animals, to note which methods are best tolerated. Once a mild method is used successfully, I find that amounts can be gradually increased and tolerance of the application is easier and easier.

For example; I may not dilute my oils – and leave them neat on my hands to pet my animals. For certain cats, diluting these oils or waiting until they are basically absorbed completely into my hands, is tolerated just fine. However, if I were to have a heavier amount of essential oils present on my hands, or be holding the bottle while I approach them, they may move away from the situation. After a few very light applications – I find I can gradually expose them to more and more oils on my hands, because they have never had an over-experience.

Food aversions are well documented in the animal kingdom. A pet nauseated from kidney disease may avoid a food that was fed during that time frame. The pet relates the particular food to the feeling of illness. An aggressive exposure and bad experience with an essential oil, can make an animal leery of all essential oil exposure.

If you look at it like cooking, it can make more sense. Let's say every time your Grandma offered you a taste of soup it was over-seasoned, you would quickly want to avoid tasting Grandma's soup. Too strong makes an impression!

Now, this is not to say that we cannot use oils more aggressively when needed; but when possible, we need to start light and be respectful of what animals "like" – to make administration (and life) with an animal easier!

METHODS OF APPLICATION

There are many ways to expose animals to essential oils. The pros and cons of each method, as well as the species they best match with will be described. You will hear me say often – use a "Species Specific" oil application. This refers to the fact that if you are researching a specific condition in humans, and find an oil that you may like to try for an animal, you will consider the type of animal in which you are applying the essential oil to, to determine the best application route.

DIFFUSION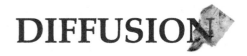

FORMS OF DIFFUSION:
There are several ways in which diffusion of essential oils into the air can occur. Mechanical diffusion utilizes a machine or propulsion of some sort to mobilize essential oil particles into the air. Passive diffusion is what I consider the evaporation of essential oils into the air on their own accord.

Within the mechanical category, three main styles can be considered. One is what I will refer to as water-based diffusion, the other an air-style diffusion, and the third utilizes a spritzer bottle. I do not recommend any type of diffusion that involves heating or "burning"– as this can damage the essential oil.

Passive diffusion can include the placement of essential oils onto cotton balls, toys, tissues, cage papers, blankets, bedding, and even humans and other animals – allowing the oils to passively waft into the area around the animal.

WATER-BASED DIFFUSION:
There are several styles of water-based diffusers on the market today. With the popularity of essential oil use booming, we are seeing a wide variety of essential oil diffusers being marketed. Unfortunately, we are bound to see some quality issues with this surge into the market place. Always make sure that the diffuser you select to use has decent reviews, and has been marketed with the intent of being used with high grade, therapeutic based aromatherapy needs. Some diffusers designed only for scent or humidifying, may be destroyed or damaged when true essential oils are used.

A few features to be mindful of when selecting a diffuser include the amount of water they are designed to use (100mL may be a very small portion, and 1000mL may be too much). Average is 300 to 500mL for what I enjoy in a diffuser. Anything more, and we may find that the volatile compounds of the essential oil are "used up" prior to the full amount of water being used. Anything less, and I find I have to fill up the diffuser more often. You can also evaluate what type of water is recommended for use with the diffuser. In general, I prefer distilled or reverse osmosis water for use with diffusion, however I will use bottled spring water as well. This removes any abnormal amounts of minerals that might interfere with my diffuser operation, as well as the chemicals associated with some tap or city water. Well water can be used, if you know the testing situation of your particular well. However, I prefer a more "sterilized" version of water for diffusion, to avoid bio-films and other contamination issues.

Other features of diffusers you may wish to explore are in regards to lights and feature settings. Some diffusers allow you to set particular pulsing features, timing of diffusion, and to turn off the lights on the diffuser completely. While I have a particular model of diffuser that I enjoy using, I still wish the "power light" would shut off for night use. The very small green glow from the "on indicator" still drives me nuts, even though I love the diffuser for functionality.

Some machines utilize all of the water added to the machine, and others may shut off at a particular "low level." Make sure to read all of the information on your diffuser prior to purchase, as some people really like one feature over another. There are some diffusers I will still purchase for the various pulsing abilities, even if they have other features I am not fond of.

With water-based diffusion, water is indeed added to the machine along with varying drops of essential oil(s). The beauty of a water-based diffuser is the variable diffusion concentrations that can be achieved. The teeniest dip of a toothpick, one drop of essential oil, or even 20 drops of essential oil can be added to a batch of water in a diffuser; allowing the utmost control in levels of exposure. Although hardly necessary – one drop or less can be added to a diffuser.

STARTING POINTS:
For most water-based diffusers – 1 to 4 drops of essential oil(s) can be added to the machine when close contact with a diffuser and an animal is planned. This includes placing a diffuser close to a caged animal, tenting an animal with the diffuser vapor, and for animals that have not had much "mapping" in essential oil use or whom are considered fragile or exotic. In this category, I would include animals such as insects (honey bees, tarantulas), Chinchillas, Sugar Gliders, etc…

Dilution of the essential oil(s) is accomplished by varying how much oil is added to the water within the diffuser. The need for dilution of essential oils with a carrier oil, is not necessary for water-based diffusion - and could actually be harmful to the diffuser.

METHODS OF APPLICATION - DIFFUSION

I always recommend smelling the diffuser vapor yourself prior to introducing it to an animal. I hadn't considered 4 to 5 drops of an essential oil blend to be a very intense concentration, until I put my face directly in the vapor for a few minutes. As I was intending to place this vapor into a cage with a dog – I wanted to know how it felt. It was actually quite intense.

When starting to diffuse for an animal – start with a light amount, start diffusing in an open area, and stay with the animal for the first five to ten minutes or more of the diffusion. If an individual animal can only tolerate 5 minutes of diffusion in an open room – they would likely not tolerate a tenting situation. In emergency situations, you may need to move towards more intense diffusion right away, but these situations are hopefully few and far between.

Another method of water-based diffusion is to add essential oils into water contained in a glass spray bottle – also referred to as a water spritzer or water-mist. This solution is shaken to disperse the essential oils within the water, and then sprayed into the air. This method is also incredibly flexible, as anywhere from a toothpick dip to 20 or more drops of essential oil(s) can be added to varying amounts of water – allowing for incredible flexibility in the concentration of essential oils that are put into the environment.

WATER DIFFUSION – OPEN ROOM:
In this situation, water-based diffusion is used in an average household room with the animal. The animal may or may not be able to leave the room, but is generally over 5 feet away from the diffuser. This method is appropriate for all animals including birds, reptiles, exotic species, fish tanks, and cats. In general, most households I work with, use this method in multiple rooms of the home, basically in a continuous nature.

WATER DIFFUSION – SMALL CLOSED ROOM:
This situation may include using a water-based diffuser in a much smaller room, such as a bathroom, with an animal. This allows for greater exposure to the essential oil vapor, and the potential for more therapeutic results to be seen.

WATER DIFFUSION – CAGING:
With this method, I would be directing the diffuser vapors into a cage or kennel of an animal. Basically placing a diffuser in close proximity with an animal who otherwise cannot move away from the vapor.

WATER DIFFUSION – TENTING:

This method is more intense and concentrated than directing diffusion vapor into an otherwise open cage. With tenting, I cover an animal's enclosure to effectively trap the diffusion vapors around the animal, and ensure a higher level of inhalation and exposure. Placing plastic wrap, plastic sheeting, or towels over both the cage and diffuser, creates a situation where generally the animal will be enveloped in a misty cloud of essential oil vapors. This method must be monitored much more intensely, and is used similarly to nebulization treatments in veterinary care. For some cases, we will use a tenting diffusion for 20 minute lengths of time, and even 3 times a day.

AIR-STYLE DIFFUSION:

There are several styles of air diffusers on the market currently. Air diffusers eject pure "neat" essential oils into the air. The concentration of essential oil is thus much higher than water-based diffusers. This method of diffusion is best reserved for larger rooms, barns, stalls, chicken coops, etc... The more "sensitive" the animal may be to essential oils, the larger the room and the farther away an air diffuser should be placed and used. For the most part, water-based diffusion should be used for homes with any sort of animal within it.

Only rarely would a tenting situation be used with an air-style diffuser. The closest to tenting would be enclosing a stall with solid walls or plastic over the doors and windows and diffusing for a horse or other large animal. This method can be particularly beneficial for Heaves and other respiratory concerns. Plastic "drop sheets" for painting can be hung over the entrance to a lean-to or run-in shelter and a horse can be held inside with a diffuser to administer essential oils in this manner.

Air-style diffusion is also used for techniques such as "bombing" – when a fogging sort of action is desired to completely permeate carpets, walls, or basements in which molds or insects have taken up residence. For these situations, all animals are removed from the room in which a "fogging" type diffusion is desired.

MONITORING DURING DIFFUSION:

Diffusion can cause discomfort in some situations. Both to humans and animals. I believe it would be unwise to assume that the things we do, could never adversely affect another living thing. An animal who is not tolerating the level of diffusion you are exposing them to, may show lethargy, increased breathing rate, panting, drooling, change in breathing pattern, squinting eyes, or any other change that you would consider to be "detrimental" or out of the ordinary.

If an animal exhibits signs of distress during diffusion, simply turn off the diffuser and increase access to plain fresh air. If the animal continues to show abnormal symptoms after 10-20 minutes of the removal of the essential oil, you should seek veterinary attention.

I believe there is an increased risk factor with the diffusion of single essential oils, and with the diffusion of any essential oil that may not be of the total and complete quality needed for animals. With single essential oils, we lose the ability to dilute individual properties of that oil, even if they are beneficial. In herbal medicine, it is often discussed that the whole herb, ameliorates any toxic or harmful effects that the herbal medicine may carry. With essential oils like Tea Tree (Melaleuca alternifolia) we recognize that while it is a widely used essential oil, it is very strong, and quite intense. Used alone, it can overwhelm animals. Much like the use of Cinnamon alone would be very intense. However, used with other more mild essential oils, we can still reap some of its powerful benefits, without the possible physical overwhelm.

With any possibility that you have purchased an essential oil that has been misrepresented to you in terms of quality – diffusion can also present a larger risk factor. As discussed earlier in this book, if you do not truly know that an essential oil has been selected for use with animals, or do not know the qualifications of the person directly responsible for sourcing that oil and designating it as safe for animals – you should proceed with full caution. Considering that even animalEO – animal screened essential oils – "could" be use incorrectly and cause harm – it is just never worth the risk of using an essential oil of questionable quality, even if it is "just for diffusion."

While we use to consider diffusion one of the safest routes of essential oil use, this outlook is starting to change. Diffusion of poorer grade oils (even those safe for humans, may not be safe for birds and amphibians) – is likely to be even more detrimental to animals when presented in this method. Airways can become irritated from chemical issues, and inflammation can cause swelling of the airway. For animals with already compromised airways (such as brachycephalic breeds) – this could prove very dangerous.

INGESTION OF OILS

Regardless of the route, any essential oil entering the mouth and being swallowed instead of absorbed by the mucous membranes should be considered ingested. To some extent, essential oils that are "consumed" during the grooming or licking process, are ingested, but a far greater percent of these oils should be considered absorbed topically to be most accurate. And absorption via the tongue, buccal membranes, or oral cavity in general, should likely be regarded as potentially more effective than the swallowing of essential oils.

For our purposes, we will consider ingestion to be via the drinking water as well – however, for some species, this route may result in more oral absorption than true ingestion. A bird drinking water, often just swallows it down. While a dog will lap it up, resulting if much more contact with the tongue and mucous membranes.

Other forms of ingestion of essential oils will include addition into foods, as well as other carrier items (coconut oil, butter, juices…), to some extent dripping directly into the mouth, or placing the essential oil(s) within a gelatin capsule and swallowing directly. There are also a few other options, such as dripping onto a treat or chewable vitamin – but you get the picture.

For all essential oils that indicate that ingestion of the oil is used for animals – you should refer back to these chapters on ingestion. Not only to gather information on how to administer for a particular species, but for the dosing recommendations. An essential oil single may include specific maximum dose usage that we know of within its description, however in general, we will apply similar dilutions and doses for all ingestible essential oils across each species.

Remember that essential oils can have a milligram (mg) designation, and while we most commonly refer to essential oils in terms of "drops" – it is far more accurate to weigh an essential oil to deliver a distinct and known quantity of a substance.

How are we going to be measuring essential oils within this book? We are still going to consider drops – however please remember that a drop is generally going to be considered to be 35mg of essential oil, or 0.03mL volume on average.

These are averages, however, it sure would be a wonderful thing if we could start to convert the world of essential oils into accurate measurements and practices!

For our purposes, and for the general public, we will still be referencing essential oils in terms of the most easily understood, and the most easily applied methods. This will actually keep the animal use of essential oils a bit safer, for the consumer front as a whole.

Let's start with individual species. What you will find in the essential oil recommendations is that a particular essential oil may be used via ingestion for the species you are interested in. The first step, is determining how you are going to deliver the ingested oil. Obviously for a bird – we are not going to add essential oils into a gel capsule and try to get them to swallow it. Only in rare circumstances (such as with raptors) do we attempt to "pill" a bird, and then it should only be in distinct veterinary or rehab work. However, we can "consider" pilling a cat or dog. With a horse, a pill is less likely again, and we may consider the better route of buccal absorption instead of focusing on distinct swallowing of the essential oil. Or for horse or livestock, we may be considering addition to the water trough – which naturally they will swallow the essential oil, but they will often not consume the entire trough of water. So our doses added within a water trough will be far different than a capsule.

When offering foods with essential oils mixed into them, we also have to consider the volume of food offered. If we mix essential oils into an entire ounce of a juice supplement as one avian protocol suggests in a different resource, it should be expected to have further instructions upon how much of that mixture is to be given, or how. I find many references to be so woefully deficient in instructions, and this can promote a very dangerous situation. When you are considering that you might want a dog to consume an entire drop of an essential oil, as recommended for its weight, then if you are adding it to food, you would not add it to an entire 40 pound bag of dog food. We would add it to a realistic meal size, that the dog would consume in one offering.

All of our animal recommendations for foods or water, take into account real and accurate veterinary information regarding what animals actually eat, consume, or will tolerate. But again, we place it into your hands to use logic as to what your animal will eat, and how much it consumes when you are considering dosages within a meal or drink.

If there is not a distinct amount recommendation within an essential oil for your species – use the general recommendations within Adding Oils to Drinking Water, Mixing Oils into Food, or Oral Administration.

Birds: In general ingestion of essential oils will begin with addition to food. Please follow the directions in the chapter Mixing Oils into Food. The second most common form of ingestion is the addition of essential oils into drinking water. Please see the chapter Adding Oils to Drinking Water for further directions.

Exotic Animals: Depending on the species you are working with, you will need to have an understanding of what items they typically eat, and how or if they drink regularly. For ingestion of essential oils with exotic animals – most commonly the addition into food items is used. These animals are uncommonly "pilled", and depending on the species and essential oil in question, addition to drinking water may not be a possibility.

Cats: If I wanted a very distinct oral ingestion of essential oils with a cat, I would typically select a small gelatin capsule for delivery. However, I rarely find that this is necessary, and the fact that a feline grooms so often, results in wonderful buccal absorption of topically applied oils. While some cats may drink water with essential oils added to it (often in dog homes, and not quite intended) – it is not a primary route we recommend. Most cats will not select to ingest essential oils readily in their drinking water, so other more effective and "cat-friendly" routes are suggested. This also applies to the addition of essential oils to their food. While some may ingest essential oils in this way – it is few and far between, and we have much easier, and very effective other options available. When a cat purposely selects to drink "dog water" with essential oils added to it, licks a dog with oils applied to it, or otherwise ingests known safe oils – this is not cause for concern. We simply do not force it upon them, when other methods are much more effective and realistic.

Dogs: Dogs become a bit easier with ingestion of essential oils. They are often quite willing to eat things within food (although taste will play a factor) or drink them in their water. They are also fairly easy to "pill" with a gelatin capsule. Depending on the essential oil you select, if ingestion is recommended you can consider your dog's particular personality as well as suggestions for the individual oil, as to how you might administer an oral dose of essential oils to your dog. I typically find that addition to food is my most common route. Dilution of the essential oils prior to adding to food (or capsule) in a carrier oil is recommended. This makes it easier to disperse the essential oil within the food item or meal – and eliminate a "direct hit" of one particular intense flavor associated with a drop of oil added right on top of a bowl of food. Mix your essential oil into a carrier oil such as raw coconut oil, for a tasty disguise. You can mix the essential oil dose into as much of the "carrier" as would be normal or safe for your dog to consume.

If your dog has never consumed raw coconut oil before, adding a ¼ cup to a meal to disguise a few drops of Peppermint within it – is likely to result in an upset tummy for your dog. Even if a tiny dog ate a tablespoon of coconut oil all of a sudden, we could see some GI upset. So use common sense, and make sure that what you "bury" your essential oil in, is logical and something that your dog can and has eaten without issue.

Horses & Livestock: With these animals, ingestion of essential oils is more commonly achieved through the drinking water. Please see the chapter on Adding Oils to Drinking Water for further instructions. With some of these animals, we may be able to mix some essential oils into grain, applesauce, or a warm bran or beet mash. Read the chapter on Mixing Oils into Food for more advice and information. For large animals who may be consuming milk from a bucket or bottle, essential oils can be added to these meals as well. For most large animals, "pilling" is not widely used, although for some animals large boluses may be created and delivered. In those circumstances essential oils can certainly be included within herbal blends or other items within the large "balling gun" capsules.

Other Considerations:
You may be thinking, "But you didn't tell me how much to give." The following chapters will give you guidelines on how much essential oil to add for each species, depending on the route of delivery you have selected. So most essential oils in the water, will be given at a rate of about 1 drop per liter or 3-4 drops per gallon. And if the item is designated as ingestible in food or capsule, follow the specific directions for your species on amounts.

Ingestion of an essential oil within a fatty substance, may also enhance its absorption directly into the lymphatic system, thus avoiding a bit of first pass metabolism that occurs.

Essential oils can also be mixed with edible and therapeutic clay powder (such as green clay, montmorillonite, illite, Redmond clay, or bentonite) or a dry herb by weight, and then placed into a capsule. For many conditions, the clay or herb will impart added benefits to the essential oil treatment. For most clay or herb capsules, 10% essential oil is added by weight. A milligram scale becomes much more important in this situation, as is a wonderful mathematical mind. Thankfully clay is less likely to require an exact dose than an herbal preparation may. Follow the directions indicated for whichever herbal or clay you plan to use in regards to dosing.

Let's look at an example. You have "Rx Clay" powder by Rx Vitamins for Pets. For an 80 pound (36kg) dog, 1 teaspoon is suggested per day. Measure out your teaspoon of clay powder, then figure out how many of your capsules it might take to give this amount. As capsule size can vary, there is no clear cut answer. Next, you can do one of two things. You can add the daily amount of essential oil you wish to give to the entire batch of powder (clay or herb) then divide this between the capsules, or fill your capsules with the clay, and drip the essential oil on top of it.

As using clay or herbals therapeutically is an art unto itself, please be fully aware of the needs and possible contraindications of these additions to essential oil therapy. Certainly some oral use of clay may cause gastrointestinal diarrhea or constipation, and some herbs may have drug interactions. However, if you are currently working with your vet, and have existing well established protocols in place, they can work wonderfully and synergistically with added essential oils.

ADDING OILS TO DRINKING WATER

Whenever considering adding essential oils to an animal's water supply – several considerations must be made.

Oil Selection:
Of course, there are some oils that are more friendly for use in drinking water than others. Adding "hot" oils such as Oregano would obviously not be as appetizing as Tangerine. Strong tastes and flavors must be a consideration in selection. Starting with items that you find pleasant to drink is a good idea.

Water Containers & Storage:
Many exotic pet water containers are made of plastic or have plastic components. As essential oils may degrade these plastics, care must be taken only to use glass, ceramic, or stainless steel water containers with the use of essential oils. In the situation of horses and large animals, troughs are commonly made of hard plastic or galvanized metals. It is difficult to avoid these materials, and in practice, it appears to cause no detrimental effects. If given a choice, I do prefer the hard plastic troughs or old ceramic bath tubs over galvanized materials when possible. Stainless steel troughs would be even more ideal.

Exposure of the Animal:
Care must also be taken in how the animal may interact with its water source. For snakes who often soak in their water dishes to birds who may bathe in them – considerations must be made to the strength, oil selection, and property of the oil added to the water. Peppermint may be considered a nice oil to drink on a hot day, however a snake soaking in water with peppermint added may find "cold irritation" from the sensation and contact.

Ensuring Adequate Water Intake:
One of the worst things we could do is to cause an animal to avoid drinking by making an essential oil solution too strong or by choosing an essential oil that the animal dislikes. Although many animals actually prefer water with essential oils – it is always wise to provide a plain water source while you offer the new water – until you are certain that the animal is drinking the essential oil water well, and in adequate amounts.

Concentrations:
Unless a situation is critical, it is wise to start with small amounts of oil added to high quality water, and gradually increase the oils over the course of a week. A concentration that is often used for animals is one drop per liter of distilled, reverse osmosis, or good quality spring water. A glass bottle is the best for mixing and storing your essential oil water. Since glass containers come in all sorts of sizes and measures – below is a chart of how to arrive at the same "1 drop per liter" concentration for multiple measures. Please note, these do not always arrive at the same exact concentration when measured in drops – but will still be safe and effective for your uses:

1 drop in 1 Liter of water (35mg/L)
1 drop in 1 quart of water (37mg/L)
1 drop in 2 pints of water (37mg/L)
3 drops in 1 Gallon of water (~28mg/L)
4 drops in 1 Gallon of water (37mg/L)
2 drops in ½ Gallon of water (37mg/L)
1 drop in 4 cups water (34mg/L)

For highly sensitive or fragile animals – such as certain species of fish, insects, snakes, and amphibians – starting with a toothpick dipped into the essential oil, then into the Liter of water is a conservative starting point.

In critical situations – adding essential oils to water is typically not a route that would be used – as often times these animals may not be drinking properly.

Species Specific Recommendations:

Birds: Birds generally have a very poor sense of taste, and it is quite easy to add essential oils to their drinking water. Care must be taken for birds who bathe in their water, and careful monitoring of water intake is important. In general, 1 drop per liter of water is commonly used.

Chickens & Poultry: Chickens are much less able to bathe in their drinking water based on the water dispensers used by most farms. Many more "hot" oils have been given via drinking water to flocks for various conditions. This is likely the easiest method for administration to flocks of chickens, turkeys, pheasants, and so forth. Care must be considered when adding the oils to drinking water systems, as high concentrations may damage plastics or certain components of automated systems. Starting with low amounts, and gradually increasing the concentrations is recommended. Knowing how much water your flock generally consumes on a daily basis – BEFORE adding essential oils to the water supply is crucial. After you know how much water should be consumed, you will be able to compare if the same amount of water (or more) is being consumed after the addition of essential oils.

Exotics: For oils recommended for use in drinking water, the general starting point is to add 1 drop per liter of water. Of course, it is always advisable to start with even more dilute concentrations (such as a toothpick dip), and gradually work your way up to the desired amount of oil.

Cats: Cats are less likely than other animals to consume essential oils within their water, although there certainly are cats that do, and sometimes with surprising oil selections. The key with cats is to start with extremely small amounts (toothpick dips), to always offer an alternate water source for drinking, and to very gradually increase concentrations. It is important to note that just because a cat may refuse to drink one particular essential oil, it does not guarantee the refusal of others. Most cats are unlikely to progress to a concentration stronger than a 1 drop per liter of water.

Dogs: Dogs are much easier to work with. Starting with small amounts and gradually increasing the concentration is still advisable, along with careful monitoring of acceptance and water intake. While 1 drop per liter of drinking water is average, there are many dogs who drink from horse troughs with much higher concentrations of essential oils added to the water.

Horses & Larger: These animals almost prefer essential oils in their water. Often many drops can be added to a trough. Start with 5 drops, and gradually increase based on responses. Agitating the water's surface after the addition of oils can help to disperse them.

Examples of the Use of Essential Oils in Drinking Water:

Birds:
As an antihistamine, antiviral – 1 drop of Melissa Essential Oil in one Liter of water. Shake well and use as drinking water.

Chickens:
1 drop or more of Three Part Blends per liter of drinking water – can help to improve health, immune system function, and can replace the need for medicated feeds.

Guinea Pigs:
1 drop of Orange, Tangerine, or other citrus oils per liter of drinking water.

Snakes:
Toothpick of Three Part Blends per liter of water used as drinking and soaking water, gradually working up in concentration.

Dogs:
Peppermint, Melissa, Copaiba, or Three Part Blends: start with 1 drop per liter, then gradually increase if needed and tolerated.

Cats:
Cats may refuse oils in drinking water more than other species. Start with toothpick amounts, then gradually increase the concentration. Use mild, "cat friendly" oils within Three Part Blends and even the Feline Supportive Blend – when selecting oils to add to their drinking water. Which oils are tolerated and accepted by our feline friends, will certainly be made clear by the individual cat.

METHODS OF APPLICATION – DRINKING WATER

Horses:
Peppermint, Lemon, Copaiba and other oils are often enjoyed. Three to Five drops or more can be added per 50-100 gallons of water. Often with horses and other large animals, we cannot avoid plastic or other materials in the troughs. The hard plastic troughs commonly available, do not appear to become degraded by the essential oils.

Cattle & Large Animals:
Peppermint on hot days is often enjoyed, and can encourage drinking during transport. Other oils can be considered as described for horses.

MIXING OILS INTO FOODS

Some species do very well with this method of using essential oils.

Birds:
Birds have very little taste buds and will accept many oils (even "hot" ones) in their foods. Most bird owners will recognize a favorite food that their bird loves. Often times something such as warm oatmeal is great to add oils to. Starting with a tablespoon of warm (not hot) mushy favorites – mix in a "toothpick dip" of the essential oil. Make sure the bird likes to eat the food item already, and it is wise to make sure they are hungry when you plan to introduce the "therapeutic" item of food. Gradually increase the amounts given as needed, unless the situation is critical. Birds have even ingested oils such as Oregano, Clove, Basil, Copaiba, Frankincense, Thyme, and Melissa in their favorite foods.

Ferrets:
Ferrets will often easily consume oils in chicken baby food, mashed banana, coconut oil, or another squishy treat or favorite food. Again, starting with small amounts added into a favorite food, and gradually increasing the amount given is recommended.

Rodents, Reptiles, and Other Exotics:
Just as described for birds and ferrets, it is a good recommendation to start with very small amounts of essential oils added to foods initially. The "name of the game" with the various species, is to find something they enjoy and consume to mix the oils into. For most of these animals, moving towards oral administration of an essential oil is often reserved for more critical cases and conditions. However, there are certain oils that certainly will benefit animals to consume on a regular basis (such as antitumoral oils for rodents).

Ideas for ingestion: For animals who eat crickets and mealworms, these critters can be "gut loaded" by being fed with essential oils added to their food source, prior to them becoming a meal. For rodent-eating exotics, small amounts of essential oils (toothpick dip) can be applied or inserted into a meal prior to serving. With companion rodents, they may also consume various mushy foods or treats that can have essential oils added to them. For animals that eat fruits, vegetables, sprouts, or leafy greens – a water mister of essential oils can be used to spray the food items with the essential oils. Often exotic animals require a creative approach to the use of essential oils, and it can be fun as well as rewarding.

Rabbits, Guinea Pigs, Chinchillas:
Care with hindgut fermenters such as Rabbits, Guinea Pigs, and Chinchillas should be taken. Exotic animals such as these, rely on gut flora for normal digestive function. Since essential oils can have strong antibacterial action – the oral routes of essential oils are often avoided unless absolutely necessary. Many times there are many other routes of application and exposure that can be used very effectively. However, in critical situations or with severe cases that are not responding to other methods of use, adding very small amounts of essential oils into fruit or vegetable baby foods and syringing them into the mouth, can be quite effective. While we use and advise caution with gut flora, more and more research is indicating that "natural antibiotic" sources such as essential oils, appear to display action upon harmful bacteria, while often sparing any damage to beneficial flora.

Dogs:
It depends on the dog as to if they will eat essential oils in their foods or not. Many dogs routinely consume Copaiba and other anti-inflammatory oils mixed into their moistened foods, twice a day for long term support and care.

Cats:
Cats are unique. They will tell you that themselves. Not many cats are interested in eating essential oils in their food, however there are some that will. Diluted Copaiba mixed in with canned food has been accepted by several cats. However, the vast majority of cats, will ingest adequate levels of essential oils via grooming or topical absorption, to not require additional administrations within their food.

Horses:
Horses easily ingest essential oils in their foods. Mixing oils into applesauce, maple syrup, agave, oats, molasses, feed, and even onto hay is well tolerated. Almost any oil can be given in this manner. Diffusing with an air-style diffuser into an enclosed hay storage room can permeate the hay with beneficial essential oils for ingestion and also for mold prevention within the hay itself.

Cattle, Others:
Cattle, small ruminants, and other forms of livestock can easily ingest essential oils within feeds. Using the suggestions for horses works well for these animals.

ORAL ADMINISTRATION

This method is generally used in debilitated animals or in more severe situations. For example; animals with hives, internal bleeding, pain, allergic reaction, cancer, internal parasites, etc... Oral use of essential oils is generally not used immediately in most situations, unless it is the easiest route of administration for that particular oil or species of animal.

It is also important to recognize that oral administration may create an aversion to essential oils in some animals. Animals will know when you open the cabinet or grab the oil bottle which was last associated with a very intense oral exposure to oil. The memory of a negative experience with oils will remain stronger than a positive experience, and may lead them to avoidance behavior to any essential oil application.

Via Capsules:
Oils can be added to empty gel capsules and given to dogs by mouth. Smaller gel capsules can be found through health food or medical supply stores and pharmacies, and are helpful for use in cats and smaller dogs. While we have not stressed this in the past, we have found that essential oils diluted first in an edible carrier oil, prior to adding to the capsule, seem to be tolerated better, and are better absorbed.

Via Buccal Route:
The buccal route refers to absorption of the essential oil through the mucous membranes of the cheek or lip area of an animal. Horses do very well with oils dripped into the bottom lip. Dogs also tolerate drops inside the cheek area fairly well. Depending on the essential oil to be administered, and the need of the animal, the essential oil may be used neat for buccal absorption, or may be diluted prior to use.

Via Oral Drops:
Cats and dogs have actually had essential oils dripped into their mouth for pain or post-operative recovery. With horses, we commonly drip oils into the lower lip. With this method, little care is placed as to where the oil drop lands, just getting it into the mouth is the main goal. While some of the oil is swallowed, it is likely that some is also absorbed via the mucous membranes (buccal). Cats often drool and salivate from strong odors or tastes. When possible, other routes

are preferred, however there are a few select urgent situations in which we drip oils directly into the mouth.

Via Gums:
This can be an effective way to get small amounts of essential oil into the oral cavity of dogs. Often a light coating of oil is placed on the fingers, then rubbed onto the gums. Oils can be neat or diluted for this application, although diluted is preferred. This route can be utilized for items such as toothpastes as well.

Via Sublingual Administration:
While recovering from anesthesia, drops of essential oils are easily placed under the tongue of animals for easy and fast absorption.

Via Grooming:
Cats will ingest small amounts of essential oils that have been applied onto their fur. This is often enough to reach therapeutic levels in many cats.

Via a Carrier:
Essential oils can be mixed into Agave, Honey, Coconut Oil, and other carriers and offered orally. Follow the directions for mixing oils into foods, for further instructions and details.

THREE PART BLENDS

I'm not going to lie. While I find blending quite easy, many people struggle with this. So sometimes, the hardest part of teaching essential oil use, is the art of blending. Some are artists, and some are not. Some people have a natural knack for baking, and some follow the recipe perfectly, and still do not end up with a great end result.

I wanted to make blends WAY EASIER for everyone! So, we are going to design Three Part Blends. What I have noticed in the past, is that while I may give a wonderful recipe, people felt they were too complex. They would leave out ingredients all the time, then wonder why they did not get optimal results. Sometimes, adding or having 10 ingredients on hand for a recipe, was just not in the cards. I get that. So if you want complex blends, with a ton of thought and experience behind them – you may wish to stick with the blends that are already made for you (by a veterinarian of course) and never be without an ingredient!

Three Part Blends are designed for you to use when you do not have a specific recipe spelled out for you. Say you read about several oils in our singles section, and just feel that you need to use these for a situation. Definitely, we've all been there. One essential oil company or Facebook post, will glorify one particular essential oil – and it is off to the races! We all want it! We all need it! We have to have it! In reality, the essential oil has been there the entire time, and usually just some new (or even old) research has been discovered or read about, and the marketing machine was turned on. It's true, I love a good research article as much as the next nerd, but we need to use caution when one particular oil becomes the "oil of all oils" and the *only* one we consider for a condition.

This became a popular thing with Frankincense. Just say the word cancer, and Frankincense is soon to come out of someone's mouth or typed on someone's keyboard. But you are really doing yourself a huge disservice when we ONLY look at Frankincense. We are missing a huge number of oils with potential benefits for cases of cancer. There is a lot of research being done on essential oils and cancer, and one only has to search www.pubmed.gov to be happily overwhelmed with research articles. And certainly not only on Frankincense! As of December 2017, a search on PubMed for Essential Oil and Cancer yielded 1146 articles. And I am certain that there are more. Usually by varying the key words in my search, I find far more information. I can find 360 articles when searching Essential Oil and Apoptosis. And only 11 of these articles pertain to Frankincense.

So, don't sell yourself short. Do not be quick to accept a single oil trend, or limit yourself to overlooking the synergy that blends provide. I for one, would much rather combine Frankincense with two other highly researched essential oils if my dog was fighting cancer. Or better yet, my favorite stance, to set myself up for the best possible chances that my dog never gets cancer in the first place! Preventive actions with essential oils are key in my eyes. Why wait to use them until our precious fur kid has cancer. I would so much rather use great diet, eliminate toxic household chemicals, reduce or eliminate over-vaccination, reduce toxic medications with side effects, and use essential oils that promote health – than ever be in the position of having to fight a bad disease.

So in this chapter, I am going to encourage you to create a 3 oil blend for any challenge that you feel you are facing. Then dilute it to the proper concentration for the species and situation you are dealing with. This will also get you some prime experience with blending for aesthetics as well. Let's face it, your dog may not care as much how they smell, but you or your roommate will! And certain mixes of essential oils, may not be all that complimentary. I made a blend one time with Valerian in it – that smelled like ANAL GLANDS! That's right – anal glands. I kept wondering who the culprit was who "blew out" in our house. Nope, it was the essential oil. Naturally, we'd still use something that smelled like anal glands if we knew it was a direct health help for our critter. But thankfully, we do not have to!

I remember years back there was a certain "new" single oil called Eucalyptus Blue released by one essential oil company. Well gosh all mighty – it smelled like cat pee when diffused! So many people thought their cats were peeing inappropriately, it was sad. But blended with a few other items, it became tolerable. Getting to know your essential oils, and having a relationship with them is half the battle of blending. Once you know your ingredients, you will understand who plays well with others, and who gets along the best with others. Starting with fewer essential oils on your plate, will greatly facilitate your learning and ability to create pleasant and effective blends.

Here's an example. You want to make a calming blend. Select at least 3 single essential oils you feel provide calming mechanisms in their description. Usually not hard to do, and you'll often come up with more like 20 oils you may wish to use. But at first, I urge you to limit yourself to about 5-8. Now go through those individual oil smells, and see which ones call to you, and seem pleasant if mixed together. There are no real rules here, and truly if you mix some oils together that smell horrible, no worries, we just try again. But for this reason, I often urge beginning blenders to create their blends initially drop by drop.

THREE PART BLENDS

Let's use the example of the calming blend. You selected the oils of Lavender (you are so un-original!), Bergamot, Valerian, German Chamomile, Frankincense, and Rose. Maybe also due to the fact that you have some of these oils on hand, will play a factor in your selections, as it should.

Now, smell all of these oils and create a mindset of which you think go well together. Some are stronger than others, such as Rose, and could be overpowering to a blend. And some are quite stinky in nature, like Valerian, and you may wish to avoid this if the blend is being used while your ultra-picky, scent-hating mother-in-law is over! All of these things come into play. Do you have a preference for what the "base" of the oil will smell like? Would you rather it be mainly German Chamomile in scent, or Frankincense?

Now pick three. You select Rose (nice), Frankincense, and Lavender. In general, I might suggest that you start with equal parts of the oils together. But in reality, your blend would probably smell only of Rose, which is great if you want a Rose only smelling blend. But, often we enjoy smelling multiple parts of the blend. So let's try 1 part Rose, 3 parts Frankincense, 2 parts Lavender. The selection is really up to you – (I personally am not as big of a fan of Lavender - so, I'm going to reduce it a bit.) Now, I suggest at first that you use these "parts" as drops.

I will often utilize an empty 2mL bottle to start my blending adventure. Make sure to write down what you put in, and any modifications you make to the blend. I also record the date I create the blend, then also how the scent may change over the next few days to weeks. So, say that you add 1 drop Rose, 3 drops Frankincense, and 2 drops Lavender to your bottle. I then screw on the cap (without the plastic orifice reducer in place yet) – and rock my solution to mix it. After mixing, I open it back up and give it a sniff. I might like it, I might hate it. Most likely, this blend may smell really strongly of Rose, so I might want to tone that down a bit. I may add 2 more drops of Frankincense then (adding this change to my blending log) – close it up, rock it, then sniff again.

This process is the art and charm of blending. Especially when we consider emotional uses of essential oils. True, a blend that smells intensely like Rose only, will still impart benefits of the other oils present. But, interestingly enough, I find that the more pleasant and rewarding the blend is to smell by the human, the better the response is in terms of continued use, and in terms of animal response. Imagine if someone applies something to you, but then acts like they are a bit disgusted with how you smell. Or they say "you're giving me a headache you stink so much!" Well, even if our animals do not speak a language, they most certainly are adept in the art of body language. Trust me, if you do not like a blend you are using for them, they will know it – and they may think they are the object of dislike, and not the oil smell.

We want everyone to have a pleasant experience, and not just a dog-calming effect. So, you continue to adjust your blend until you think it has reached its Goldie Locks Zone of "just-right" – now you can decide if you want to diffuse this blend (leave it undiluted or neat then) or if you want to dilute it in a carrier oil for other uses. And, amazingly enough, you can do both! Follow the instructions on how to dilute for certain concentrations in the Essential Oil Dilution Rates chapter.

Another thing to consider when blending, is curing time. Not the time to help an animal, but the amount of time you allow your blend to sit together and "marry". I do find that blends change and take on new characteristics after a length of time, than when they are freshly blended. Some blends "peak" at 3 days, some seem to be at their best after 2 weeks. There is no harm in using a fresh blend, however, you may find with experience that you will prefer a certain "baking time" for your custom creation. I personally enjoy the unique personality each of my blends possess, and finding their particular "sweet spot" in blending time is intriguing.

Below is a sample of a blending log. You can really make it anything you want – but you should always include the date you blend it, the names and sources of the oils you put in (this can include a brand name, supplier, and/or country of origin), some sort of lot number or tracking number so that you know when the oil you added to your blend was created, or how to trace it back to which bottle it came from, how much you add, and if a repeat recipe log – if you added it (the check mark area). If you are creating blends for others – record below the blending log which bottles were filled from this batch, or which animal they were made for, etc.

Basically – you want to be able to account for all parts of your blend, not only where the ingredients have come from, but where those ingredients are going. You can include other things like your own blend name, a bottle ID, different measurements, the date in which your blend is "ready", when and if you transfer this blend to another bottle, that bottle's ID, and so forth. Basically, the more information the better. And if you are in the veterinary field, think of it much like a compounding pharmacy. We want an accurate record of the ingredients, amounts, instructions, and patient information to be complete. You may also wish to have a place for notes about what you do and do not like about a new creation. When first adding drops into your new creation, you may want to use the tally mark system to keep track of any additions you make to the blend.

Sample Blending Log:

Date Blended: 12-31-2017   Bottle ID: A

Essential Oil	Source	Lot #	Amount Added	√
Rose Otto	Bulgaria	123456	3 drops	
Frankincense	Ethiopia	78910	9 drops	
Lavender	France	34521	6 drops	
Coconut Oil	Grocery	12-2017	36 drops	

A few more examples are often helpful. I have a dog with a cruciate injury, and would like to create a blend for the knee. I have selected Copaiba, Black Spruce, and Lemongrass for my blend. In reading about these oils, I find they have good support for inflammation, pain, bones, and ligaments. But, I also see the Lemongrass can be a bit intense topically. I read the carrier oil and dilution information, and know that most dogs use topical oils between 5-50% concentration, and I'll be using Fractionated Coconut Oil to dilute my creation. Knowing that there is information on Lemongrass being a bit hotter, I might add either less total drops of this oil to my creation, or I will make sure the entire blend is diluted a bit more than the "top range" of the recommendations.

This is where you have to apply a little bit of final art and knowledge to your blending. There is no other way around it if you wish to create your own blends, without a spelled out recipe. So, pull the trigger, and just decide. I add 10 drops Copaiba, 10 drops Black Spruce, and 5 drops Lemongrass to my 2mL bottle. Cap it, rock it, open it, smell it. How does that seem? Pleasant enough? Overpowering in one way or another? Do you want to change it? Nope. Perfect. Now let's add some carrier oil. You have added 25 drops total to your 2mL bottle, so to make a 50:50 blend, you would be adding 25 drops of the carrier oil. But, we decided we want to make it a bit more dilute, and will start at a 10% concentration.

This is where math starts to come into play. You go back to the chapter Dilution Rates, and find this chart.

10% Concentration:

Essential Oil	Carrier
18 drops	5mL (1 tsp)
35 drops	10mL (2 tsp)
53 drops	15mL (½ oz)
105 drops	30mL (1 oz)

But, you have added 25 drops into your bottle. How do you figure out how much carrier oil to add? The easiest thing to do, is to just measure out your drops from your newly created blend, and add that to your carrier oil in the exact measurements listed in the chart. So, using a pipette, add 18 drops of your Three Part Blend to 5mL of carrier oil. Simple as that. If you wanted to make 10mL of your new blend, then you will obviously need more than 25 drops of your Three Part Blend base. The simplest thing to do, is to just make a second batch in the same proportions that you just created. So, since I like the mixture of 10, 10, and 5 drops. I will just add that again to my base bottle. Ending up with a total of 50 drops of my base Three Part Blend.

You may have left over "neat" Three Part Blend, but that is okay. You can use it for a future creation, or keep it if you feel that the 10% concentration Three Part Blend that you made, is not quite strong enough for the animal you are helping. After using a 10% concentration for a few days, you feel that maybe "just a little bit stronger" might be nice. Open up your base (neat) Three Part Blend, and simply add another drop to your 10% solution. Naturally, with this method, we may not know how much of the original solution you have used up, or be able to calculate the "new" actual percentage of the blends concentration. But, in a practical sense, you are unlikely to alter or change the concentration so drastically, as to be dangerous or irresponsible in any way. Use common sense. If you had made up 10mL of a diluted blend, and it is almost gone – and then you start adding additional drops of neat oil to it, you will be affecting the concentration in a much more aggressive manner. And whenever in doubt, just make up a full new recipe bottle, with a 15% concentration or whatever your desired concentration may be.

Life is flexible. And blending can be as well. However, just like with baking, you cannot modify recipes and suggestions too much before you no longer get a successful outcome. You will always be rewarded by not cutting corners. If you are a beginner, or struggle with math, then always start over from the beginning. You will be well rewarded for your additional labors.

TOPICAL APPLICATIONS

There are many different methods to apply oils topically to animals. Each species has methods that are more suitable to their particular needs.

Direct Topical Application:
This involves applying drops of oil directly to the skin or fur of an animal – often in a "drop" form. This can include neat or diluted oils. Dripping the oils directly from the bottle onto the animal, is considered a Direct Topical Application. Another form of Direct Topical Application would be if you placed a puddle of essential oil (blend, neat, or diluted) into the palm of your hand, put a bit on the tip of your finger, then dabbed it onto a location of concern (say a lump or skin tag).

This method certainly is used in what we call the "Drip & Rub Technique", and is used quite often for easy applications of blends created for full body support. In the case of the dog's knee – a lighter application that covers the entire knee area instead of a one drop location, will likely be better tolerated by the skin and the dog, and may be more effective as it spreads the essential oil over more hair follicles and enhances the absorption of the oil. In this situation, we change to a different version of topical application we call "Petting".

Direct Topical Application may also be used when dripping oils directly into a wound or abscess, onto a site where acupuncture is to be performed, onto a hoof, or onto another site of intense need.

Animals such as dogs, horses, cows, goats, and other large animals accept this form of application very well. For cats and smaller, when direct application of oils is used, it is generally in a diluted form, such as the Body Supporting Blends. For some cats, directly dripping the oils onto them works better than approaching them for a Petting Application. And for very small animals such as a gerbil, Petting Applications are more appropriate due to the difficult nature of getting a drop to fall onto the animal easily and in the proper locations.

Petting Applications:

This method involves applying essential oils (neat or diluted) to your hands. Your hands are then rubbed together, and a varying amount of essential oil is allowed to remain on your palms. This may vary from completely absorbed (for say a rabbit) to an obviously light coating of oil spread out over your hands. Your hands are then used to pet the animal in question. This technique could also involve petting a specific location – such as the knee of a dog.

This method is well tolerated by almost every form of animal. The technique can be modified for small rodents, amphibians, or animals that may be difficult to handle, simply by having the oils absorbed into your hands, and then "cupping" and holding the animal within your hands.

Even the largest horse or even elephant, can benefit from this method of application. The larger the animal, the more film of essential oil is allowed to remain on our hands prior to petting. Remember, that just because an animal is very large, it may still require a diluted application of essential oil. This is very much an individual variation, and if you are ever in question as to how to proceed, start with the diluted oil, see how the animal does, then use more concentrated oils later.

With cats, we need to consider their individual personality when deciding whether to drip oils directly onto them, or to use a Petting technique. There are some cats who truly do better if a blend is just dripped up their back, without a lot of fanfare. As in the case of my feral farm cat population, sometimes drops of the diluted Body Support Blend, will just fall out of the "sky" while they are eating. I will not be able to massage it into them, as I cannot touch them. But the benefits will still be there. For them, Petting Applications are not a possibility. For cats with the ability to be pet, I also consider if Petting or dripping will be more appropriate for them or not. When I grab a bottle, coat my hands, then start to approach my cat with what I term "the big smelly hand syndrome" – they know something is up. I'm like a hawk on the attack. Just like the moment I grab the cat claw scissors for a nail trim, my cats turn into Houdini, and quickly disappear.

While some cats enjoy petting techniques with oils, some cats will need more of the "drops from heaven" approach, or even a bit of encouragement or restraint to accept their application. After all, none of my cats ever volunteer for a nail trim, however, we do it anyway. While I will always strive to make an application as pleasant and appropriate for the animal, there are situations in which we just have to get the job done for the better of the animal.

Tipping the Ears:

This method is a variation of the petting technique to some extent. It involves applying varying amounts of neat or diluted essential oils to your fingertips, then stroking the animal's ear. Although it has often been considered a superior location to apply oils due to increased ability for absorption, I do not believe this to be accurate. Many animals' ears are a bit sensitive to touch and to oil application, and as I have seen obvious responses to petting the body surfaces with oils, I have quickly found that I prefer the overall petting method to the body – as do many of my patients.

There is a differentiation to be made from "Tipping" as an overall application, than with applying oils to the ear as a treatment to the ear itself. Certainly, if I am applying oils to a cut on the ear, or a skin tag or tumor, we consider the application to be to the wound or tissue itself, and disregard the fact that the location just happens to be on the ear. Rubbing a bunch of oils onto the ear flap in an effort to calm a dog, is far different than dabbing a bit of oil onto a wound located on the ear. General petting of an oil onto the body area for an emotional blend, will be far more appropriate than "Tipping the Ears".

Applying to Pads & Feet:

When I first started using aromatherapy - a definite statement was made that applying essential oils to the bottom of a person's feet - was the safest and most tolerated location. People who could not tolerate oils on various locations of their body, could tolerate even "hot" oils rubbed onto their feet. I have heard many different explanations of why the bottom of your foot is an excellent location for application - from the skin is tougher to that we have larger pores for absorption ability. Regardless of the "why" - it can be true that many humans tolerate oils very well when applied to the bottom of their feet. However, the same does not hold true for many animals.

As you start reading this - please, do not feel badly. Many, many people (including myself) have applied essential oils to their animal's pads and feet. And, sometimes this application goes just fine! However, I am going to tell you my opinion based on treating thousands of different animals with essential oils. I rarely recommend applying essential oils to the bottom of dog, cat, ferret, rabbit, rodent, or exotic animals' feet.

Horses, Livestock, Primates, and in some circumstances Birds - are exceptions - and we will apply various oil preparations to their feet. Since hoof-stock really have hooves - it is a much different thing. Bird and primate feet seem to be a bit more like human feet in their acceptance of oil - although I would still say that this application is not usually the absolute first route recommended.

There were multiple issues we could see regarding applying to pads and feet. Many times, if someone is dipping a paw into a puddle of oil in their hand, simply too much oil is being used. Second, some will apply a neat oil in this manner, which will never be appropriate unless we are attempting a direct topical application to a tumor on a foot (such as Bumblefoot). For the most part, animals rarely like their feet messed with, and finally, easier methods and locations of application are available, that yield the same if not better results.

For many animals, we see a distinct irritation both emotionally and physically with general applications of oils to feet or pads. I would term this sort of thing as an "overly aggressive application." The essential oil may not cause permanent harm to the dog or cat - however - the skin may have burned, itched, or become inflamed and reddened. Even with no changes to the skin's appearance, oils can create a warm, cool, or even burning sensation. We never need to create discomfort for an oil application to be effective.

We need to differentiate the application of oils in general to the feet, versus treating an actual condition located on the feet. A dog with a yeast infection between the toes, may warrant the application of a diluted blend onto the location. This again is treating the issue, not necessarily the foot or pad as a location entity. If there is a wound on a pad, or infection in between the toes, then yes, we apply essential oils to the feet.

It is also important to recognize that the pads of animals (dogs and cats) possess their sweat glands. There can be quite a difference between the sensitivity of a human armpit and the bottom of a human foot. So in making blends or dilutions in regards to foot applications, this sort of sensitive nature of the tissues should be taken into account. For most foot applications, a 5% concentration or less of a blend should be considered.

While "detoxification" of chemicals and irritants in the feet are often given as the reason for a "reaction" – I do not see this as a beneficial thing, or a necessary one. And, we could indeed be increasing the absorption of toxic chemicals into the feet of our animals with overly aggressive applications of essential oils.

Water Misting Applications:

This method involves diluting an essential oil or blend, generally in distilled water, shaking well, and spritzing the mixture onto the animal, wound, location of injury, or application site. This method can also be used to spritz leafy greens, vegetables, fruits, sprouts, and other foods when we would like an animal to ingest certain essential oils.

Although we are taught that essential oils and water do not mix, this is an effective way to disperse a light and even amount of essential oil over a large area or onto an animal that is difficult to apply oils to. This method will generally include various bug repellant recipes as well as the Feather Spray for birds. Read the chapter Forms of Dilution for more information on dispersment versus dilution.

The oils should be added to a glass spray bottle, especially if they are to be stored for more than a day or two. Essential oils can degrade plastics, so the least amount of contact an oil can make with plastic, the better. The plastic tube and sprayer components seem to do just fine, however, I try to avoid entirely plastic spray bottles.

There are various essential oil spray recipes that will recommend the addition of detergents, shampoos, or other agents and surfactants to the essential oil and water mixture. These items act to help the essential oil mix with the water more completely and for a longer period of time, before separating. I do not recommend their use for sprays intended for use on animals. These items are not necessary for an essential oil mist to be functional, effective, and safe – and I find that a good shake of the bottle before use, is quite effective in mixing plain solutions.

We are also taught that if we want to drive an oil into the skin, that applying a water compress can help to do that. Additionally, we are told that if you need to "take the heat away" from an oil, or "rinse" it from an eye – to not use water and use a diluting carrier oil. Many people have expressed concern that by applying a spray application of essential oils in water, that we would make them more intense. I'll set your mind at ease. Because we are applying these oils with the idea of absorption in mind – it would actually be beneficial for the water to drive the oils "into the animal." Furthermore, the oils are generally being used at quite a low concentration, so water enhancing the absorption is actually a good thing!

Some have concerns of intensity, as we are misting a "neat" oil onto application sites. However, the fact that the droplets are so finely dispersed through the mist, really acts just as a heavily diluted essential oil solution would.

For some locations that we wish to not get "greasy" or have additional residual moisture, a water mist remains a good option for application. A condition such as a hotspot on a dog, is already a moist and infected dermatitis. So using an essential oil blend within a carrier oil, may add excessive and additional moisture to a location we would like to see dry out and crust over. In this way, a water mist is more ideal as the water will dry and evaporate off of the area of concern, faster and more effectively than coconut oil, while still allowing us to get a nice coating of minute amounts of essential oil over the wound.

When spritzing an animal such as a bird, I have found that they blink their eyes very effectively. When I first used spritzers in birds, I tried to avoid their head and eyes, and aimed only for their feet. The birds quickly showed me who was in control of where the spray landed, and they often made sure that it came in contact with their head, face, and mouth. Unless there is neurologic damage or functional issues with the blink reflex, normal misting towards an animal would rarely, if ever, result in eye irritation.

Situations in which Water Misting is highly useful include the following: misting birds with the Feather Spray, misting large proud flesh wounds in horses, misting wounds (such as hot spots in dogs) in which ointments would provide too much moisture, misting into the air when diffusion is needed, misting bedding, fabrics, or other areas in need of odor control, and the list goes on and on.

When selecting the oils to add to a spritzer – you should consider which oils are the best choices for this use. Certainly, for a horse with proud flesh, any of the oils indicated for this condition could be applied with this technique, and in a fairly high concentration; 20-40 drops or more in 4 ounces (120 mL) of water. However, if we plan to spritz a bird with a water mist – selecting an oil such as Oregano would not be a good idea. When spritzing a bird or small animal, I would consider what it would feel like if I sprayed myself in the face or eyes with the mist, and I often do just that, to test out what I have created. After all, I would never expect that I should be able to spritz a bird with a solution that I cannot spray directly into my own face.

It would always be the wisest to start with very low concentrations of oils in the water mist. 1 drop of essential oil in 4 ounces (120 mL) of water is a very low concentration, one that is unlikely to cause discomfort in even the most sensitive of species. You can always start with this concentration for a few applications, and then add an additional drop into your solution – ending up with 2 drops in 4 ounces (120 mL) of water. Then apply this concentration for a few more applications. Increase the concentration again by adding another drop of essential oil to your 4 ounces (120 mL) of water, and so on, and so on. This is how we "titrate" a concentration to a specific animal or species.

A great rule of thumb to remember is "While you can always use more, you can never take away what you have already applied!"

Swimming Pools, Ponds, Soaking Water, and Aquariums:

Any animal entering water containing essential oils will absorb some of the essential oils topically. Dispersing agents can be utilized if desired and appropriate – such as adding essential oils first to carrier oils, natural cleaning solutions, or to natural animal shampoos – which will help spread the essential oils throughout the water, instead of just floating on the surface. Adding essential oils to salts is sometimes recommended, but may result in more essential oil floating on the surface of the water, than truly mixed throughout. There are some who practice herbal packs or salt based soaks, and adding essential oils to these often offer great synergy.

Adding essential oils to salts, sugar poultices, or cleaner may be most appropriate for soaking a horse's hoof, for example. Dogs have especially enjoyed having a few drops of Peppermint oil added to their "wading pools" in the heat of the summer. Not only to they lay in it, but they also drink it. Many owners have reported incredible improvements in arthritis pain when their older dogs soaked in a Peppermint pool!

While adding essential oils into water may raise concern for many in the aromatherapy community, it has indeed been used by a large number of essential oil consumers. In practice, adding essential oils to water remains a reasonable option for exposure to essential oils. However, based on today's knowledge, we can offer a few tips to allow for a more safe exposure.

In human aromatherapy, safe bathing with essential oils promotes the addition of essential oils to items such as castile soap, shampoo, shower gel, fractionated coconut oil, aloe jelly, polysorbate 20, polysorbate 80, or products such as Solubol or Natrasorb Bath. On the not recommended list is milk, Epsom salt, baking soda, cornstarch, witch hazel, glycerin, and aloe gel (according to Tisserand Institute). For animals, we must select more non-toxic and non-irritating substances, that also make sense for the animal who will be exposed to them. Adding essential oils within fractionated coconut oil to a fish tank – is more likely to be harmful to a fish – as we are created a fatty "oil spill". Likewise for birds – bathing in water containing fractionated coconut oil, would be far more harmful than the likely contact with the essential oil when in minute amounts.

For all animals – I would only suggest the appropriate use of mainly edible and non-toxic ingredients. If a dog were to soak in a tub of water, certainly adding essential oils to a shampoo or fractionated coconut oil would be well tolerated. However, I would urge everyone to avoid the use of polysorbate 20, polysorbate 80, Solubol, or Natrasorb with animals.

Certainly oils can be added to any body of water from Koi ponds, habitats for Hippopotamus, ponds for Tigers in zoos, glass aquariums and fish bowls, dolphin holding tanks, dog wading pools, physical therapy pools, underwater treadmills, and more. The key is to start with small amounts of oils, agitate the water's surface to disperse the oils when possible, and to gradually increase the level of concentration of the essential oil exposure. Even when very small amounts of oils are used, there will be benefits to the exposure.

Shampoos, Ointments, and Other Products:

We shouldn't forget how convenient it is to add additional essential oils to products that are routinely used for our animals. If you plan to bathe your dog with a natural shampoo, why not add a few extra drops of Frankincense oil to the shampoo for Cognitive Dysfunction, or add a few drops of Copaiba oil for Arthritis. Including essential oils into other items can be an easy and wonderful way to provide preventive measures to your animal. I marvel at the idea that if every time you gave your dog a bath, by adding Frankincense to the shampoo, you may be preventing cancer in the future. I for one, will always support prevention over treatment, any day of the week!

Adding additional essential oils to natural ointments is also a wonderful technique. For example, adding 1 drop of Balsam Fir to 1 tablespoon of ointment, and mixing it together, can be a wonderful way to apply the Balsam Fir onto the feet of a chicken or bird. When using ointments on animals, it is important to not overuse it, especially with our feathered friends, where we could get them too "greasy." With animals such as Dogs, Horses, and other Large Animals, many more drops can be added to a natural ointment making it quite strong and potent when needed. The technique is incredibly flexible.

Oil Misting Application:

This is similar to water misting, however in place of the water, fractionated coconut oil is used. I have found that this carrier oil will spray through certain misting bottles, and results in a longer contact time and "oil presence." Situations where I use this method the most, is to repel insects and for topical parasites such as lice.

For example, I have found that by mixing up strong bug recipes within fractionated coconut oil instead of water for my cow, that I am more effective and have a longer lasting repellant action. This is also a great way to mix and spray on recipes for lice.

This application could be used for any large area that you would like to apply diluted oils to and have a longer contact time, with less evaporation of the essential oils. Avoiding an oil spray may be warranted in conditions where you desire the skin to stay dry (rain rot in a horse, hot spots in a dog, or scabs that are healing up).

Diffusion:

Although this method is not often considered as a topical application, I would beg to differ. Essential oils have the ability to penetrate into surfaces of walls and other materials when being diffused, which can actually act to kill toxic molds in the environment. Think of some homes absorbing the smell of frequent cooking with fragrant spices. The essential oils and essences of these spices, often permeate into walls and ceilings, leaving rental units wondering how to eliminate the odors. Diffusion of essential oil chemicals into the air, is most certainly a form of topical application.

Since animals absorb oils through hair follicles, diffusion alone can indeed create a level of systemic or topical absorptions of the essential oils. Situations such as Ringworm can be contained and certainly aided by the diffusion of anti-fungal oils that will contact the hairs and skin. Although diffusion may not be the only technique we would utilize for a certain condition, it is certainly not to be excluded in a layered approach to the use of essential oils. Diffusion for physical conditions such as arthritis discomfort, will often not be enough to notice sizeable improvement, however we never neglect the opportunity for additional layers of easy and helpful exposure.

When diffusing for an animal, it is important to select appropriate oils and concentrations in which to diffuse. The instructions discussed in this book for diffusion should still be followed, even if topical exposure to the oils is the goal in mind.

Indirect Applications:

Indirect application of oils topically is considered to be situations such as rubbing essential oils (neat or diluted) onto a perch or onto your hands, and allowing the animal to come in contact with it. A bird perching on a wooden branch would naturally be exposed to small amounts of essential oils found within the tree. When we rub essential oils onto perches or branches, we recreate this indirect transfer of essential oils to the body.

ESSENTIAL OILS & EYES

Although this chapter is sure to meet with some controversy, there is much good that has come from certain uses of essential oils in and around eyes. Since many people are in fact using this method, and many people and animals have reaped benefits from it, I feel it is an important topic to cover.

We are taught continually, to avoid getting essential oils into our eyes. This as a whole, is advice well heeded. However, there are many cases in which the proper use of essential oils can benefit various eye conditions.

I urge you to only use these common and well-tolerated methods, and to always err on the side of caution when considering use of this method. I also recommend that before applying any essential oil spray to an animal's face or eye area, that you try it on yourself first. After all, one should never do something to an animal that they wouldn't do first on themselves.

The most common start of the use of what I will term a "water spritzer" for the eyes, started with people experiencing dry eye, most commonly associated with Lasik Surgery. Someone apparently placed 4 drops of Lavender in 4 ounces (120 mL) of distilled water, misted this into their eyes and found amazing comfort. Not only was comfort found, but increased healing as well.

Upon witnessing someone spraying their eyes with a mister – I was immediately curious. Wondering what they were misting, I investigated further. It turns out they were spraying this very diluted lavender solution into their eyes. Well, since her eyes were not red, swollen, watering, and she was not writhing on the ground in pain...I had to try it! It was wonderful. Very soothing and felt moisturizing.

As time passed on, I would use this eye spritzing technique for my own children during a pink eye scare, for one of my dogs with a corneal abrasion, for friends and patients with dry eye, for eye infections, and so much more. The application has not only become a way to use oils for the eye itself, but for the delicate tissues surrounding the eyes. Styes, conjunctivitis, eyelid tumors, blocked tear ducts, lacerations or surgeries of tissues near the eye – all became accessible to oils via this "mister."

Misting the eye and eye area, has quickly become a favorite tool of mine. It has been used in many animals and humans, however, I would still urge you to use caution and common sense, and never risk any individual's safety if you do not feel comfortable using this method.

Always have a carrier oil on hand when planning to use essential oils near the eyes, face, or head. Especially when you intentionally plan to use oils for the eye area. If any discomfort would ever be noted, you can flush the area with a carrier oil, such as fractionated coconut oil until the area is comfortable. Signs that an animal may be experiencing discomfort with an eye application could be; pawing at the face or eyes, blinking or tearing, increased reddening of eyes or surrounding tissues, squinting, whining, or any other behavior that is out of the ordinary. It is worthy to mention, that these responses have not been noted at this time with responsible and appropriate use.

Since cats have different views of the world unique to being a feline, they often do not appreciate any form of a spritzer being used on them. The use of this method for cats will have to be considered with individual personality and acceptance in mind. I do not recommend "traumatizing" a cat by forcing the spray into their face, unless a critical eye situation demanded the attempt. If any animal greatly dislikes this misting procedure, I recommend finding less stressful ways to expose them to the essential oils. Even water diffusion, via caging or tenting, can be effective in exposing the eye's surface to beneficial essential oils.

Tried & True Recipes:
I will present for you several recipes that have been used repeatedly and with great success. I do not encourage anyone to go outside of these recommendations without the advice of a veterinary aromatherapist or very experienced medical aromatherapist. The only alterations that should be made to these recipes are ones of greater dilution – i.e. adding less essential oils to the water.

Lavender Eye Spritzer:

This is the basic eye recipe, and has been used for tens of years or more in humans and animals. It is the recipe I recommend starting with, then only if results are not seen with this recipe, moving onto others. This spritzer can be misted into the eyes even 4 or more times per day. Long term use has not been evaluated, but many have used this spritzer for 2 months or more, without harm. Do not aggressively attempt to squirt this mixture directly into the eye, the goal is to lightly mist the area, and if possible hold the eye open slightly while doing so. Even the mist contacting the areas directly next to the open lids, will be beneficial.

- Add 4 drops of Lavandula angustifolia to 4 ounces (120 mL) of distilled water. Use a glass spray bottle. Shake well, mist into eyes or surrounding eye tissues.

Therapeutic Eye Spritzer:

This recipe is wonderful for many reasons. It adds the many other benefits of Copaiba, Frankincense, and Helichrysum Essential Oils to Lavender. This recipe is a powerhouse for situations such as eyelid tumors, inflammation, corneal ulcers, corneal abrasions, post-surgical sites, and more. I still recommend starting with the basic Lavender Eye Spritzer, but this recipe is being used more and more, with wonderful results. This spritzer is recommended to be used up to 4 times per day. Long term use has not been evaluated, but we have used this particular spritzer for 2-3 week intervals without harm. Do not aggressively attempt to squirt this mixture directly into the eye, the goal is to lightly mist the area, and if possible hold the eye open slightly while doing so. Even the mist contacting the areas directly next to the open lids, will be beneficial.

- Add 4 drops of Lavandula angustifolia, 2 drops of Copaiba, 2 drops of Frankincense (Boswellia carterii), and 2 drops of Helichrysum to 4 ounces (120 mL) of distilled water. Use a glass spray bottle. Shake well, mist into eyes or surrounding eye tissues.

ESSENTIAL OILS & EARS

Like eyes, ears also carry a bit of controversy and warning associated with essential oils. Similarly, I have found that there are again some ways we can use essential oils in and around ears, and there are ways we should not. Contacting the ears, and specifically the ear drum or tympanic membrane, with an essential oil can be excruciatingly painful.

Even with these precautions, the veterinary market is flooded with ear washes, flushes, cleaners, treatment solutions, and ointments containing essential oils. Many holistic veterinarians will get negative feedback when knowingly adding an essential oil to an animal product, but yet, when it is "snuck" into the ingredient list as a fractionated and un-natural constituent within a mainstream veterinary product, nobody raises concern.

What I have found to be true is that in the proper ways, in the proper dilutions, and in the proper methods essential oils can be incredibly helpful for ear conditions of all sorts. Ear infections that are resistant to traditional veterinary drugs are often completely eliminated or greatly helped with the use of essential oils in our veterinary practice. Many times these dogs are facing surgical removal of the ear (Total Ear Canal Ablation or TECA) to deal with the resistant and chronic infection. Certainly, the use of essential oils within the ear canal, is a far better solution than the surgical removal of the problem area.

Described will be various methods in which essential oils are used in animal ears, and for which animal each method is recommended for. It is important to note, that most animal's ear canals are "L" shaped, especially dogs. This means that the tunnel that runs from the outside of their ear, to the ear drum, takes a sharp turn near the bottom. This also provides a level of "security" from essential oils being able to drip directly onto the ear drum. Before an essential oil could reach this sensitive surface, it would have to get past a long track of skin without becoming completely absorbed first. Thankfully, this is actually a fairly difficult task.

The basic rules that I follow for ears are:
- Always consult with a veterinarian concerning ear related problems. Situations, such as ruptured ear drums are common, and even a veterinary ear cleaner without essential oils can cause damage in this situation.
- Never place neat essential oils directly into the ear or ear canal.
- Never "drip" neat oils, concentrated oil solutions, or even diluted oil solutions into the ear with the intention of "reaching the bottom."
- Monitor the skin of the ear canal and of the ear flap for irritation to essential oil use.
- Always dilute your essential oils, and never attempt to fill the ear canal with an essential oil solution completely.
- Essential oils may be used within a liquid ear cleaning recipe, which may fill the ear canal. It is suggested that when the cleaning solution will be filling the ear, a maximum 1-3% concentration should be used unless specifically indicated by your veterinarian.

Cotton Ball Application:

This method involves placing drops of diluted essential oil(s) (1-15% concentration) onto a non-colored, 100% pure cotton, cotton ball. This cotton ball is then inserted into the ear canal of the animal, and left in place for a varying amount of time – usually 12-24 hours. Many animals dislike the cotton ball in their ear, and readily shake it out – so it is not a favorite method of mine. Care must be taken that the cotton ball does not travel too far down into the ear canal of a large dog or horse, which could require extraction by a veterinarian. Cats and small animals do not enjoy this method much. Overall, it is only a method I use when I absolutely have no other options.

Essential Oils in Carrier Oils:

Essential oils can be mixed into raw or fractionated coconut oil, and then applied to the ears. The focus of this application is not to fill the ear canal with the diluted essential oil, but to allow a coating of the ear tissues with the diluted mixture. Raw coconut oil is often solid at most room temperatures, and will melt and become liquid once in contact with the animal's warmer body temperature inside of the ear and on the tissues. Raw Coconut Oil carries its own antibacterial, antifungal, and anti-inflammatory actions, making it a wonderful tool for cleaning ear debris as well as carrying the essential oils to their place of need.

New & Improved Ear Spray:

This is a helpful recipe for many dogs who struggle with ear issues. I mainly recommend this recipe for use in dogs, and I generally would not use it for cats. Dogs are the main animal that experience ear infections that require this sort of remedy.

- Add the following ingredients to a 1 ounce (30 mL) glass spray bottle.
- 7-8 mL of grain alcohol (Everclear)
- 1 Tablespoon of Fractionated Coconut Oil
- 1 drop of Clove Essential Oil
- 2 drops of Melaleuca alternifolia Essential Oil
- 3 drops of Lemongrass Essential Oil
- 4 drops of Copaiba Essential Oil
- 5 drops of Lavender Essential Oil
- Then fill the rest of the bottle with Distilled Water.

Shake well and spray 1-3 pumps into the ear(s), once to twice a day. You are not trying to saturate the ear canal or drip this solution into the ear canal directly. Coating the infected outer surface area of the ear and upper part of the exposed ear canal, will result in the "traveling" of this solution to deeper parts of the ear. Monitor the ear tissues for any signs of irritation. This recipe has been used long term, for several months at a time or more. However, if irritation occurs, the solution may be diluted further or discontinued and other methods used. Irritation seems rare with this recipe, however alcohol could always be drying or irritating to sensitive dogs. Discontinue use immediately with any sign of redness or irritation.

This spray can act to break up debris, and make cleaning of the ears easier. When indicated, this spray has been used in the ears of horses and other large animals as well.

Ear Cleaning Solutions:

Plain Raw Coconut Oil, Fractionated Coconut Oil, or Fractionated Coconut Oil mixed with small amounts of essential oils, make wonderful and soothing ear cleaning concoctions. Placing a "glob" of Raw Coconut Oil into the ear canal, and allowing it to soften wax and debris, creates a gentle cleaning action. Gently wiping the ear clean with a cotton-tipped swab, works wonderfully after the Raw Coconut Oil has been instilled into the ear. As Raw Coconut Oil carries its own antibacterial, antifungal, and anti-inflammatory actions, it is a wonderful medium to use to break up wax and debris. This remains one of my most favorite methods for cleaning cat ears especially. Essential oils can be added to the coconut oil, even when intended for use as a cleaner. Approximately 5-10 drops of essential oils are added to 1 Tablespoon of coconut oil.

Several DIY ear cleaning recipes for dogs may be found as well. Dr. Karen Becker (Mercola Healthy Pets) created this recipe, which is suggested to be used on cotton wipes, and not as a flooding solution for the ear canal:
- 1/3 cup Witch Hazel
- 3 Tablespoons Hydrogen Peroxide
- 1 Tablespoon Apple Cider Vinegar

Additional ingredients can be added such as 1 Tablespoon of colloidal silver. 3 drops of essential oils (especially a Three Part Blend) can also be added to this solution if desired.

RECTAL INSTILLATION

Rectal suppositories of essential oils may be quite effective for several situations. The lining of the rectum and colon are rich in blood supply, and approximately 2/3rds of the items which are absorbed rectally, will be carried to the lungs prior to metabolism by the liver. This may be useful for conditions such as lung cancer, bronchitis, pneumonia, and various lung infections. More essential oil is available to reach the lung tissue following rectal instillation, than by ingestion.

Rectal insertion of essential oil suppositories has been reported to be very helpful in prostatic conditions. There are several methods in which to instill essential oils rectally, and generally these application methods must take into account the ability to administer them to the individual animal. Animals such as dogs, horses, cattle, and other large animals will obviously be easier to administer to than say a cat. Ferrets are commonly affected with prostatic issues, and using the indicated oils externally (over the prostate area) first, is a wise decision. However, if the protocols are not revealing enough results, one can attempt rectal instillation as well.

Effective methods of rectal instillation include diluting the essential oil within carrier oils (generally starting with 1 drop of oil in 20 drops of carrier or more), and using a needle-less syringe to introduce the liquid into the rectum. Ample lubrication of the syringe with a lubricating jelly is highly recommended. For small animals such as ferrets, cats, or small dogs (less than 20 pounds), instilling 0.5 mL or less of the diluted solution is a recommended starting point. For larger dogs, between 1-3 mL of the dilution could easily be instilled. Exact dosing amounts for rectal administration is less known for animals, and starting with small amounts and increasing the concentration is recommended. Too frequent administration of oils rectally, can lead to irritation of the anus and mucus membranes. In general this therapy is recommended for short term use, usually no more than twice a day. However, for severe cases that respond well to this remedy, more frequent and longer term use can be considered.

Suppositories can also be made for rectal instillation. Raw organic Coconut Oil will generally be solid in form at most room temperatures, melting at over 76 degrees Fahrenheit (24 degrees Celsius). Essential oils can be mixed into the liquid raw Coconut Oil at approximately 5 drops per tablespoon. The solution is thoroughly mixed, and then placed into a refrigerator or freezer temporarily to start the hardening of the coconut oil. Once the coconut oil mixture is a bit solid, a teaspoon or more of the mixture can be formed into a "bullet shape" on a piece of plastic wrap. You may have to return your bullet to the cold environment several times to perfect your suppository, but once it is in a form that you feel you could insert in to a rectum, place the suppository into the freezer until it is completely frozen and solid. It is this frozen suppository that will be inserted into the rectum. Insertion with a gloved and lubricated finger is generally the easiest method.

The human world of aromatherapy has indeed, quite perfected the art of rectal suppositories and instillation. For most humans, the general dosing for rectal administration of essential oils is about 175mg (or approximately 5 drops) two to three times a day. Items such as Witepsol and Cocoa Butter are often used to "build a better suppository" – along with suppository molds and creation aids. I strongly urge you to research human suppository information if you decide you will pursue rectal instillation of essential oils.

For larger animals, there is no set guideline for how much or how we instill the essential oil. Starting with amounts suitable for oral ingestion is suggested, however there are no hard and fast rules. Dilution of the essential oil is recommended (approximately 10-20 drops per tablespoon), and any carrier can be utilized. Larger volumes of liquid are sometimes easier to instill in horses or cows, and the removal of large amounts of fecal material from the rectum is recommended prior to instillation.

HOW MUCH, HOW OFTEN

No matter what the application method, one common question that is constantly raised, always focuses on the questions "how much do I give?" and "how often do I give it?" My best answer is to teach you a common sense approach to empower you to be able to navigate these questions for yourself. As every animal is an individual, you will be far better equipped to logically evaluate a situation and make reasonable changes, if you first understand how to evaluate the situation.

Whether you are starting to use an oil orally, topically, via diffusion, or by administering a Drip & Rub Technique – the basics are all the same. We can start with a small amount and gradually increase the amounts that an animal is exposed to.

Start by using a small amount of the recommended oil. Did you see a response? How long did it last for? Did the animal show some sort of negative response? I never use an essential oil with the immediate goal of using it twice a day, three times a day, or four times a day. How often I use an application method, will largely hinge on how long the animal received comfort from that application. This idea also holds true for determining the correct amount or concentration of an oil application. Starting with a lesser amount, and seeing if there were any results, allows me to decide whether the next application be stronger, the same, or less concentrated.

If I have administered too little oil, I may see no response at all. In this situation, I can repeat the same dose or increase the amount given. It often depends on how critical the situation is as well. More critical health concerns may need to have larger amounts given faster than in other situations.

It is possible to have also administered too much oil. Seeing any sort of negative effect, will tell me that I should use less of the essential oil or vary my approach for the future. Various negative signs could include soft stools, poor appetite, scratching or rubbing at the site of application, reddened skin, rolling on the ground, running around the room, sneezing, coughing, squinting, or other behaviors that are out of the ordinary. We must remember that we never have to make an animal uncomfortable through the use of essential oils, to have them be effective! In some situations, I may accept a runnier nose as an acceptable response to a treatment, however if the animal appears to be breathing with difficulty, this would not be satisfactory.

A good note to be aware of, is that some animals (dogs in particular) may be prone to rubbing an application off of their fur or skin, no matter what the concentration. We have tested this theory by applying simply plain fractionated coconut oil, and indeed some dogs commence "surfing" along couches and carpets to rid themselves of the offending item applied to their body. My personal dogs, do this even after being outside in the rain. While I will always respect that an essential oil application may have been too intense for an animal, we may also have to do a bit of an evaluation, to see if it is truly the essential oils causing the response.

Another consideration is if the animal caretaker is able to dose the animal once a day, twice a day, or more. Sometimes human factors will dictate how often essential oils will be used. Possibly, a farmer can only access a certain animal once a day. Then, this will be the frequency of the treatments.

It is wise to give a little time to evaluate each change you make to a protocol. If you decided to increase an oral essential oil administration by one drop, then waiting approximately 3 days to evaluate the response to that increase is suggested. Of course in critical situations, waiting 3 days is usually not possible nor recommended.

How we time the next dose being given, is related to how long the treatment lasted for. For example, if a dog gets a whole body support blend application and itches less for 3 days; however, on day 4 the itching has recurred, then repeating the application every 3 days would be suggested. This allows for the comfort and benefits to continue, at an interval that is dictated by the body's own needs. If the itching subsides for 12 hours, then returns, twice a day applications may be more appropriate. And it may not always stay to that interval. After a few days of applications, we may see that daily applications are now capable of maintaining comfort instead of needing twice daily applications.

For an animal who is not showing benefits long enough – it is not always true that more concentrated oils will equal a longer lasting result. Sometimes the use of a stronger oil concentration, still results in the same length of response. In this situation, it becomes wasteful to give more oils than you need. Increasing the frequency of the use of the essential oil is often the correct choice in these situations.

Most importantly, whether you are using an essential oil or a supplement, start with one thing at a time, use them in very low amounts initially, and wait 3 days between each increase or addition. Do not overwhelm an animal with 20 different oils or supplements all at once.

PREVIOUS TECHNIQUES

Once upon a time, there were brand specific recommendations for application techniques which do warrant a bit of discussion and update, some 6+ years later. "Raindrop Technique" is one of those things. There were entire chapters dedicated to this method of essential oil application in the first edition of The Animal Desk Reference, and so I do believe an explanation of the changes to what we know are in order.

"Raindrop Technique" was coined and developed for humans by a popular multi-level marketing (MLM) essential oil company many years ago. The technique basically involves the neat application of Oregano, Thyme, Basil, Cypress, Wintergreen, Marjoram, and Peppermint oils (with some variations) along the spine of a human, followed with a variety of stroke and massage techniques. This application was later transferred to use with animals. Many companies developed their own version of this application in response to its popularity, so you can find names such as "AromaTouch", "Waterfall Technique", and yes, in some ways, "AromaBoost".

Here are the short answers to these techniques and why there may be portions we should retain for use with animals, and reasons we should leave them for humans only.

Initially, I used "Raindrop Technique" clinically for cases for which we had no further answers or options. Euthanasia versus trying some controversial essential oils, did not seem like a complicated decision. And, in truth, we found some quite amazing responses. There were just some things about this intense "Raindrop Technique" that did bring benefits to animals. However, we also saw some harm. Horses developed welts where the oils were dripped on, some horses threw themselves onto the ground and rolled between each application sequence, people applied the "Raindrop Technique" to cats in completely inappropriate manners, and dogs and other animals received chemical burns and severe irritations from the oil applications.

When things went well, it went very well. But when things went badly, well, that is not something we would like to see – ever. No matter if it is the "Raindrop Technique", "Waterfall Technique", or "AromaTouch" – these applications were created for humans. Only the "AromaBoost" technique has been specifically created for animals. All of these techniques involve applications of proprietary blends along with some single essential oils commonly. So it is important when considering the use of any proprietary blend, to ensure that it has been created specifically with animal use in mind.

In practice – certain very difficult conditions would respond well to the aggressive nature of this application process. And, animals seemed to enjoy the action of dripping several oils up the spine, then massaging them in. In actuality, it does not appear to matter what types of strokes or massage is used to rub in the oils. It likely does not even matter that the oils are dripped from a certain distance above the spine, or that they are dripped tail to head. But, in the truth of it all – we become a bit addicted to routine. So for me, it became an enjoyable sequence of applications for myself and my patients. I would meditate a bit with some calming oils with my patient. I would drip the oils up their back, and massage them in. And honestly, most of my patients, along with myself, greatly enjoyed this calm "down-time" in our clinic. My own personal dog will sit for hours to be massaged in this manner!

So, because it gives us something new to focus on, and because it has been so enjoyable – I will retain some of the recommendations of dripping oils up the spine, from tail to head, and also rubbing them in – often "against the grain" from tail to head.

There are interesting facts that can go along with the massage and with rubbing the oils in "against the grain". With chronic pain and inflammatory signals, it is possible to interrupt these messages with things like massage. So if you will humor me for a moment, consider a cat with chronic arthritis or hyperesthesia. The body has been sending, and the brain receiving, the message of "my body hurts" on a chronic basis. By initiating an essential oil massage, we not only have the physical and emotional effects that essential oils can bring, but we can interrupt the sensations this cat is experiencing. In a way, we "distract" the cat from the message of pain. The massage becomes a bit of the dominant sensation the cat is feeling, and we can effect more pain relief for that time.

This would be accurate as well for dogs, horses, and other animals. So for those reasons, I like to keep the "technique" as a viable option to help the entire body in ways other than just contact with an essential oil, and the physical properties that this may impart. For each animal, there is often a bit of a different technique or essential oil solution that will be used. For cats, in the past we modified this "Raindrop Technique" into what was termed "Kitty Raindrop Technique" or KRDT. For the feline version, a blend of essential oils would be diluted within a carrier oil, and then dripped up the spine and rubbed in (yes backwards strokes for the cat too!). I do truly believe that the combination of oils along with massage that is not the typical "petting" in nature – still provides great benefits.

For this book – since we are non-brand specific – I will rename this technique and its descriptions. For lack of anything better, let's call it the Drip & Rub Technique. Couldn't get any more basic than that!

You will find a chapter dedicated to Drip & Rub Techniques and recipes for all animal species.

DRIP & RUB TECHNIQUES

For cats and smaller animals – generally all of the oils you wish to use are combined into a single diluted solution. Although each individual oil could be diluted then applied in the same individual manner – small creatures tend to not sit still for very long periods of time. So it can be more difficult to complete the technique in this manner. In truth, blended and diluted oils remain quite effective for a variety of animals. So for convenience, and because it works, why make things harder on ourselves.

Basic Drip & Rub Procedures:

Balancing, Grounding, & Calming:
Prior to dripping a body supportive blend up the spine, a balancing step has traditionally been performed. This step can be optional, however reducing stress and aligning your energy with the animal in a calm manner, can result in even more benefits. Balancing is performed by placing a diluted calming blend into each hand. Depending on the species of animal you are working with, you may rub your hands together to obtain the diluted oil as a light film, or the oils may be absorbed completely into your hands.

With the appropriate oils on the palms of your hands, you will then hold each hand over the shoulder and rump area of the animal (some species may have different recommendations for balancing.) You may also find that you are drawn to balancing with your hands over the heart and front of the chest. All of these locations are fine, and allow your intuition to guide you. As you hold your hands in these locations – breathe deeply and meditate with your companion. If you are experienced in energy work, such as Reiki, this is a perfect time to insert this method. Continue for as long as this feels comfortable for you and the animal. Often times, you will feel a release of tension in both yourself and the animal, and deep sighs are often noted. If you feel a difference in hot or cold, or tingling between right and left hands, you may hold the balancing step until both hands feel equal.

Do not be alarmed if you feel nothing at all. Many of us experience this. Just strive for relaxation, and holding the position for a few minutes or as you feel guided. There is no perfect or specific way this is meant to feel. This step has also been omitted without detriment when time constraints or ability to handle a certain animal makes it necessary. The medical benefits that can be had with the essential oil application are still present.

We need to relax and recognize that essential oil applications can be adapted and grow with us. Starting with a method that is easy to understand, and gradually adding "skills" into it, makes the most sense in how we actually learn things. If you practice canine massage, equine chiropractic, or one of the animal specific practices of healing energy, you can create and modify these techniques for your own individual personality and needs. Just follow basic blending and dilution techniques described for your species, and don't be afraid to forge your own trail. Apply oils before a massage, after a massage, before an adjustment, after an adjustment, the choices are really yours. And you may find that for you, or for an animal in your care, one may work better than another. Don't be afraid to experiment and observe.

What about the feet?

In humans, applying essential oils to the feet along with reflexology is definitely promoted and used. While animals do have reflexology points in their feet, that coordinate similarly, I most commonly found that the application of oils to the paw was either difficult for my clients to perform or that it was less tolerated by the animal. Due to these elements, I recommend doing reflexology without additional application of essential oils to the feet. If you are practicing reflexology, allow a diluted blend to be almost completely absorbed into your hands and fingers, prior to activating your sites. The main exception to this recommendation lies with horses, especially if they are exhibiting any signs of lameness, hoof, or leg issues. For these animals, applying the oils to the hoof and/or leg area is a definite benefit – and while you can combine reflexology with these applications, I would qualify these applications as topical or massage based to the leg itself.

Applying Oils:

If balancing has been done, the next step is just simply applying your selected diluted oil or oil blends. Please be sure to consult the section for your particular animal species – as each species may have recommendations specific to their individual needs.

Application of the diluted essential oils will generally be on the spine, from the start of the tail to the base of the head (for horses or livestock, stopping at the withers is also acceptable). When applying oils to the spine, dripping from approximately 6 inches above the animal was recommended in the past, with a 3 inch distance for very small animals such as rats. Thankfully, in clinical work, we have recognized that there was no perfect spacing or distance necessary. Do not fret if you do not drip the oils directly on the spine, or if your spacing above the spine is not ideal. There are many situations that have to be modified when we work with animals. Some animals will roll to the side, or may be "recumbent" while ill, making it harder to drip oils onto the spine itself. It really is fine, and even dripping oils along the side of a rib cage and then massaging in, works very well.

The dripping of the oils from a distance above the animal, is thought to allow the drops to pass through the animal's energetic field. There may be benefits to this occurrence, ones that science will likely not be able to explain or document for some time. If you are artful in energy work, work with chakras, or auric fields, you may find particular distances or techniques that speak to you within oil applications. Allow yourself to explore this, and adapt to your particular needs.

Drip your diluted oil or oil blends, up the spine, generally from tail to head. Be cautious as you drip oils up the neck, nearing the base of the head. I have many cats and dogs that choose to "look up" and discover what I am doing - right as an oil drop falls towards them. Since animals are often moving targets, I may stop the location of the drip a bit farther down the neck to avoid accidently dripping an oil droplet onto their face or near their eyes. If an animal or your work dictates that oils are dripped from neck to tail, or even both directions during an application – relax. This is all just fine. Occasionally, I have dripped oils onto a kitten starting at the tail, moving up to the neck, and then back down to the tail again. Thankfully – there is no wrong application.

Although it might seem necessary, shaving the back or parting the fur is not needed for essential oil applications to be effective in animals. Some references actually recommended care givers to "shave the spine area for direct application of the oil" - with the thought that "you will use less oil". However, shaving the hair may actually cause mircoabrasions to the skin, little cuts which increase the possibility of excessive absorption, irritation, or sensitization of the skin. Shaving of a location for essential oil applications is not necessary, required, or needed. As discussed in the chapter "Sensitivity to Oils" – hair follicles are likely involved with enhanced absorption of essential oils.

Stroking in the Oils:
After oils are dripped up the back, they are stroked into the animal. Various feathering and massage techniques have been described, but in reality, any method has remained effective. There are no hard and fast rules. And you may utilize just basic petting or more advanced massage techniques as you see fit, or as the animal enjoys. One cautionary statement – please be aware that while stroking short coats in the opposite direction of the way the hair lies – you may create a flicking of the oils into the air. Altering your technique by using a lighter touch, less aggressive stroke, or in some circumstances a more "full contact" stroke can often eliminate this flicking action. As a human, this flicking oil can accidentally land in your face or eyes, and it is not pleasant.

Applying a Carrier Oil:
In the past, aggressive oil applications were made, then a carrier oil was applied after or within the application to provide comfort. Our goal with current techniques, is to apply an oil that is already properly diluted, instead of trying to "re-capture" comfort after an insult to the skin. Applying aggressive oils to the hair or skin first, then trying to remedy that situation just does not make sense. The body is far better off not ever having to deal with irritation in the first place. So applying an overly concentrated oil on purpose, with the intent of applying a carrier oil afterward is never recommended.

For additionally sensitive dogs or animals, applying carrier oil prior to any Drip & Rub recipe can be a better way to ensure a more mild absorption and tolerance of the skin. Drip your plain fractionated coconut oil, or carrier oil of choice, along the spine to create a "landing strip" prior to dripping on your already diluted blend. This can be an easier way to apply an already created and diluted blend, without having to additionally dilute it further for one animal versus another. So for your Great Dane, you may drip a 10% concentration of a blend along their spine directly from the bottle. But for your Chihuahua, you apply a carrier oil to the spine first, then drip the same 10% blend along his spine. Effectively creating a bit more of a diluted application for one dog, versus another. Without having to have a 5%, 8%, and 10% concentration on hand.

It is also wise to note that just because a horse is a horse, or that they are a large animal, does not mean that it can necessarily tolerate neat oils or more concentrated oils better. If it became apparent that a particularly sensitive horse needs oils additionally diluted, then this should be what is done for that horse.

Modifications of the Recipes:

One important aspect of using the body supporting recipes, is the ability to modify it. This can mean a number of things including the use of completely different oils, to omitting or adding various essential oils from the recipe.

For a dog with cancer, you may wish to include additional oils that are indicated for the situation. Several other oils for cancer could be added to the recipe, as you see fit for that individual dog.

However, the main concentration of the body supportive blend, should generally remain the same. If you are using the Feline Body Supportive Blend, but feel that you would like to add additional cistus to the blend for a saddle thrombus, you should add it to your blend in one of a few ways. First, you could predilute the cistus with coconut oil, then mix this into your body supportive blend. Alternately, you could mix all of the neat oils recommended for the body supportive blend together, then add your neat cistus to this blend. With your "new" neat blend, you could then follow the directions on how to dilute to your final desired concentration for your species.

Be aware that if you create a full body supportive recipe, but then add neat drops of oils to that bottle, you will be increasing the concentration of the entire blend. This is much harder to accurately track and calculate, so starting with a base neat oil blend, and then diluting that to a proper percentage is usually recommended for accuracy and safety, especially with smaller animals.

BODY SUPPORTIVE BLENDS

These recipes will give you a nice base blend to start off with for a variety of species. Think of these blends as a smoothie. If you take all that you will eat within a day, and mix it into a blender, you will now have a body supportive blend. I also think of this in terms of how my body or emotions might respond to the blend as well.

While a smoothie will still give me all of the nutrition from the foods within it, there is a bit lacking in the fact that I do not get to eat my dessert separate from my steak. For me, there can be a distinct difference between the application of several custom created blends, versus those blends being all combined together. Not that any certain one was wrong, they are just different.

I relate the application of several blends to be more like a 5 course meal. You enjoy some soup, then salad, then an entrée, etc... There is sometimes just a different feeling, sensation, or emotion behind the soup than the chocolate cake for dessert. We can respect that a body may "prefer" to deal with one course at a time, or find particular differences in enjoyment (for lack of a better word) for each application. Even if the applications are performed within minutes of each other, there can be a different feel to each individual blend.

However, all of the oils we wish to use, CAN be mixed into one very appropriate, and very effective blend as well. It is just your weeknight meal, instead of your Sunday Dinner. For our purposes, I recommend that most people just create and use the recipes as described. There are many intricacies to if you add or subtract oils, and if you change concentrations in doing so, that make the use of a base recipe the safest and best recommendation for overall use.

When adding additional oils to the recipes, add them to the neat base blend, then dilute that blend to your desired end concentration. Most additional oils are added similarly, in equal parts. However, more aggressive oils (as noted in their single oil description) – may be selected to add in lesser amounts to the base.

BODY SUPPORTIVE BLENDS

Small Animal Supportive Blend:

This blend will be appropriate for rabbits, guinea pigs, rodents, birds, and most animals smaller or more fragile than cats. This blend will generally be diluted in fractionated coconut oil, so care must be considered to not apply to feathers, or specific delicate coats of fur such as a chinchilla. Blends diluted in coconut oil may not be appropriate for fish, amphibians, and certain reptiles. The oils within this blend are particularly mild in nature, while still providing amazing benefits. This blend can certainly be applied to larger animals as well. In general, I recommend a final 1-3% concentration to be used for these animals.

- To create a base neat blend; combine equal parts Copaiba, Frankincense, Lavender, Lemongrass, Helichrysum, Tangerine, Ginger, Basil, and Marjoram
- Add to carrier oil to create the concentration desired.

Alternately, add one drop each of Copaiba, Frankincense, Lavender, Lemongrass, Helichrysum, Tangerine, Ginger, Basil, and Marjoram to 30 mL of Fractionated Coconut Oil. Apply 3-6 drops of this solution up the back, and stroke in. This blend may be applied to other locations of need as well.

Feline Supportive Blend:

This blend is most appropriate for cats, but can be used for larger birds such as chickens and ducks, ferrets, and is also wonderful for small dogs, puppies, large dogs, and even horses and other large animals. In general, I recommend a 3-5% final concentration.

- To create a base neat blend; combine equal parts Oregano, Thyme, Basil, Cypress, Marjoram, Lavender, Copaiba, Helichrysum, and Peppermint.
- Add to carrier oil to create the concentration desired.
- Additional oils often considered to add to the base blend include Frankincense, Myrrh, Catnip, Ginger, Juniper, Ledum, and Melissa.

Alternately, add four drops each of Oregano, Thyme, Basil, Cypress, Marjoram, Lavender, Copaiba, Helichrysum, and Peppermint to 30mL of Fractionated Coconut Oil. Apply 5-8 drops of this solution up the back, and stroke in. This blend may also be applied using the Petting Technique.

Canine Supportive Blend:

This blend is more appropriate for dogs and larger animals. While cats will be safe if exposed to it by laying with a dog, or even grooming it, the concentration and oils contained within are not as suitable for use directly on a feline. In general, this blend is often used between a 10-30% concentration.

- To create a base neat blend; combine equal parts Oregano, Thyme, Basil, Cypress, Marjoram, Lavender, Copaiba, Helichrysum, and Peppermint.
- Add to carrier oil to create the concentration desired.
- Additional oils often considered to add to the base blend include Frankincense, Myrtle, Catnip, Ginger, Juniper, Ledum, and Melissa.

Alternately, add 10 drops each of Oregano, Thyme, Basil, Cypress, Marjoram, Lavender, Copaiba, Helichrysum, and Peppermint to 30mL of Fractionated Coconut Oil. Apply 8-10 drops of this solution up the back, and stroke in. This blend may also be applied using the Petting Technique.

Large Animal Supportive Blend:

This blend is just a bit more powerful for larger animals such as horses or livestock. In general, this blend is often used between a 20-50% concentration.

- To create a base neat blend; combine equal parts Oregano, Thyme, Basil, Cypress, Marjoram, Lavender, Black Spruce, Copaiba, Helichrysum, Ginger, and Peppermint.
- Add to carrier oil to create the concentration desired.
- Additional oils often considered to add to the base blend include Frankincense, Melissa, Catnip, Balsam Fir, German Chamomile, Ledum, or additional portions of Copaiba, Helichrysum, or Marjoram.

Alternately, add 25 drops each of Oregano, Thyme, Basil, Cypress, Marjoram, Lavender, Black Spruce, Copaiba, Helichrysum, Ginger, and Peppermint to 25mL of Fractionated Coconut Oil. Apply 12-15 drops of this solution up the back and stroke in. This blend may also be applied using the Petting Technique.

EMOTIONAL WORK WITH OILS

Emotional work with animals is an area that has been neglected for far too long. In an age of rescue dogs, puppy mills, hoarders, and over-run rescues...the emotional health of our animal population is tragic. My patients have taught me so many things once I started to use essential oils. It wasn't that I didn't recognize how important their emotional health was – but just that I never saw how powerful it could be to correct it, until I started using essential oils.

Essential oils are the most holistic modality that I know of. Not only can I get powerful health benefits and responses by the body – but even without trying, I see behavioral and emotional benefits in patients. Essential oils treat mind, body, and spirit – and with this – we can change the face of how animals will benefit from medical treatments in the future. No longer will a pill of amoxicillin be shoved down a cat's throat, creating distrust, upset stomachs, and hiding behaviors. My dream is to incorporate aromatherapy into medical treatments that make everyone happy – as well as healthy.

It is important to recognize that there is no "wrong way" in working with essential oils and emotions. If you feel guided to do one thing versus another – please do so. However, I will guide you on a few recommendations that are worthy of notice.

In the past, it was usually recommended to separate an animal from others when working on emotional clearing. This would mean separating a dog from other dogs or cats in the household, or separating a horse away from herd mates. Imagine yourself going through an emotional release. We usually are not very comfortable doing this in front of others. In the animal kingdom – the odd ball is often shunned, rejected, or even attacked for bringing attention to the pack, herd, or flock. We would not want to create this experience for any animal we are working with. While this advice is still worthy of notice, in practice it became more obvious that this was an issue mainly in cases of over-use of essential oils. The application of neat oils, or extreme or aggressive exposures, created animals that were on-edge more than relaxed. Or who smelled drastically different than others in the household. With use of diluted blends, water-based diffusion instead of air-style diffusion, or with the application of blends to all of the animals in the home; we note distinct improvement in overall responses.

Mixing of Emotional or Physical Blends:

There is no law that says that you cannot mix blends. Everyone can also take heart in the fact that you will not create something harmful, if you do choose to mix blends together. What does hold true, is that the energy and frequency that was intended in the original recipe of an emotional blend, may be changed by the co-mingling. Sometimes this can result in a beautiful thing, and sometimes it results in an unattractive odor. The basic idea of not blending blends, truly exists in the fact that you may lose the intention or reduce the effects of the original blend if you combine them.

Quite often in our veterinary hospital and home, my husband will add a drop of a totally unrelated blend, into an emotional blend we have created. Naturally I scold him. Scoffing at what is sure to be a marked failure! Instead, we often find that it works. And it ends up being a beautiful and effective way to emotionally support hospitalized patients, while still ensuring good odor control, respiratory support, and reduction of transmissible agents. Any combination could be used in this manner. The intent is not to change the effects of either oil being used, however we wish to enhance the situation ever so slightly, and it has worked wonderfully for our patients.

Common Methods for Emotional Work

Again, there are no right or wrong methods. However, these are the ones that we have found most useful. It is important to recognize, that the humans administering the emotional blends to the animals, will often benefit as well. It may be fair warning to alert the humans in the household of this fact.

Nightly Diffusion: This should be done with water-based diffusion, which will be well tolerated for the entire household, not only the animal it is intended for. Often, if an emotional blend is used more intensely than a human in the household "can stand," the emotional work goes by the wayside, and no one benefits. Emotions are powerful things, and the resistance of a human to the use of a certain odor can be strong when emotions come into play. Nightly diffusion is just that; the diffusion of a selected oil during the night, while animals and humans sleep. The diffuser is generally set up in the same room as the animal, and allowed to run all night. Between 1-4 drops is generally added to a diffuser (to approximately 1 cup of water). Diffusion can occur every night, once a week, once a month, or whatever is deemed necessary by the situation. The same oil can be diffused, or a rotation of different oils can be selected for each new diffuser batch. Many times, the diffuser would be left running all night long, but shorter time frames can also be used.

Rotational Diffusion: We have had situations in our veterinary hospital, where a dog rescued from a puppy mill would benefit greatly from emotional support. However, it is a common situation that we will only have the dog in the hospital for 2 days or less. In these situations, or in others where emotional work is desired to occur on a faster schedule, a different emotional selection can be diffused every hour or two. There is no set recipe, but one scenario may include diffusing one selection for 20 minutes, then in 2 hours, a different blend is selected and diffused for 20 minutes. One could rotate through as many blend selections as they like, but in general, a magic number of around 7 seems to be a good suggestion. Do not throw out a batch of diffuser water, just because you want to change essential oils. Store the oily water in a covered glass bottle, and use it later.

Alternately, and possibly in response to our own laziness, we have taken to "batch" diffusion rotation. In this set up – we fill our diffuser with water, add one particular emotional blend or oil, and then diffuse it until the water is gone or the diffuser shuts off. When we fill the diffuser next, we add the next emotional oil we wish to use. The amount of time may vary with diffuser settings you select. Every time I fill up the diffuser, I just change to a new essential oil or blend. I now practice this with physical as well as emotionally intended oils – with great success.

Petting Application: This technique can be performed with any frequency you desire. Nightly, hourly, daily, or monthly; the choice is purely individual. Several drops of a diluted essential oil blend are placed into your hand. Depending on your species of animal, you will select the appropriate concentration, and may have a fair amount of the oil still "wet" on your hand (as for horses and dogs), or you may have the oil completely absorbed into your hands (as for birds, rodents, and exotics) prior to Petting them. It is always amazing how much an animal will smell like the essential oil after Petting, even when the oils have seemingly been completely absorbed into your hands.

Locations of Petting: This too, is a completely subjective matter. Yet, there are some oils that just seem to call to application at various sites. Common locations that people are drawn to apply to include over the heart area, over the shoulder area, and over the brain stem area. Any location is fine, and you will not do any harm by applying a "heart" oil over the "liver." Remember, any suggestions on location are purely opinion, and if you feel drawn to apply an oil in a certain location, then by all means, please do!

Emotional Drip & Rub Technique
This is an amazing technique for using emotional blends. Single oils can certainly be included as well, so never feel that a single has to be excluded from any form of emotional work.

Basically, between 6-8 pre-diluted emotional blends or singles are selected for an animal (sometimes less), and they are applied over the spine in a series. This application is not limited to spinal application, and you may find you would like to group certain oils to compliment a chakra or organ area.

Chakra Emotional Techniques
This is an incredibly powerful application technique both physically and emotionally. As all essential oils carry an emotional and a physical aspect to them, we can overlap these qualities for some very powerful results. For example, neurologic supporting oils, which always also carry emotional benefits, may be selected to be applied at the spinal region at the base of the head - corresponding with the Crown or Third Eye Chakra. Next, we might select a blend that supports the thyroid, while also imparting its natural emotional aspects, this blend could be applied over the neck or Throat Chakra. Cardiac supportive oil (also emotionally significant in their own right) – may be applied over the chest area or Heart Chakra. Liver supporting oils, which tend to also be helpful in areas of anger, may be applied over the Solar Plexus Chakra. Adrenal supportive oils and even urologic supportive oils can be considered for use over the Solar Plexus or Sacral Chakra areas. And often endocrine and metabolism supportive oils will be used over the Root Chakra (base of spine).

Certain essential oils are often linked with the different Chakras as well. These oils are particularly wonderful for use with animals:
- Crown Chakra – Myrrh, Frankincense, Spikenard
- Third Eye Chakra – Ylang Ylang, Clary Sage, Helichrysum
- Throat Chakra – German Chamomile, Hyssop, Cypress
- Heart Chakra – Rose, Eucalyptus, Cistus, Melissa
- Solar Plexus Chakra – Basil, Ginger, Bergamot, Nutmeg
- Sacral Chakra – Geranium, Patchouli, Grapefruit
- Root Chakra – Vetiver, Copaiba, Sandalwood, Black Spruce

Favorite Oils and Properties

There are a few favorite oils that contribute greatly to emotional work with animals. With emotional work, it is also a wonderful thing to explore Zoopharmacognosy. Please see that chapter for references and a bit more information regarding Zoopharmacognosy or Self Selection of oils.

There are several oils that jump to mind when we consider what tends to work best with animals, and for animal related situations. Certainly anxiety and fear are common considerations, and one of the most asked about in terms of essential oil use. Standard oils such as Lavender may aid in calming aspects, but even oils such as Anise have been shown to relieve anxiety. When considering which oil you might use, it is also important to consider the species you will be using it with, and which route you plan to use it.

For a cat household, it is likely that water-based diffusion will always be a viable option for exposure to a certain oil. However, if you plan to make a topical blend, it is unlikely that your cat will appreciate smelling like Anise solely. Cats may like the grounding and earthy scent of Valerian or the herbal aspect of Catnip, while a dog may accept just about anything. When selecting your oils, take into account the "aesthetics" of use, functionality and physical properties, as well emotional offerings.

ZOOPHARMACOGNOSY

This term is more commonly called self-selection and can relate to things other than just essential oils. Herbs, minerals, clays, and other items can also be selected by the animal to allow them to "self-medicate" themselves.

Unfortunately, some who have trained or studied in this area, may take an approach that ONLY if an animal self-selects an essential oil, should it be used. In the veterinary field, we obviously recognize the limitations to this sort of thinking. In reviewing the information set forth by the creator of Applied Zoopharmacognosy – Caroline Ingraham – I don't truly believe that this would be her full stance on the position – to withhold veterinary care if it is not "selected." However, I do plan to take coursework with her directly in July 2018, to fully gain an appreciation for her beliefs and methods.

What I can tell you of Zoopharmacognosy, is that I do think it is a wonderful and powerful thing. In some ways, we have practiced this on many levels during the many years I have worked with essential oils and animals. A cat may select to lay right next to a diffuser, diffusing citrus oils. Which in the past, were most certainly on the list of oils to avoid for felines. I always saw benefits to items that animals seemed to select on their own to be exposed to.

Even my own Bengal cat, would lick essential oils off of me! Very strong oils in fact, containing things like Oregano, Thyme, Frankincense, etc... These most certainly would not be items I would expect a cat to purposely "groom" off of my skin, however, she sure did. And she would come back for more! She'd even lick and make some faces and actions of disgust, but then come back for some more licking. I do whole heartedly believe that when given the opportunity and exposure to items, animals can make some amazing decisions about what their own bodies need or require.

But as a trained veterinarian, I am certainly not going to only operate in this manner. My entire career focuses on the use of items that are highly unlikely to be selected by an animal, but may be entirely necessary for their well-being. Anesthesia, antibiotics, medications, etc. certainly are not selected by animals, but sometimes we have to use them. And I do look at essential oils in this way. I am fine with the fact that if your animal self-selects an essential oil for use, and it is effective – then by all means – it is amazing and wonderful. But if your cat is facing full mouth extractions due to stomatitis that cannot be brought under control, and I know of a blend that when applied to cats, really seems to help. I will recommend using it, even if the cat fails to select that particular blend or oil. That is just me.

I am not saying that the practice of zoopharmacognosy is wrong. And although I do come across those who say that I am wrong for applying oils to an animal without their "consent" – I would never say that someone practicing zoopharmacognosy is wrong. It is just different. Powerful and meaningful when it happens and if it is effective; but, I am most certainly still going to recommend the use of items that I know to be beneficial for a condition, regardless to if the animal selects it or not.

With emotional concerns, I do think that self-selection is a powerful entity. More powerful than we can likely decide upon, based on what we "think" we know about essential oils. With children especially, I am always telling parents to allow their child to have access to many oils or blends, and allow them to decide what works or smells wonderful to them. They are amazing in their ability to judge how an oil makes them feel. And we should respect that emotions will go far beyond what a basic rule of "this oil is good for this".

ADVANCED TECHNIQUES

Essential oils can be combined with techniques such as Acupuncture, Acupressure, Massage Therapy, Chiropractic Adjustment, Electro-stimulation, Homeopathy, Flower Essences, Reiki, Animal Communication, Reflexology, Tapping, Emotional Release Technique, and more. I find that every modality that is used in the animal world today, is greatly enhanced by the addition of essential oils.

There are a few techniques that are worthy of discussion and explanation – as they provide additional benefits to the way we can administer essential oils to animals.

Reflexology:
There are many forms of reflexology, and pressure points of significance in the ears, feet, and other energetic meridians of the body. If you are trained in reflexology, incorporating essential oils into your work can really be quite amazing. Most reflexologists simply apply some essential oils to their fingers or if using a manipulation tool or glass rod, to that item. You really could select any oil or blend, and generally use it diluted for your species. A Three Part Blend is an excellent consideration, and you could even tailor the blend to reflect the organ or effects you are most hoping to affect with your therapy.

Acupressure:
This can be performed just as described for Reflexology. You can match oils to their meridian or organ base, or more based on the function of the condition you are trying to affect. For example – you can use Liver supporting oils for a Liver meridian point. Or if that particular Liver point is for another condition (cardiac for example) then you could apply a cardiac supportive oil or blend to that location. There is no right or wrong, and we see huge synergistic effects when essential oils are used in conjunction with Acupressure.

Chiropractic:
Chiropractic adjustments can often be made easier with the use of essential oils. We especially hear this for large animals such as horses. The use of oils that benefit the musculoskeletal system in general, of course can be a natural physical help. But, oils such as Bergamot have been specifically noted to ease a chiropractic adjustment. Oils such as Marjoram, Lavender, and Basil may have a relaxant effect on muscles, facilitating easier manipulation. Oils such as Clary Sage, Dill, Fennel, Frankincense, and Nutmeg have shown effects on muscle contraction with nerve stimulation in research. Applications of appropriately diluted blends can be made directly to the patient prior to adjustment, or after an adjustment. Oil blends could also be on the chiropractic hands prior to manipulation.

Massage:
Almost every massage can be better with the use of essential oils. If there is any one modality in which aromatic medicine shines the most, it is likely to be in combination with massage. Depending on your goals, you could select oils to increase lymphatic circulation such as Cypress, or decrease inflammation with Copaiba. Any of the essential oils, and their related properties that you feel will benefit the massage subject, can be used in diluted topical forms (of course when it is an oil suggested for topical use.) For most animal massage, the Three Part Blend or your own custom creation will be diluted to the concentration recommended for your species. Then a coating of this diluted blend is applied to the hands delivering the massage. Alternately, you could also apply oils to the animal in a Petting manner prior to the massage.

Acupuncture:
To use essential oils with acupuncture in animals, several methods have been used. Some acupuncturists will dip the acupuncture needle into a clean and dedicated bottle of essential oil, coating the needle prior to insertion. Others choose to apply the essential oil of choice (neat or diluted) to the skin at the site of needle insertion. While still others may only have the option of applying an essential oil to the acupuncture site after the needles are withdrawn. Whichever method is used, essential oils have enhanced acupuncture greatly. After continued conversations with animal acupuncturists and through veterinary experience, I currently recommend the application of diluted essential oils to the acupuncture site prior to needle insertion. While I will not say that an individual acupuncturist is necessarily wrong with whatever method they select,

I will caution that some people have reported adverse skin reactions and irritations when the needles were dipped into essential oils prior to insertion. Whether this is a contamination problem, essential oil quality issue, or direct irritation – we do not know for sure. However, it may be wise to avoid this practice. Alternately, a diluted essential oil or blend could be Pet over the areas in which Acupuncture will be received, prior to needling.

Reiki:

As my husband and I are Reiki Masters and also trained in many versions of energy work, we have an affection for the relationship essential oils and energy work display. Truly, almost any essential oil will enhance animal communication, Reiki, or any other energy work you may do. I encourage you to form your own relationships and experiences with oils in your growth – you will most certainly find those which resonate most for you. Favorites we have include Melissa, Spikenard, Black Spruce, and Frankincense. But this list, in no way, should limit your exploration.

INJECTIONS & IV'S

While injecting essential oils or administering them intravenously (IV) was becoming a popular craze, I doubt that many of the people promoting these practices had fully witnessed some of the harm being done. Unfortunately, when people are faced with horrible conditions such as Cancer, the fear factor surely plays a role in what someone is willing to try to save their beloved animal.

Currently, there are a variety of ways essential oils are being introduced which I would classify as only appropriate for research. Yet, truly the lay person population has attempted these things, due to their glorifications. While it is true, that you can often do anything you would like in terms of treatment of your own animal – I do believe that injecting caustic substances into an animal should be classified as abusive. It is incredibly painful – and should be considered much like doing surgery without anesthesia or pain medications in terms of importance.

I personally know humans who have injected essential oils into tumors or moles, and who have had IV administrations of essential oils. There have been far more reports of complications, than there has been of clear medical evidence of results. And this is clearly no modality to be messed with, or considered lightly.

While I have witnessed a few amazing cases where essential oils were injected into tumors such as sarcoids on horses, it is important to realize that the injection is truly causing mass harm and destruction to the tumor – initiating a massive inflammatory and immune response. This can stimulate resolution of a tumor – that is true. But, it is highly important then, that what you inject you intend to fully die, become necrotic, or fall off. Injecting essential oils into an internal tumor or a lymph node – may create a large toxic mass of dying tissue, which is unhealthy to be within a body. I have heard accounts of a woman who injected Frankincense into her breast tumor, and it turned necrotic, black, and almost killed her. And I consulted on a case of a cat in which Frankincense was injected into a large injection-site sarcoma. The cat showed distinct signs of adverse reactions, and the tumor created an abscess-like situation, rejecting the Frankincense from the body in what was surely not only painful but quite toxic.

While in research, I often come across IP (intraperitoneal) injections of essential oils into mice or rats, or other routes…this rarely equates to any sort of safety in my opinion. The caustic and irritating factor of this injection should not be under-appreciated.

With intravenous use (IV), essential oils and "water" or the intravenous fluids still do not mix. Agents must be included within the solutions in order to administer the essential oils, hopefully creating some sort of dispersal or emulsification. This in its own right, may prove harmful depending on the agents selected and doses administered. These techniques have mainly been created and promoted by people who have no actual medical training, and while some veterinarians are starting to explore these administrations, it is still based on the advice and techniques that were initiated with very poor understanding of chemistry, pharmacology, and fluid therapy.

In interviewing those actually in attendance of classes promoting infusions and injections of essential oils into animals, the general take away was a feeling of paranoia and irresponsibility. The room was screened for recording devices, and people were encouraged to not take any notes. If this was a practice worthy of veterinary training, we would most certainly be encouraged to write down notes so that we could retain the information correctly. Not be forced to remember an odd point here or there.

These practices are most certainly not within veterinary standards of care, and should only be considered when full pain management can be in place and monitored closely, and when being done in a closely monitored and effective arena of medical research investigation. While I won't say there may not be potential someday for the use of essential oils in this manner, I abandoned my own research into these modalities for lack of responses and increases in adverse events.

INTO THE FUTURE

The future of essential oil use with animals is profound in my eyes. Not only is there a modality that can potentially replace some of our uses of traditional pharmacology, but likely we will witness that this modality far surpasses it.

I am incredibly excited to be a part of shaping this new frontier. From when I first started using "medical aromatherapy" – I have grown to dedicate my entire veterinary work to Veterinary Aromatic Medicine. The present sees me sharing my knowledge at major veterinary conferences and to the new generation of veterinary students still in college. The future does indeed look promising.

There is always a concern for regulation of essential oils to become much more stringent. Not that I completely see this as a bad thing, but recently certain natural remedies were made unavailable to veterinarians and consumers alike. Access to natural products should remain an option for the world, and we have to be cautious with how we proceed in the world of veterinary aromatic medicine, if we are to avoid excessive regulatory measures.

The ways you speak of and practice aromatic medicine, can indeed determine the future. In 2014, the FDA sent letters of warning to two major essential oil companies, warning them of infractions. Basically, these companies and their large number of distributors have acted inappropriately with product claims and labeling. For example, you cannot say that an essential oil will treat anything basically. And while I might site research that claims an essential oil may kill bacteria, it is a far cry from calling it an antibiotic. Labels must also clearly indicate if an essential oil is for topical use, or oral use, but not for both. So that is why you will see a whole new "line" of the same exact essential oil, labeled and sold for consumption now.

So the accurate statement also about these new labels is not that they are FDA approved essential oils, but that the label is merely FDA compliant. There is some confusion within the general marketplace there.

While I see natural medicine as a way to definitely improve health, let's make no mistake about it – THE BODY HEALS THE BODY. There is no "cure" for cancer, except to get the body into maximal health, so that it can fight off the cancer. Even surgery and chemotherapy do not cure cancer. They eliminate it enough so that the body's own immune system can wipe out any remaining cells. This will be true for anti-viral medications, antibiotics, and anti-fungals. Rarely in medicine do we anticipate or expect for a drug to do all things for the body, and eliminate a pathogen. A functional immune system is by far the most important item one can maintain in their arsenal of health.

And while traditional medications can greatly help certain conditions, it may also be at a detriment to other parts of the body. The use of steroids for severe inflammation can be a necessary treatment course. However, we also suppress the immune system in the process. So in the case of skin allergies, when steroids are prescribed, we WILL see decrease of itching and inflammation. However, while we also suppress the immune system's ability to fight infections, we may see a huge flair of fungal or bacterial skin issues once the course of steroids is finished.

With natural medicines, we are much less likely to see the abnormal suppression of one area of the body, while we are helping another. I think of essential oils much as I do food (shocking I know, especially if you have read the other chapters of this book already). Food can nourish you, and help maintain a healthy immune response. We rarely would say, "Well now that you have cancer; we are going to cut it out, irradiate you, and poison you... Therefore, you should only eat fast food. Good foods such as blueberries, you should avoid; as these may counteract the damage we are trying to implement upon your body."

The avoidance of antioxidants, vitamins, herbs, and other natural remedies is often recommended to those undergoing chemotherapy or who may be on therapies designed to disrupt our immune system. I guess I will never subscribe to this philosophy.

But, back to the future. We need to carry a different communication about our natural remedies. Never should we say a remedy "cures" anything. The body cures a condition, let's not hold our offerings in too high a regard. However, a remedy most certainly may support the body to do a better job. While some essential oils may have research that shows that they can reduce or even kill bacteria, we need to have the understanding that if we apply this essential oil to the skin, it is merely reducing the bacterial load the body has to deal with. Helpful, most certainly. The other nice part about using an essential oil for a skin infection, is that we may have other pathogens or even inflammation present that makes it even harder for the body to heal itself. Thankfully, this is where essential oils shine. Because they are a natural substance, and not a "test-tube baby" – they are not a one trick pony either! Our traditional antibiotics, are ONLY traditional antibiotics. They kill bacteria, and generally only a certain kind of bacteria – such as gram positive rods, etc. We do not see traditional antibiotics that also reduce inflammation, or are antifungal at the same time. And with natural remedies, we can see multiple functions.

Essential oils carry with them multiple functions. Most will show anti-inflammatory, antibacterial, and antifungal actions to varying degrees. Then, add that some may modulate an immune response or even be anti-viral – and you have an amazing ability to support the body on so many levels. Continue with the fact that essential oils also address a multitude of emotions – and we really could not ask for a better natural "medicine".

But, calling it a medicine or a drug by definition – limits our ability to maintain use of these items in actuality. If you say "xyz essential oil is an antibiotic" – oops – now you have claimed a function. You have made a "product claim" – and the FDA recognizes that as a new drug.

Essential oils to me, are like good nutrition. Let thy food be thy medicine. However, I do NOT want the FDA calling my chicken soup a new drug and regulating it. You have been warned. If you love essential oils, and you want them to remain available to the public – you will need to be cautious in how you speak, write, or communicate their apparent benefits to others. The hard part, is that even the FDA does not relay their information on how to communicate very well.

In short, it remains a good suggestion to never say "copaiba is for arthritis" or a similar sort of phrase. This would make copaiba a drug, designated to treat a specific condition or disease. Which is why the FDA got involved in the first place. While aromatherapy books everywhere will list conditions for which certain essential oils are indicated, it should always be in a manner of support for the body, when that diagnosis has been made by a qualified health care professional.

As a veterinarian, this can be especially hard for someone trained to diagnose and prescribe. It is just part of my nature to think in these terms. But as much as I think of diet at the primary "medication" I will prescribe when any animal is ill – I parallel essential oils in importance. I would not want to practice veterinary medicine without the ability to suggest dietary improvements. And I would also feel that a significant portion of my ability to help animals would be removed without the ability to practice Veterinary Aromatic Medicine.

Let's use essential oils and good health practices to aid in the prevention of illness. In this way, we can exclude any "claims" to benefits in the first place.

FUTURE RESEARCH

As we move forward into the future, I would love to see some data collection, research, and publication of some of the following subjects. And yes, it is true that I personally have a lot of data that I have yet to publish. Some may accuse me of not providing my work, but honestly, none of them ever ask! It is quite hard to answer someone's question, if you never even know it is a question in the first place!

So, yes, I have decided that I will still continue to be a Mother, and enjoy some personal time, instead of devoting a huge portion of time to publishing works at this time. I'm sorry for that. But, if anyone who actually asks (and let's face it, has the medical knowledge to understand what I throw at them)...I am happy to submit some answers to them. However, if I am being honest, most people ask for the sake of asking. I do not have hours to dedicate to "proving" to one person that what my data shows is actually there or teach them what it means. I just won't do it for any old request, for which there could be thousands!

Areas of research that I hope to help coordinate in the future include accumulation of health data of all animals within homes using oils. There is a huge pool of data to be evaluated. With the millions of people using oils in their homes daily – statistics say that 63% of those homes contain animals. This is a vast amount of information that can be collected and presented, to show us more about blood work and safety in animals being exposed to many quality levels, and many routes of essential oil exposure. I hope to complete some of this work in 2018.

Then, I am hopeful to coordinate some essential oil metabolism and excretion studies, especially specific to cats. This will most likely be coordinated with some of the veterinary colleges I have relationships with. I hope we can finally have some answers and documentations to truly put the controversy and questions to rest. This will hopefully give us a better understanding on true dosage and administration frequency.

Researching cortisol level responses to essential oils has long been on my list of things to do. With new saliva-based cortisol testing kits hopefully becoming available through researchers in Italy, I hope that we can easily coordinate some elegant studies in stress responses in animals.

ESSENTIAL OIL SINGLES

It is so important to recognize that information does change. What we used or said years ago, may not be as widely true today. You may find this when comparing this edition, with the first edition of the book. While some oils were written about to the knowledge base that we had at the time, over the next 7 years, it may have become obvious that a certain oil has not been used very commonly. Or that other oils were far more animal friendly than others. Some oils entered the market as a "trend" – and were quick to leave, and while some were beginning to be used with possible promise, they just didn't hold up to their reports.

This chapter is written with what I consider my current veterinary recommendations in 2017. Our goal with a book for the public, is safety and efficacy for the majority, not for the 1% of people who have used a certain essential oil and have "been just fine". While some oils may indeed be being used with some animals, I will state whether I would use the essential oil within my own personal work with Veterinary Aromatic Medicine. The list will never be all inclusive, and is intended to be dynamic. One essential oil may just be starting its journey in my clinical applications, and within a few years, I may think it is the most amazing essential oil on earth! This is the way of research, use, and education. Please value this information for what it is. A current report on single essential oils.

For more information on the chemical constituents, historical data, medical properties, and research information please see the references at the back of this book.

For each essential oil, I will list the best routes to use the essential oil, not necessarily every possible use of it. In the past, I listed all known information about how an essential oil had been used. However, I would like to change the recommendations to the best possible, and safest routes to expose each species to. All oils take into account if they are able to be ingested by routine contact with licking or grooming. So if it is not directly stated for oral ingestion, you can still assume that the percentages listed for your species, and the use-type recommended for your species will be appropriate if they may ingest it during daily life activities.

This is by no means a complete representation of what each oil can do, or how it can be used – however, it will provide you with a current knowledge of how we are using these oils in the animal kingdom.

At this time, I did not feel it was necessary to list all of the chemical constituents or expected compositions of the oils. There are amazing resources such as *Medicinal Essential Oils: The Science and Practice of Evidence-Based Essential Oil Therapy* by Dr. Scott Johnson (a naturopathic human doctor) – has over 1000 pages of material on each essential oil, their constituents, research references, and reported uses. It is a highly valuable text, and I do not see the value in repeating things that have been so well done elsewhere.

In regards to conditions and properties of the oils; often it will be indicated if an individual essential oil would be selected for use with a certain condition. This is anticipated to be suggested with the understanding that you are working with a veterinarian and have obtained a medical diagnosis. As it is difficult to describe a certain illness without the use of the name – you may see a condition or disease listing. Know that the oils suggested for a particular disease are not intended for use in the diagnosis, cure, mitigation, treatment, or prevention of disease. They support the body – just as proper nutrition would.

Agarwood (Aquilaria malaccensis)
Also called aloes wood, and ood – this essential oil is incredibly expensive as it is only extracted from fungus-infected wood. It is also a CITES protected species, with a high rate of adulteration. It is not recommended for use with animals.

Ajowain (Trachyspermum ammi)
This essential oil is also known as Ajowan, Bishop's Weed, Wild Celery Seed, or Sprague. It is not currently used with animals beyond research, but shows potential beneficial properties including antibacterial, antifungal, antiviral, antispasmodic, and analgesic actions. It may be particularly helpful for neuropathy pain and symptoms.

Allspice Berry (Pimenta officinalis)
This essential oil may show promise as an antioxidant and with metal chelation. It may also show properties beneficial for fungal and microbial conditions, as well as aid in digestion. It is not currently recommended for use with animals.

Allspice Leaf (Pimenta dioica)
Also called Pimento Leaf, it also shows properties for fungal and microbial conditions, and digestive concerns. Usually high in Eugenol content, it is not currently recommended for use with animals.

Amyris (Amyris balsamifera)
Also called Amyris Sandalwood or Torchwood; Amyris is not currently recommended for use with animals.

Angelica Root (Angelica archangelica)
Angelica Root is a photosensitizing oil; do not apply to areas that will be exposed to direct sunlight or full spectrum UV lights within 12 hours after application. Angelica is not commonly used with animals at this time, however it may show promise with emotional work, and can be considered for water-based diffusion within blends.

Angelica Seed (Angelica archangelica)
While the seed source of Angelica essential oil is not photosensitizing, it contains high levels of constituents that readily oxidize, and may be more prone to causing irritation when improperly stored or older. Angelica Seed essential oil is not currently used with animals.

Anise (Pimpinella anisum)
Also called Aniseed, this essential oil is often used for digestive concerns, however it is useful for many situations. Anise is antibacterial, antifungal, analgesic, anti-inflammatory, antiparasitic, and antispasmodic. With a distinct line up such as that, it is clear why Anise is excellent for use with Inflammatory Bowel Disease, and is commonly added to blends created for intestinal health. Anise is also reported to have decongestant and expectorant actions, making it useful for coughs and respiratory conditions. Anise can also be quite calming, and can be useful for cases of anxiety as well. As you may know, the brain and gut are highly connected, and both gastrointestinal inflammation and the stress of anxiety feed off of each other. Anise has the wonderful ability to affect both of these issues.

Anise can be used with most animal species, and can be utilized topically, diffused, or ingested. Most commonly Anise would be added to a Three Part Blend, and used with the Species Specific recommendations for the application method you are selecting.

Birds & Exotics: Use as a single or within a Three Part Blend for water-based diffusion or dilute for addition to foods. Use species recommendations for appropriate topical (Petting) use of a Three Part Blend. Anise can also be considered for addition into the Small Animal Supportive Blend.

Cats: Can be used as a single or within Three Part Blends for water-based diffusion. Can be added to Feline Supportive Blend. Should be used with dilution for topical and Petting applications, and generally within Three Part Blends.

Dogs & Larger: Used as a single or within Three Part Blends with water-based diffusion, or diluted for topical or Petting applications. Anise may also be diluted and added to foods. See the chapter on adding and dosing essential oils within foods for further directions.

Anise, Star (Illicium verum)
Star Anise is commonly adulterated and should not be used with animals at this time.

Aniseed Myrtle (Syzygium anisatum)
Also known as Anise-scented myrtle (Backhousia anisata). This essential oil is similar to Sweet Fennel in composition, and contains a high level of Anethole which is prone to oxidation. It is likely to have similar effects and properties to Sweet Fennel, and is mainly used with diffusion in the animal kingdom at this time.

Balsam Fir (Abies balsamea)
Also called Fir Needle or Fir Balsam; Balsam Fir is great for bone conditions, muscle and joint conditions, respiratory conditions, emotional work, inflammatory conditions, lowering cortisol levels, and more. It is an oil that is commonly incorporated into animal protocols.

Birds & Exotics: Commonly water diffused, mixed with carrier oils for topical applications, diluted and applied topically via petting, especially within Three Part Blends.

Cats: Used in all of the methods listed for Birds & Exotics, as well as added in small amounts to blends, applied via petting (diluted), or added to litterbox blends. This oil is not the most "cat-friendly" in terms of smell, or for grooming/ingestion. There are certainly other oils we may select, which give similar results for felines. Diffusion is a wonderful consideration for feline exposure.

Dogs & Larger: Used in all of the mentioned methods, in water-based diffusion, direct topical applications (diluted), Petting applications (diluted). While we know of some safe use of Balsam Fir orally in dogs, our current recommendation is that it is not always necessary for effectiveness. In the past, oral use in dogs consisted of the following amounts. 1 part Balsam Fir was diluted in 3 parts fatty carrier oil. Up to 4 drops of this solution, for each 20 pounds (9 kg) of body weight, was given orally to a dog. For horses and others, 1 drop per 100-200 pounds (45-90 kg) of body weight, was given orally twice a day. Monitoring responses with a veterinarian, and adjust according to individual need was always recommended. For reduction in cortisol levels, Balsam Fir is most commonly recommended to be used at night before bed.

The reasoning behind the lessening of oral use of Balsam Fir is simple. We purely see enough effects and results through diffusion and topical use of this particular oil, eliminating the need to jump towards oral administration. There are other essential oils which are highly effective, and lend more safety toward their use.

Basil, Holy (Ocimum tenuiflorum)
Also called Sacred Basil or Tulsi, this oil may be anti-oxidant and hepato-protective in nature. It may also have some anti-cancer type actions. However, it is not commonly used with animals at this time.

Basil, Lemon (Ocimum x citriodorum)
Lemon Basil is an oil that may have actions on insulin levels and blood glucose handling in animals. It is not commonly used in the animal kingdom at this time.

Basil, Linalool Chemotype (Ocimum basilicum L.)

This basil is high in the constituent Linalool, and carries with it some different properties than the basil we are most commonly presented with. In research, it has been shown to induce glutathione S-transferase, making it anti-oxidant in nature and likely protective to the liver (hepato-protective). It is used sparingly within the animal kingdom at this time.

Basil, Sweet (Ocimum basilicum)

Also known as Sweet Basil, or the Estragole or Methyl Chavicol chemotype of Basil (Estragole and Methyl Chavicol are different words for the same thing). As a single oil, we mainly use Basil for anti-histamine properties in animals. There are sometimes cautionary statements against the use of Basil in those with epilepsy in certain references, however current research and the collection of data within Tisserand and Young's *Essential Oil Safety* (2nd Edition) does not include Basil as an oil of concern for those with seizures. In practice many animals who are afflicted with seizures are exposed to Basil on a regular basis, with no ill effects. Basil is a well-rounded oil with properties that include analgesia, antispasmodic, and muscle relaxing. It is well indicated for muscular concerns, coughs, itches, and histamine related inflammation.

Birds & Exotics: Can be used with water-based diffusion, added to drinking water for anti-histamine actions (1 drop per liter of water), added to foods (starting with a toothpick dip), used in Species Specific dilutions and blends topically.

Cats: Basil can be used in the methods mentioned for Birds & Exotics, with cats being less likely to consume the oil in water or foods. With cats, Basil is most commonly used within the Feline Supportive Blend. It could also be mixed into natural ointments (1 drop or more mixed into 1 tablespoon), diluted in carrier oils (4 drops in 30 mL), applied via Petting, or added to litter box recipes.

Dogs & Larger: Basil can be used in all of the mentioned ways, within the Drip & Rub Techniques, direct topical applications, Petting applications (diluted), added to drinking water, and oral administration. For oral use in dogs – dilute 1 part Basil with 3-10 parts carrier oil – use approximately 2 drops of this solution, for each 20 pounds (9 kg) of body weight. Some dogs may require more or less of this solution. For horses and others, starting with 1 drop of neat oil per 300 pounds (135 kg) of body weight, given orally twice a day is a good starting point. Diluting the oil within food or oil prior to giving to large animals is still recommended. Monitor responses with a veterinarian, and adjust according to individual need.

Bay Laurel – see Laurus nobilis

Bay Rum (Pimenta racemosa)
Also called Bay, or West Indian Bay. This essential oil is not commonly used with animals.

Benzoin (Styrax benzoin)
This essential oil is most commonly an absolute, and should not be used with animals. A hydrodistilled version may be available, however the constituents of this oil are converted to salicylic acid when ingested, and so is not recommended for use with animals due to ulcer and toxicity concerns.

Bergamot (Citrus bergamia)
Bergamot is generally a photosensitizing oil, however a fractionated version of this oil is also available, removing the causative constituent (bergaptene). For some, the whole and original oil containing the bergaptene is considered superior. Bergamot in general is considered helpful for easing chiropractic adjustments of animals, and is also wonderful for emotional concerns such as depression and anxiety. It is less commonly used as a single for animals and is most often added to blends.

Other reported properties of Bergamot include support of cardiovascular health, lowering of high blood pressure, as a digestive aid, anti-cancer properties (especially neuroblastoma), cognitive function, and it may especially be indicated to reduce insecurity and loneliness. It is also said to help release negative emotions.

Birds & Exotics: Commonly used via water diffusion, added to drinking water, added to foods, used within a water spritzer.

Cats: Most commonly used via water diffusion. It can be considered for addition to Three Part Blends, or to the Feline Supportive Blend when desired.

Dogs & Larger: Commonly used in all of the mentioned ways, as well as included Three Part Blends, Drip & Rub Recipes, direct topical application, Petting applications, sprayed on via water spritzer, and diffusion.

Bergamot Mint (Mentha aquatica)
Reported to have antispasmodic, wound healing, and anxiety relieving actions, this oil is not widely used with animals at this time.

Birch (Betula lenta)
Also called Sweet Birch, it has been nearly impossible to find a true and non-synthetic or adulterated source on the market. There are far more animal-appropriate oils to use, when the properties of Birch are suggested (such as Copaiba). The use of Birch is not recommended with animals, not only due to adulteration issues, but due to the high methyl salicylate content.

Bitter Orange (Citrus aurantium)
This oil may cause photosensitivity, so caution should be used with sun exposure for 12 hours after a topical application. While Bitter Orange has not been used widely with animals at this time, there is a plethora of research to support a variety of benefits. Protection and healing from gastric ulcers, reduction of anxiety, improvement of cognitive function, anti-inflammatory properties and more can be found attached to this oil. Most likely, we can consider its use much in the way we would other citrus oils.

Black Cumin Seed Oil (Nigella sativa)
This oil is most commonly regarded as a carrier or fixed oil, and is cold pressed from the seed. While there may be some CO_2 extracts or distilled oils available, it is most common to find this oil as a carrier oil. Please see the information under carrier oils for additional information. Caution should be used to make sure that solvent extraction has not occurred with this oil, prior to any distillation when considering its use for therapeutic purposes in animals.

As an oil, Black Cumin or Nigella carries with it some amazing properties. A source of Thymoquinone, this constituent is highly researched. Anti-cancer, antiviral, sugar balancing, supportive of liver and kidney function, analgesic, protective of cognitive function, and so much more – it is a broad spectrum consideration in Veterinary Aromatic Medicine. It is well indicated in cases of cancer, asthma, COPD and Heaves, high blood pressure and cardiovascular issues, diabetes, liver and kidney disease, cognitive dysfunction, immune support, and so much more.

Because of its mainly fatty attributes as a cold pressed oil, we use caution when adding into blends intended for diffusion; it may cause hardships upon a diffuser if used in high enough percentages. Most use would be concentrated on ingestion, topical use, or within litter box blends.

Black Pepper (see Pepper, Black)

Blue Cypress (see Cypress, Blue)

Black Spruce (see Spruce, Black)

Cajeput (Melaleuca minor)
Not commonly used with animals at this time.

Caraway Seed (Carum carvi)
Not commonly used as a single with animals at this time.

Cardamom (Elettaria cardamomum)
Not commonly used as a single with animals at this time.

Carrot Seed (Daucus carota)
Not commonly used as a single with animals at this time.

Cassia (Cinnamomum cassia)
Cassia is a "hot" oil with powerful anti-bacterial properties. It is mainly used within blends for animals, and is sometimes used within diffusion blends for a cinnamon-like aroma. Its use as a single for difficult abscesses in Horses and Large Animals could be considered topically.

Catnip (Nepeta cataria)

Catnip is an essential oil with many up and coming uses. As we all recognize, the catnip herb has long been cherished by cats, creating euphoria and sometimes a bit of mania. Some cats do not have the genetics to be affected by catnip, and it does remain an individual trait as to if your cat loves catnip, gets a bit crazy, or basically does nothing at all. The essential oil of catnip, does appear to evoke a different response than the catnip herb in general. In my use of catnip oil with hundreds of cats, I will see attraction, happiness, calmness, or playfulness. Thankfully, the "manic" sort of behavior that sometimes is seen with catnip herb (the one where your cat attacks you!) is not as apparent with proper use of the essential oil.

As an undiluted essential oil, catnip is incredibly strong. Use for cats is likely to be at 1% concentration and lower for most applications and uses. For other animals and humans, catnip is proving to be a powerful oil in regards to insects, and can be used at the recommended concentration ranges. Use the lowest concentration that is effective for your species. Nepatalactone within the catnip oil, has been shown in research to be more effective than DEET. Catnip essential oil is a wonderful oil to consider for use with ear mites, fleas, ticks, skin mites (mange), mosquitos, gnats, and other insect repelling needs.

The addition of tiny amount of Catnip to a litter box blend, can aid to attract cats to the box, and encourage its use. Again, if too much is added, whether to the blends total concentration or to the litter box in general, we have witnessed cats loving their box a little "too much" – laying in it, and rolling in it. This is a sure sign that less is more. Also, coating a scratching tree with diluted catnip blends may encourage appropriate clawing where we would like to direct it.

Catnip is not limited to insect repellent and feline euphoria however. It actually contains β-Caryophyllene, so is quite anti-inflammatory, as well as antimicrobial. It has research to show it has been quite beneficial for oral health and reduction of dental disease, which is a huge bonus to me. How many products can we apply to our animals in attempts to keep fleas and ticks off of them, which will actually promote dental health if it is licked or groomed off!? Not many.

Catnip has been found to have effects against resistant bacteria (MRSA) and fungi, reduces spasm and promotes muscle relaxation, and reduces pain and inflammation. The incredible layers that Catnip essential oil offers for health and insect repellent actions, warrants great respect.

Birds & Exotics: Mainly used with water-based diffusion. Very dilute topical use may be considered for external parasites and insects – generally within a Three Part Blend or within addition to a Small Animal Supportive Blend. For some exotics, addition to shampoo or ointments may also be appropriate.

Cats: Used within water-based diffusion, Three Part Blends, added to Feline Supportive Blend, used within litter box recipes, added to shampoos or ointments.

Dogs & Larger: Used within water-based diffusion, in water-mists, direct topical application (diluted), via Petting (diluted), within Three Part Blends, added to Canine or Large Animal Supportive Blends, added to ointments or shampoos.

Catnip, Lemon (Nepeta cataria var. citriodora)
Lemon Catnip is also reported to have insect repelling properties, among others. However, this oil is not commonly used with animals at this time.

Cedar, Western Red (Thuja plicata)
Not commonly used as a single in animals at this time, however emotionally this oil has been indicated for work with PTSD (Post Traumatic Stress Disorder). Addition to blends intended for diffusion or diluted topical applications is recommended at 5% or less of the total blend.

Cedarwood (Cedrus atlantica)
Cedarwood is an oil that is extremely high in sesquiterpene content, supporting the body with increased ability to oxygenate. It is commonly used to increase circulation and support the body when oxygenation needs will be higher such as work at higher altitudes, support prior to anesthetic events, increased athletic performance, and increased brain function. Cedarwood is often used in insect repellant recipes available on the commercial market, and could be included in any insect repelling spray or recipe you would like to create. Cedarwood is also reported to aide in a full night's sleep and to help with stress and anxiety.

Birds & Exotics: Water diffusion, mainly within Three Part Blends, especially starting 2 weeks prior to anesthesia events.

Cats: Water-based diffusion, and can be considered for addition to Three Part Blends or Feline Supportive Blend. For the most part, this oil is rarely used on its own with felines. It can be considered for addition to litter box blends. While it is considered a popular addition to shampoos, it is not the most feline friendly of ingredients. Other options are more ideal (add Feline Supportive Blend plus Catnip to a shampoo.)

Dogs & Larger: Used with water-based diffusion, by water-misting, direct topical application (diluted), within Three Part Blends, added to the Canine or Large Animal Supportive Blends, via Petting applications (diluted), or included within natural ointments or shampoos.

Cedarwood, Himalayan (Cedrus deodara)

This oil is not commonly used with animals at this time, however, research shows some value in the potential to reduce inflammation in the stomach, and protect against gastric ulcers. It also may have actions on mast cells, reducing inflammation and allergic response, as well as aiding in autoimmune disease.

Celery Seed (Apium graveolens)

Not commonly used as a single oil in animals at this time. It is beneficial for the liver and to increase milk production. Research shows it may be protective against gastric ulcers. Inclusion in blends for diffusion, or within blends for diluted topical applications can be considered.

Chamomile, German (Matricaria recutita)

A wonderful oil that has come into its own in Veterinary Aromatic Medicine. High quality oil is important to obtain, and there are a lot of tainted and untrue oils on the market. Also called Blue Chamomile, this oil has wonderful promise for fatty liver disease, hepatitis, liver, and digestive issues, emotional concerns, and skin conditions. German Chamomile is rather strong, and even when used with water-based diffusion, you are likely to need half or less of the normal amount of oil you will use in your diffuser.

Birds & Exotics: Mainly used with water-based diffusion. Use for topical use at 1-3% or within Three Part Blends. Use via oral or water administration is likely as well, especially for liver and digestive concerns.

Cats: This oil can be used via water-based diffusion, added to Three Part Blends, Feline Supportive Blend, applied via Petting (diluted), or added to litter box blends.

Dogs & Larger: This oil can be used in all of the mentioned methods as well as direct topical application (diluted), included in Three Part Blends, Canine and Large Animal Supportive Blends, applied via Petting. Ingestion of diluted blends through grooming or licking may actually be desired.

Chamomile, Roman (Chamaemelum nobile, Anthemis nobilis)
Roman Chamomile has wonderful properties indicated for behavioral concerns and anxieties, skin conditions, nerve regeneration, and detoxification of the blood and liver (such as detoxification from vaccination insult.)

Birds & Exotics: Recommended for use with water-based diffusion, and for use topically (diluted for your species) within Three Part Blends, or added to the Small Animal Supportive Blend.

Cats: Roman Chamomile can be diffused via water-based diffusion, included in Three Part Blends for diffusion or diluted topical applications, added to Feline Supportive Blends, and added to litter box recipes.

Dogs & Larger: Roman Chamomile can be used easily in many methods for these animals. Water-based diffusion as a single or within Three Part Blends, applied via water-mists, topically (diluted) as a single or within Three Part Blends, or added to Canine or Large Animal Supportive Blends. While Roman Chamomile is safe for average ingestion and has been used orally, it is not commonly administered or recommended for direct oral use.

Chaste Tree Berry (See Vitex)

Cilantro (Coriandrum sativum)
Also called Coriander Leaf, Cilantro as an herb, has long been valued for its ability to bind and chelate potential toxins and heavy metals. This would indicate it as an excellent selection for damage due to over-vaccination or poisoning. Cilantro has a distinct odor, which may or may not make it appropriate for topical use with cats and smaller animals. Its use within Three

Part Blends for water-based diffusion or diluted topical applications can be considered. I find this oil a very pleasant addition to diffusion blends as well as cleaning recipes for a bright and fresh scent. Cilantro essential oil has GRAS status.

Cinnamon Bark (Cinnamomum verum)

Cinnamon oil contains a moderate level of Eugenol, which is often implicated in toxic situations in animals and especially cats. Although quite a hot oil and rarely indicated for direct single use in animals, there are actually many situations in which Cinnamon oil is used successfully, and without ill effects. Blends containing small percentages of Cinnamon Bark oil are often water diffused in households with cats, birds, and other exotics.

Care must be taken with Cinnamon oil in animals who are bleeding, have a tendency to bleed, or are on any sort of anti-coagulant therapy. The over use of essential oil(s) that have anti-coagulant actions, especially in oral administration, can produce a temporary and dose dependent, increases in bleeding and reduction of clotting.

Cinnamon Bark is commonly adulterated, and care should be taken to ensure synthetic cinnamaldehyde is not present. Many companies have been "caught" with lesser grade Cinnamon Bark oil, even when they claim it to be pure and natural. Cinnamon Bark has GRAS Status.

Birds & Exotics: As a single oil, this oil would rarely be used. It may be considered for use within blends for diffusion. No more than 10% of the final blend should be Cinnamon Bark.

Cats: As a single oil, this oil would rarely be used. It may be considered for use within blends for diffusion. No more than 10% of the final blend should be Cinnamon Bark.

Dogs: As a single oil, cinnamon would likely only be indicated for severe abscesses that were resistant to other first line therapies. It may be considered for use within blends for diffusion. No more than 10% of the final blend should be Cinnamon Bark.

Horses & Large Animals: Cinnamon oil is often indicated for large abscesses, applied diluted, directly to the site. Cinnamon is a wonderful oil for hoof abscesses, and other conditions such as Canker, Thrush, warts, or other lesions which do best with a "burning" sort of action to eliminate them from the body. Cinnamon is often implicated in the balancing of blood sugars – and used diluted could be given (especially to horses) orally for this effect. However, since there are many other oils which also perform this action, their use may be better indicated.

Cinnamon, Leaf (Cinnamomum zeylanica)

Cinnamon Leaf varies from Cinnamon Bark in the fact that it is quite high in Eugenol, while lower in Cinnamaldehyde. While often considered to be safer than Cinnamon Bark by human aromatherapists, this does not exclude Cinnamon Leaf from distinct caution. Cinnamon Leaf oil will still carry with it the ability to decrease clotting ability, and caution should be used with any animal on anti-coagulants or with a bleeding concern. Cinnamon Leaf oil has GRAS Status. Cinnamon Leaf can be considered for use similarly to Cinnamon Bark, with water-based diffusion being the most common route of use.

Cistus (Cistus ladanifer)

Cistus is also known as Labdanum, Rose of Sharon, or Rock Rose. The most common use for Cistus in the veterinary field is for conditions of blood clots and hemorrhage. Cistus is by far the leading oil indicated in conditions of internal hemorrhage (bleeding). This oil has been successfully used in many cases of internal hemorrhage and weeping after an Ovariohysterectomy or Spay surgery.

Due to the content of α-pinene in Cistus, oxidation is more likely – and care should be taken with storage and age of oil. Increased skin irritation can occur with oxidized oil.

Birds & Exotics: Cistus would likely only be used in emergency situations of hemorrhage or of blood clots. 1 drop of Cistus diluted in 2 mL of carrier oil, would be used for oral administration. 1 drop of the diluted solution would be given orally, and repeated every 20 minutes or more until internal bleeding was controlled. Cistus can be applied neat or diluted directly to a bleeding toe nail, or broken blood feather to help stop the bleeding. Water diffusion could also be utilized, especially in situations where lung penetration is desired. Cistus may be considered for use within Three Part Blends, or with one drop added to the Small Animal Supportive Blend recipe.

Cats: Cistus would commonly be used by adding it to the Feline Supportive Blend or in a Three Part Blend. The diluted blend may be applied via Petting or a Drip & Rub Technique. Cistus can be considered for addition to litter box blends, and in a severe emergency situation given orally. Depending on the severity of the bleeding, Cistus could be used orally either neat or diluted with an equal part of carrier oil. Whether diluted or neat, the Cistus would be given orally, one drop at a time, repeating every 20 minutes or more until the bleeding was controlled. Cistus would also be well indicated for situations of blood clots in cats, such as Saddle Thrombus. Water-based diffusion could also be used, especially in situations where lung penetration is desired.

Dogs & Larger: Cistus can be used in many ways; water-based diffusion, addition to Three Part Blends or Canine or Large Animal Supportive Blends, direct topical application (neat or diluted), via Petting (diluted), and orally. In situations of internal hemorrhage approximately 3 drops per 50 pounds (22kg) of dog is given under the tongue or directly into the mouth. This can be repeated if necessary, usually about every 20 minutes. However, the frequency is usually based upon the severity of the situation. A maximum dosage has not been determined, but after repeat dosing, dogs have received approximately 7-10 drops per 20 pounds (9kg) in total oils, without concern.

Citronella (Cymbopogon nardus)
This essential oil has been widely used for insect repellant properties in animals and humans. Citronella is mainly recommended for use within blends or products such as shampoos, and often intended as insect repellant, for ear mites, mange, and other forms of external parasites and insects. Citronella has a nice deodorizing quality to its scent. Undiluted Citronella can be irritating to skin.

Birds & Exotics: Citronella has mainly been used with blends intended for water-based diffusion. Addition into the Small Animal Supportive Blend or Three Part Blends, can be considered.

Cats: Citronella is recommended to be used within Three Part Blends for water-based diffusion or diluted topical applications. Citronella may be added to the Feline Supportive Blend. Petting with the single oil (diluted) will likely be tolerated, however the majority of information on the use of this oil with cats has been through its use within blends or products.

Dogs & Larger: Citronella can be used within Three Part Blends for water-based diffusion, water-mists, addition to shampoos and ointments, or for diluted topical applications. Citronella can also be added to the Canine or Large Animal Supportive Blends.

Clary Sage (Salvia sclarea)

Clary Sage is most commonly thought of for hormonal balancing. This oil can be used in both male and female animals, and would be indicated for any condition where hormones are the suspected culprit. Situations where we use Clary Sage include excessive egg laying, poor egg production, lack of singing in Canaries, hormonal and cranky mares, excessive stud behavior in stallions and other males, lack of cycling, false pregnancies, cystic ovaries, feather picking, and more. Basically anything that is hormonally driven, Clary Sage is indicated for. Clary Sage has GRAS Status.

Birds & Exotics: Water-based diffusion is the most indicated and well used method of administration at this time. Clary Sage within Three Part Blends has been used within water spritzer applications – generally at a dilution of 4 drops per 4 ounces (120 mL) of distilled water – misted onto the bird or animal directly. Clary Sage can also be considered for addition to the Small Animal Supportive Blend or the Feather Spray recipes. Direct Oral administration has not been widely used at this time.

Cats: Cat friendly methods of use include water-based diffusion of the single oil or within a Three Part Blend, use within Three Part Blends (diluted) for topical applications, within Feline Supportive Blends, via Drip & Rub or Petting Techniques, and adding to litter box recipes. Rarely would we use this oil orally in a cat, beyond the grooming off of diluted recipes.

Dogs & Larger: Water-based diffusion, direct application of Three Part Blends, Petting application (diluted), addition into Canine or Large Animal Supportive Blends is most recommended. Oral administration has been used in the past, however is rarely necessary. With oral administration – a starting amount of 1 drop per 20 pounds (9 kg) of dog, and 1 drop per 200 pounds (91 kg) of larger animals can be used. Careful monitoring for response will allow you to adjust the amounts up or down for the individual needs of the animal.

Clove, Bud (Syzygium aromaticum)

Clove oil contains a very high level of Eugenol, which is often implicated in cases of toxicity reported in small companion animals, especially in cats. Many times I have been asked to evaluate animal products which contain Clove oil. I consistently find that these products are poorly designed, and that the creator of the product has very little understanding of essential oils or of animal physiology. It seems that many companies jump on the "natural" band wagon, produce a flea and tick spray, label it for use in cats, and then add poor quality, fractionated, or synthetic constituents of Clove or other essential oils. Clove oil is clearly not the enemy, as it is used successfully in the animal kingdom every day. However, the quality level of the Clove oil used, and its appropriate use for an individual species, are the most important factors with any sort of toxicity issue.

Clove oil is one of the highest anti-oxidant substances on earth. Its health benefits are quite amazing. Clove is commonly used in the animal kingdom for conditions such as warts, canker, abscesses, dental disease, gastric ulcers, preventing blood clots or thinning the blood, and deworming. Clove oil is most commonly used within blends and rarely as a single oil. Clove oil would be classified as "hot" and distinct care should be taken with it.

Diffusion of Clove oil in a home has greatly reduced human and animal responses to airborne allergens. Diffusing for a few hours prior to a "sensitive" human visitor, can leave them wondering if you even have the pets they are usually allergic to. Diffusion should be water-based and is generally within a Three Part Blend.

Care must be taken with Clove oil in animals who are bleeding, have a tendency to bleed, or are on any sort of anti-coagulant therapy. The over use of essential oil(s) that have anti-coagulant actions, especially in oral administration, can produce a temporary and dose dependent increase in bleeding and reduction of clotting.

Birds & Exotics: Clove is used most often within blends intended for diffusion. Clove oil has been used as a single in birds with severe Papillomatosis (warts). The Clove oil was mixed into soft foods, and gradually increased in concentration. This method was used with the theory that the essential oil would come into contact the lining of the gastrointestinal tract that was affected with the papilloma. As bird digestive systems are quite different from others, the essential oils are capable of contacting the internal linings of certain parts of the digestive tract.

Cats: Clove oil is rarely used as a single oil in cats. However its use within Three Part Blends for water-based diffusion is common.

Dogs: Clove oil is most commonly used within other products and blends for dogs. Clove oil can be used topically (neat or diluted) for difficult abscesses or dental abscesses and pain. Clove can also be given orally for anti-coagulant actions and can also be added to various pain protocols. Use within Three Part Blends for water-based diffusion is common. Clove is known to be topically numbing – so we utilize this feature within diffusion for conditions such as collapsing trachea. When there is much irritation to an airway – Clove may be included to calm and "numb" the irritated and spasming tissues.

Horses & Large Animals: Clove oil is used most commonly in these species, and can be used as a single or within blends. Direct topical application (often in the neat form) is used for abscesses, thrush, hoof conditions, canker, warts, and other similar conditions. Oral use of Clove oil has been used with horses and is generally well tolerated. Clove oil should be diluted in some type of carrier or food prior to administration. Clove may aid in healing and health through its massive anti-oxidant effects, and appears to decrease pain significantly when used orally. Starting with 5 total drops of Clove (diluted to at least 50% concentration) can be dripped into the lip pocket. Evaluate the response, and determine when to repeat the administration or if increased amounts are needed. Some horses have received 20 or more drops of Clove oil orally to aid with severe pain, although this is likely to be an excessive amount. Use caution with high oral amounts, if other anti-inflammatory drugs are being used which may decrease clotting ability. The use of Clove, and other oral essential oils, have been used at the same time as traditional medications with no apparent interactions.

Clove, Leaf (Syzigium aromaticum)
This oil is less commonly used with animals, however may be considered similar to Clove Bud. The use of Clove Bud is preferred for Veterinary Aromatic Medicine.

Copaiba, distilled (Copaifera officinalis/langsdorfii)
Copaiba has to be one of my favorite oils. With barely any scent or flavor, it is a powerhouse in the animal world. One of the highest anti-inflammatory oils, it replaces Non-Steroidal Anti-Inflammatory Drugs (NSAID's) in my practice regularly. The beauty of this oil is that it can be given simultaneously with

traditional NSAID's until symptoms improve and a weaning of the NSAID can begin. Since inflammation is a component of any dis-ease, Copaiba is always indicated in a protocol.

There are two forms of Copaiba you should know about. This one we are currently discussing is the steam distilled version. The other type will also be discussed again in its own heading. Copaiba is tapped from a tree, much like sap for maple syrup. This sap is called an oleoresin or resin. Some people prefer one over the other for a variety of reasons. The oleoresin is unprocessed, so therefore thought to be more natural, and also contains the diterpenes from the tree, that do not carry over in steam distillation. With steam distillation, the resin is distilled, leaving a slightly different product. Steam distilled Copaiba will generally be higher in β-Caryophyllene, however lacking the diterpenes within the initial resin. I find both to be useful, but sometimes one is indicated over another for either an individual animal, or for a specific condition.

β-Caryophyllene (and therefore Copaiba) recently came under great promotion in the aromatherapy world. Funny, how I have always loved it, and was even made fun of with my view of "Copaiba for everything!" – but given time, other aromatherapists and unfortunately mass-marketing machines have caught onto my love for and the effective nature of Copaiba. For sure we will be seeing corners cut, and poor grade Copaiba on the market in response to this popularity flare.

Why is Copaiba being promoted? Because someone found a research article such as this one from 2014 *"The cannabinoid CB_2 receptor-selective phytocannabinoid beta-caryophyllene exerts analgesic effects in mouse models of inflammatory and neuropathic pain."* By Klauke et al. (Eur. Neuropsychopharmacol. Apr;24(4):608-20.) So yes, we now have some evidence or explanation of why Copaiba is so great. It contains a very high level of β-Caryophyllene, basically the highest level of any of the essential oils. So with the current Cannabis, Hemp Oil, and CBD craze, the essential oil companies were bound to put a spin on it, and create a desire to use Copaiba instead of CBD oil. They are really quite different, however, and I would never attempt to replace CBD with Copaiba. But I most certainly would use them together.

Copaiba is reported to contain usually between approximately 25 to almost 70% β-Caryophyllene. With higher percentages being within the Steam Distilled oil rather than the oleoresin. It can just depend on what our goals and needs are, as to which oil I will select.

Copaiba is wonderful to use with many conditions; arthritis, gastric ulcers, dental disease, gingivitis, stomatitis, skin conditions, inflammation of any sort, gastro-intestinal disorders, pain, cystitis, urinary incontinence, urinary disorders, and more. Copaiba also appears to "magnify" the effects other essential oils that it is used with. This could be a direct synergistic effect, but also since all dis-ease contains inflammation, the act of the Copaiba to reduce the inflammation is a considerable contribution to healing and the effects seen in general.

Birds & Exotics: Copaiba is used in many, many ways, and is an oil that I consider an important addition to any regimen. Water-based diffusion can be used in open rooms, small rooms, in caging, and tented. Often 3-4 drops are added to a water-based diffuser to start. Copaiba can also be added to drinking water, starting with 1 drop in 1 liter of water, and gradually increasing as needed. Copaiba is also added to foods quite easily. Beginning with a "toothpick dip" of the essential oil added to a tablespoon of food, the amount can gradually be increased based on response. Please see the chapter How Much, How Often for a more complete explanation of how to monitor and increase or decrease amounts of essential oils used. Copaiba has also been used topically – 1 drop mixed into a tablespoon of natural ointments, within diluted Three Part Blends, and within Small Animal Supportive Blends. Water mists can also be considered, with 4-5 drops added to 4 ounces (120 mL) of distilled water and misted onto the bird or animal. Addition to soaking water for reptiles, as well as to fish tanks has also been used. Application by Petting (diluted) and transfer from perches or hands is also used. Copaiba can also be added to any Three Part Blend with amazing benefits and results.

Please also see the Myrrh essential oil description for more information on a Pain Recipe, which combines Copaiba, Helichrysum, and Myrrh.

Cats: Again, Copaiba is a worthy addition to any feline regimen. Situations where Copaiba is especially indicated: Cystitis, FLUTD, Inflammatory Bowel Disease, Pancreatitis, Stomatitis, and Arthritis. Copaiba can be used in all of the previously mentioned ways for cats. Some cats may or may not drink Copaiba in their water – so this option may not work for everyone. Also, when adding Copaiba to the food of a cat, this may also be rejected. Starting with very small "toothpick" amounts, and gradually increasing the amounts they are exposed to, seems to work well for most cats, effectively getting them used to the flavor or smell that surely they detect. The most well accepted and common ways to use Copaiba for cats is with water-based diffusion, within the Feline Supportive

Blend, within Three Part Blends, via Petting (diluted), or by adding to litter box recipes. It is important to recognize that for cats, normal grooming of Copaiba within appropriate and diluted blends, is one of the best ways to help oral tissues, as well as provide for ingestion.

Dogs & Larger: All of the previously mentioned techniques and benefits apply to dogs and larger animals as well. The most well accepted and common ways to use Copaiba is with water-based diffusion, within the Canine or Large Animal Supportive Blends, within Three Part Blends, via Petting (diluted), or by adding into foods. For female dogs with urinary incontinence, Copaiba is often used twice a day within food, with great responses.

For horses, Copaiba is an important essential oil for the replacement of harmful NSAID's which are known to promote gastric ulcer formation. Not only is Copaiba highly anti-inflammatory, but it also protects against the formation of gastric ulcers, eliminating the need for expensive ulcer guarding medications.

The following are recommendations for the oral use of Copaiba, however remember that some individuals may require more or less.
- For dogs up to 20 pounds (9 kg): 1 part of Copaiba oil can be mixed with 3 parts of carrier oil, and 1-2 drops of this dilution can be given twice a day, either mixed with food, given directly in the mouth, or even applied topically.
- For dogs 20-50 pounds (9-22 kg): 1 part of Copaiba oil can be mixed with 1 part carrier oil, and 1-2 drops of this dilution can be given twice a day.
- For dogs over 50 pounds (23 kg) generally 1 drop of undiluted Copaiba oil can be used twice a day, although you may still find it better accepted if diluted first prior to administration.
- For Horses and other Large Animals: Copaiba can be used orally undiluted either directly or mixed with foods or water. Approximately 1 drop of Copaiba can be used per 100-200 pounds (45-90 kg) of animal body weight. With horses, starting with approximately 5 drops twice a day is typical.

Copaiba, oleoresin (Copaifera officinalis/langsdorfii)
This version of Copaiba is the resin that is directly tapped from the tree. This oleoresin will generally have a lower level of β-Caryophyllene than the steam distilled oil. It is reported that approximately 25% of the oleoresin can be made

up of diterpenes. For now, the diterpenes are often reported generically on GC evaluations of the oleoresin. There is some research showing that the diterpenes within Copaiba oleoresin are effective against Leishmaniasis and periodontal bacteria.

The diterpenes most commonly found within copaiba oleoresins are copalic, polyalthic, hardwickiic, kaurenoic and ent-kaurenoic acids, together with their derivatives 3-hydroxy-copalic, 3-acetoxy-copalic, and ent-agathic acid. (Leandro LM et al. Molecules. 2012 Mar 30;17(4):3866-89. *"Chemistry and biological activities of terpenoids from copaiba (Copaifera spp.) oleoresins."*) At this time, while diterpenes are most certainly biologically active, we do not understand the extent or importance at this time. Clinically, we often find greater actions for what we desire, with use of the Steam Distilled Copaiba. However, we look forward to evaluating the differences between the essential oil and the oleoresin, and hope to clarify in which instances; each may be beneficial in their own right.

It is likely that Copaiba Oleoresin may be used in all of the ways described for steam distilled Copaiba. However, the Oleoresin is not as widely used with animals at this time.

Coriander Leaf (see Cilantro)

Coriander Seed (Coriandrum sativum)

Coriander is a lovely oil that is mainly used for diabetes, blood sugar control, metabolic syndromes, and supporting pancreatic function. It is most commonly used in horses with Cushing's, Insulin Resistance, and Metabolic Syndromes. It would also be indicated for Ferrets with insulinoma. Coriander Seed oil may also help to stimulate appetite and aid in digestion.

Close monitoring with a veterinarian is important when using any essential oil with animals receiving Insulin or oral hypoglycemic drugs. As correction of the body occurs, there may be less need for the Insulin, and a dangerous situation can occur when more Insulin is given to an animal than they currently need. The veterinarian needs to be aware that natural remedies are being used that may reduce your animal's need for diabetic medications. Even the pure action of dietary improvement in cats, has eliminated the need for Insulin in many patients. So, taking a slow and careful position with animals on these medications is important.

Coriander Seed essential oil has GRAS status, and is high in Linalool. It may also contain low levels of camphor, so we typically pick to use this oil in lower amounts, and within blends.

Birds & Exotics: Coriander oil has mainly been used with water-based diffusion or with addition into Three Part Blends or Small Animal Supportive Blends. Oral use of Coriander may be considered, either mixed with foods or added to water would be recommended starting places.

Cats: Coriander has mainly been used with water-based diffusion or with addition into the Feline Supportive Blend. Three Part Blends are recommended for diffusion, topical application (diluted) and for other uses such as litter box recipes.

Dogs: All of the methods mentioned previously can be used for dogs. Oral use of Coriander directly or in food, could start with 1 part Coriander mixed with 3 parts carrier oil – with 1 drop of this solution, being given twice a day, for each 20 pounds (9 kg) of body weight. Addition into the Canine Supportive Blend, use within Three Part Blends for diffusion or topical application (diluted) would also be appropriate.

Horses & Large Animals: Coriander is most commonly used in horses for blood sugar balancing. Direct topical application within Three Part Blends or the Large Animal Supportive Blend is suggested. Adding to food or water, and direct oral administration are also common. Starting with 1 drop per 100-200 pounds (45-90 kg) of body weight, given orally twice a day is a good starting point. Monitor with a veterinarian, and adjust accordingly based on need and response.

Cornmint (Mentha arvensis)
Often used as an adulterant or substitute for true Peppermint essential oil, Cornmint is not recommended for use in Veterinary Aromatic Medicine.

Cumin (Cuminum cyminum)
Cumin definitely carries with it a distinct aroma. This is often regarded as unpleasant when used within blends for diffusion or topical application. Cumin is often indicated for aiding with digestion or for detoxification purposes. While Cumin has GRAS status, it is also photosensitizing. For the most part, there are far more appropriate oils to use when the properties of Cumin is desired.

Cypress (Cupressus sempervirens)

Cypress is often used to increase circulation in animals, and aids every condition with this quality. Resorption of bruises, improvement of circulation, and circulatory disorders are main reasons to use this oil. Cypress may also contribute to a diuretic action. While Cypress is high in α-pinene and may be considered by some to be within the "avoidance for cats" category, with proper usage and with veterinary documentation, the oil has been widely used with felines without detriment, even in long term use and with grooming ingestion.

Birds & Exotics: Most commonly used with water-based diffusion. Cypress can be considered within Three Part Blends or within the Small Animal Supportive Blend. 1 drop could also be mixed with 1 tablespoon of a natural ointment for topical applications.

Cats: The previous methods could also be used for cats, although use in cats is most commonly used within the Feline Supportive Blend. Petting (diluted), direct topical application (diluted 4 drops to 30 mL of carrier oil), and litter box recipes could also be used. Ingestion of Cypress is most likely to occur from grooming after Petting or Feline Supportive Blend applications.

Dogs & Larger: Most commonly Cypress will be used within the Canine or Large Animal Supporting Blends, or within Three Part Blends for water-based diffusion or topical applications. Oral use has been used with these animals via drinking water, addition to foods, or direct oral administration; however is considered unnecessary in most circumstances. For oral use in dogs – dilute 1 part Cypress with 5 parts carrier oil – use 1 drop of this solution twice a day, for each 20 pounds (9 kg) of body weight. For horses and others starting with 1 drop per 300 pounds (135 kg) of body weight, given orally twice a day is a good starting point. Monitor responses with a veterinarian, and adjust according to individual need.

Cypress, Blue (Callitris intratropica)

This oil from Australia has a gorgeous blue tone due to its unique content of guaiazulene, which is typically not found in wood oils. It is a thick oil, which reflects its ability to be a fixative for perfumery and blending. It has a great woody base note, with a grounding character. The anti-viral potential of this oil seems high, as well as anti-inflammatory, antifungal, and calming effects. Conditions such as warts (papilloma), herpes, and other viral situations will likely benefit from this oil. While grooming of this oil within blends has been very safe, we have little data on larger amounts being given orally to animals. It is recommended to use this oil within blends, and at the lower ends of the concentrations recommended for the species.

Birds & Exotics: Use within Three Part Blends with water-based diffusion or with species appropriate diluted topical applications.

Cats: Blue Cypress will most commonly be used within Three Part Blends for diffusion or for diluted topical applications and litter box recipes. The addition of 1 drop of Blue Cypress to the Feline Supportive Blend could be considered.

Dogs & Larger: All of the previously mentioned methods can be used. Dilution of this oil by using 1 part (or drop) to 5 parts of carrier oil is recommended for initial use as a single. Blue Cypress will most commonly be used within Three Part Blends for water-based diffusion, misting, or diluted topical applications. The addition to the Canine or Large Animal Supportive Blends may be considered.

Davana (Artemesia pallens)
Traditionally used to balance menstruation, menopause, and other issues "female", Davana may also show some ability to purge intestinal parasites. Emotionally, Davana may be calming, and is often used within the perfumery industry. Davana is not widely used with animals at this time, but appears to have a fairly safe profile.

Dill Seed (Anethum graveolens)
Dill Seed is higher in Limonene than Dill Weed in chemical profile. Dill Weed is preferred for use with Veterinary Aromatic Medicine.

Dill Weed (Anethum graveolens)
Dill is used mainly for diabetes, blood sugar and insulin regulation, and for pancreatic conditions in animals. Due to the "pickle" smell associated with this oil, it is not often applied topically to animals as a single or as a large contribution to a blend. Dill is indicated especially in horses with Cushing's, Insulin Resistance, or Metabolic Syndrome, and is used in the oral route and topically for this species.

Close monitoring with a veterinarian is important when using any essential oil with animals receiving Insulin or oral hypoglycemic drugs. As correction of the body occurs, there may be less need for the Insulin, and a dangerous situation can occur when more Insulin is given to an animal than they currently need. The veterinarian needs to be aware that natural remedies are being used that may reduce your animal's need for diabetic medications. Even the singular action of dietary improvement in cats has eliminated the need for Insulin in many patients, so taking a slow and careful position with animals on these medications is important.

Birds & Exotics: Dill can be added to drinking water at 1 drop per liter, and can also be added to foods. Dill can also be added to Three Part Blends for water-based diffusion or topical applications, or it may be included within the Small Animal Supportive Blend.

Cats: Dill will mainly be used within Three Part Blends for water-based diffusion or topical applications, or by adding to the Feline Supportive Blend. Addition to litter box recipes can also be considered. Use Dill in small portions at first, increasing slowly to avoid overwhelming "pickle smell".

Dogs & Larger: Any method of use of Dill is acceptable, as long as the smell is not offensive to the animal caretaker. Within Three Part Blends for water-based diffusion or topical applications (diluted), inclusion within Canine or Large Animal Supportive Blends, via Petting (diluted), direct topical application (diluted), adding to drinking water, adding to foods, and direct oral use are acceptable application methods. For oral use in dogs – dilute 1 part Dill with 3 parts carrier – use 1 drop of this solution twice a day, for each 20 pounds (9 kg) of body weight. For horses and others starting with 1 drop per 100-200 pounds (45-90 kg) of body weight, given orally twice a day is a good starting point. Monitor responses with a veterinarian, and adjust according to individual need.

Dorado Azul (Hyptis suaveolens)

Dorado Azul is a trademarked and exclusive oil to one essential oil company. It had only recently been introduced into the market when the first edition of this book was published. Dorado Azul is reported to have actions for asthma, bronchitis, pneumonia, heaves, and hormonal concerns. Information on the direct use of this oil with animals, has not progressed adequately to warrant its use in Veterinary Aromatic Medicine. There are oils with far more use and safety data, that provide similar if not better results. The 1,8-cineole content in

Dorado Azul is likely to contribute to its respiratory effects, which can be found in many species of Eucalyptus oil.

Douglas Fir (Pseudotsuga menziesii)
Douglas Fir is likely to be able to be used much in the same way of Balsam Fir or Black Spruce. Douglas Fir has not been as widely used with animals at this time, although it is likely to carry the same characteristics of the other oils, including support for respiratory and bone concerns, as well as analgesic and immune supportive properties. Douglas Fir has shown antifungal properties in research.

Elemi (Canarium luzonicum)
Often described as "poor man's Frankincense", Elemi is an often overlooked essential oil. It has not been used as extensively in the animal kingdom as it likely should. More information is definitely needed on this oil, but reports have been very favorable for respiratory concerns and symptoms of Feline Herpes Virus. It is also reported to have benefits for cystitis (FLUTD), urinary issues, muscle and nerve pain, scar tissue, and the reduction of sebaceous secretions from skin. It is likely that this oil would be indicated for animals with sebaceous cysts, seborrhea oleosa (greasy flakey skin), excessive skin oil production, proud flesh, and scarring. Elemi is respected as an oil which is excellent for wound healing, skin regeneration, and also for emotional concerns and meditation. Research has shown Elemol, a chemical constituent within Elemi, reduced serum IgE levels, which could play an important part in reducing inflammation and mast cell infiltration in the skin. Possibly, this oil could be indicated for use with Mast Cell Tumors.

Birds & Exotics: Although this oil has not been used with many exotic pets at this time, it is likely its use within Three Part Blends for water-based diffusion, dilution for topical applications, or addition into the Small Animal Supportive Blend are reasonable.

Cats: All of the previous methods of application can be used for cats, with the most common application to be via addition to the Feline Supportive Blend or with inclusion in a litter box recipes.

Dogs & Larger: All of the previous methods can be utilized for these animals. The most common ways to use this oil would include water-based diffusion or diluted topical applications within a Three Part Blend, addition into the Canine or Large Animal Supportive Blends, topical applications by Petting (diluted), or direct topical application (diluted), or within water-misting recipes.

Eucalyptus Blue (Eucalyptus bicostata)
This eucalyptus comes from Ecuador, and is reported to be much milder than most eucalyptus oils. When the first edition of this book was first published, Eucalyptus Blue was just entering the public market. While the oil was helpful for respiratory infections and conditions, and was reported to have good insect repellant properties, it has not been documented adequately for safety and use with animals as of 2018. As it has been recommended in the past, that this oil should not be consumed or ingested – I would not recommend its use for Veterinary Aromatic Medicine at this time.

It is also worthy to note that Eucalyptus Blue has "top note" that reminds many people of cat urine. This can be an unpleasant thing, and has tricked some people into thinking that their cat had been urinating all over their home, even when simply diffusing the oil. Any other Eucalyptus species with more safety and use information with animals, is suggested for use instead of Eucalyptus Blue.

Eucalyptus citriodora
Also called Lemon Eucalyptus or Lemon-Scented Gum, this oil has a wonderful lemon scent. It has recently become quite popular for its content of PMD (p-Menthane-3,8-diol), which has been shown in research to rival DEET in insect repellency. It has quite a wide safety margin in animals, however used undiluted is irritating to the skin. Appropriate uses for Eucalyptus citriodora include within water-mists, oil-based mists, within Three Part Blends for water-based diffusion or diluted topical applications, and by addition to species appropriate Supportive Blends. Blends containing this oil, are being used quite successfully in all species, especially for insect control.

Birds & Exotics: Appropriate uses include addition to Three Part Blends for water-based diffusion and diluted topical applications. Addition to Small Animal Supportive Blend, natural shampoos, and ointments are also recommended. With chickens and other poultry, this oil has been added to water-mists for lice and mite control – however it has not been used widely as a mist with parrots and other avian species at this time.

Cats: Use within Three Part Blends for water-based diffusion and diluted topical applications is appropriate. Addition into the Feline Supportive Blend can be considered for cases of ear mites, fleas, lice, and other insect concerns. Three Part Blends for ear mite treatment, often contain this essential oil. A blend containing this essential oil, diluted to 5-10% within carrier oil, and applied sparingly to ears; has shown clinical efficacy against ear mite infections – however it is important to recognize that ear mites do not only reside in the ear, so applications to the cat as described for Feline Supportive Blend is also advised. This oil can also be added to natural shampoos, ointments, or to litter box recipes. If a cat is agreeable, use within a water-mist may be appropriate in some situations.

Dogs & Larger Animals: Use within Three Part Blends for water-based diffusion or diluted topical applications is appropriate. Addition to Canine and Large Animal Supportive Blends is a wonderful option for routine insect control. The addition of this oil to natural shampoos or ointments is often recommended, and ointments can be made quite strong for larger animals who need protection from flies, gnats, or other biting insects within ears or to local areas of concern. Combining this oil within Three Part Blends prior to addition into recipes, appears most synergistic. Water-mists and oil-mists can be considered for applications as well.

Eucalyptus Dives (Eucalyptus dives)

Also called Peppermint Eucalyptus, Broadleaf Eucalyptus, Broad-leaved Peppermint Gum, Blue Peppermint, and a few variations within these – it would be most proper to continue to specify Eucalyptus dives when referring to this oil. This Eucalyptus is much lower in 1,8-cineole content, and seems to avoid much of the warnings associated with this constituent. Rich in Piperitone, it appears to have a relatively good safety margin, and is reported to be indicated for respiratory conditions, sinusitis, and may possibly have insect repelling actions. It is not widely used with animals at this time.

Eucalyptus Globulus (Eucalyptus globulus)

Eucalyptus globulus is indicated for use in respiratory conditions, asthma, bronchitis, fungal conditions, insect repellant, internal parasites, and flu conditions. Care should be taken when exposing an asthmatic or small children to this oil in high concentrations or in its neat form, as there are relationships with high 1,8-cineole levels causing breathing issues. However, there is ample research to show that Eucalyptus globulus is very helpful in all sorts of respiratory conditions, including asthma. Eucalyptus globulus is reported to be beneficial for purifying and cleansing the air. See the chapter on Sensitivity to Oils for more on the theory of breathing issues and Eucalyptus oils.

Birds & Exotics: Use within Three Part Blends via water-based diffusion in an open room, small room, caging, or tenting can be used, and is especially indicated to help cleanse the air in quarantine situations. Eucalyptus is less commonly used for topical applications for these species.

Cats: Eucalyptus globulus is mainly recommended for use within Three Part Blends for water-based diffusion. Considerations may be made to adding it into litter box recipes. However, Eucalyptus is less likely to be added into blends used for topical applications in cats. While it was previously reported that Eucalyptus globulus had been used orally for cats with urinary tract infections, current data does not support this use at this time. While wonderful for respiratory conditions in cats, when water diffused, Eucalyptus is less "feline friendly" in general in terms of topical applications.

Dogs & Larger: All of the previously mentioned techniques can be used as well as: use within Three Part Blends for diluted topical applications, use within water-mists, direct application (diluted), addition into the Canine or Large Animal Supportive Blends, and addition into insect repellant recipes. At this time Eucalyptus globulus has not been used extensively by the oral route in animals.

Eucalyptus Polybractea (Eucalyptus polybractea)
This Eucalyptus is also high in 1,8-cineole and will carry with it the same discussion as stated within Eucalyptus globulus. Eucalyptus polybractea is reported to be indicated for urinary tract infections, Herpes infections, respiratory conditions, and also has insect repellant properties.

Birds & Exotics: Use within Three Part Blends via water-based diffusion in an open room is suggested, and is especially indicated to help cleanse the air in quarantine situations. For issues requiring diffusion in a small room, caging, or tenting situation, the use of Eucalyptus globulus or radiata is suggested. Eucalyptus polybractea has been less used in confined situations than these oils. Eucalyptus in general, is less commonly used for topical applications for these species.

Cats: Eucalyptus polybractea would mainly be used within Three Part Blends for water-based diffusion. Considerations may be made to adding it into litter box recipes. However, Eucalyptus is less likely to be added into blends used for topical applications in cats. While wonderful for respiratory conditions in cats, when water diffused, Eucalyptus species are less "feline friendly" in general in terms of topical applications.

Dogs & Larger: All of the previously mentioned techniques can be used as well as: use of Three Part Blends topically (diluted), direct application (diluted), and inclusion into Canine or Large Animal Supportive Blends. At this time Eucalyptus polybractea has not been used extensively by the oral route in animals.

Eucalyptus Radiata (Eucalyptus radiata)

Eucalyptus radiata is also high in 1,8-cineole and will carry with it the same discussion as stated within Eucalyptus globulus. While it does carry a different constituent profile, Eucalyptus radiata is often used interchangeably with Eucalyptus globulus. Eucalyptus radiata is especially indicated for vaginitis, Herpes infections, asthma, bronchitis, viral respiratory conditions, and sinusitis. It is reported to be especially effective against Herpes when combined with Bergamot. Eucalyptus radiata is also beneficial for purifying and cleansing the air.

Birds & Exotics: Use within Three Part Blends via water-based diffusion in an open room, small room, caging, or tenting can be used, and is especially indicated to help cleanse the air in quarantine situations. Eucalyptus is less commonly used for topical applications for these species.

Cats: Eucalyptus radiata is mainly recommended for use within Three Part Blends for water-based diffusion. Considerations may be made to adding it into litter box recipes. However, Eucalyptus is less likely to be added into blends used for topical applications in cats. While wonderful for respiratory conditions in cats, when water diffused, Eucalyptus is less "feline friendly" in general in terms of topical applications.

Dogs & Larger: All of the previously mentioned techniques can be used as well as: use within Three Part Blends for diluted topical applications, use within water-mists, direct application (diluted), addition into the Canine or Large Animal Supportive Blends, and addition into insect repellant recipes. At this time Eucalyptus radiata has not been used extensively by the oral route in animals.

Fennel, Sweet (Foeniculum vulgare)

Fennel essential oil is commonly used with animals for diabetes, blood sugar balancing, hormone balancing, intestinal parasites, urinary tract infection, stimulating milk production, and for gastrointestinal concerns. There are some references which caution against the use of Fennel in those with epilepsy. Although this precaution is wise to adhere to, in practice many animals with seizure conditions have used blends containing Fennel. In Tisserand & Young's *Essential Oil Safety* (2nd Edition) – there are no precautionary statements regarding use with seizures or epilepsy. Adulteration of Fennel with synthetic anethole, is likely to contain a more toxic isomer – so strict quality should be obtained.

Birds & Exotics: Fennel has most commonly been used within Three Part Blends for water-based diffusion and diluted topical applications. Addition to drinking water (1 drop per liter of water), addition into foods, and addition to Small Animal Supportive Blends can be considered.

Cats: Methods most commonly used for cats would be within Three Part Blends for water-based diffusion and diluted topical applications. Addition to Feline Supportive Blend can also be considered, as well as into litter box recipes. Oral use in cats is commonly accomplished by the use of topical applications of blends, and the resultant grooming which may occur.

Dogs & Larger: Fennel can be used in all of the ways stated, as well as direct application (diluted), addition into Canine or Large Animal Supportive Blends, and by oral administration. For lactating animals, Fennel can be included in various udder washes and teat dip recipes for easy and routine exposure to the oil and to support milk production. Unless milk is contaminated with the essential oil itself, residual flavor of the essential oil does not transfer into the milk. For oral use in dogs – dilute 1 part Fennel with 10 parts carrier oil – use 1 drop or more of this solution twice a day, for each 20 pounds (9 kg) of body weight. For horses and others starting with 1 drop per 500 pounds (225 kg) of body weight, given orally twice a day is a good starting point. Monitor responses and adjust according to individual need.

Frankincense (Boswellia carterii)

Frankincense of the carterii variety is often referred to as "regular Frankincense" as opposed to Sacred Frankincense. However, in actuality many aromatherapists and chemists believe Boswellia sacra, is likely to be the same plant, just possibly a different grade, grown in a different region, distilled with other species of Frankincense resin, or simply misidentified in resin markets. Beyond any controversy or marketing, Sacred Frankincense is often reported to be higher in α-pinene than carterii, with a few other minor differences in other constituents. Overall, I have found that I prefer the use of what is reported to be Boswellia carterii, for use with Veterinary Aromatic Medicine. Even if Sacred Frankincense is different from carterii, the apparent different constituent panel appears less desired for work with animals.

Regardless, Frankincense remains to be one of the most important and well used oils in the animal world. It has been used with every species, in almost every way imaginable. It is incredibly safe, well tolerated, versatile, and effective. Major conditions in which Frankincense is used include all forms of cancer, tumors, cysts, behavioral conditions, depression, brain disorders, seizures, immune system stimulation and regulation, autoimmune disorders, DNA repair, and more. Frankincense is considered a "life force" oil and has been used extensively in critical cases in our veterinary hospital. The use of Frankincense in times of transition and death is incredibly helpful to animal and caretaker.

Often times with cases of cancer, animals present to my practice at a point we would refer to as "end-stage." This means that the cancer is so progressed, that it is unlikely that the body can recover from the dis-ease. When owners desire to try everything, and to use aggressive methods in an attempt to reverse the cancer, the use of Frankincense oil is highly sought after. For these often terminal animals, even if Frankincense was unable to aid their body in a reversal of their condition, it is always reported by the animal caretaker to have eased the transition tremendously.

I feel it is important that we do not get into a trap however, of "only" desiring the use of Frankincense for cases of tumors and cancer. It has become a knee-jerk response, for anyone within the essential oils world to shout out "Frankincense" as soon as these conditions are mentioned. But, we are greatly cheating ourselves when we focus on its use as a single. By combining Frankincense with other essential oils that are high in potential anti-cancer benefits, we will exponentially increase our possibility for results.

In clinical practice, Frankincense has been used with newborns of every species, even when they are only minutes old. We have literally had Frankincense on the towels and hands of those who are handed a puppy from a C-Section procedure – making Frankincense one of the first things they are exposed to once they are removed from their mother's womb. It is purely magnificent to be able to change an abnormal birth situation, into a thing of beauty. Anointing the umbilical cords of kittens, puppies, foals, calves, and chickens has become routine for our farm, but instead of with Frankincense alone, now includes use within a diluted Body Supportive Blend or Three Part Blend. Water-based diffusion of Frankincense as a single or within a Three Part Blend can be performed around eggs, nests, and birthing areas to further expose animals. It is a general guideline for me, that if it is a baby of any sort, Frankincense should be included in its life!

Frankincense also appears to magnify and enhance the effects of other essential oils when they are used concurrently. Synergy of essential oils is commonly discussed these days, and it is true what Aristotle is quoted to have said, "The whole is greater than the sum of its parts."

Birds & Exotics: Frankincense has been used in many, many ways in all animals: butterflies have dipped their feet into it, honey bees have had cotton ball diffusers placed within their bee hives, birds have been misted with water-based solutions, fish have had it added to their aquariums, it has been ingested in large amounts in many species, rabbits and guinea pigs have been pet with it, and it has been diffused in a variety of ways.

The most suggested ways to use Frankincense with these species include the use within Three Part Blends for water-based diffusion and for diluted topical applications. Use within the Small Animal Supportive Blend is also highly recommended. Other methods include adding 1 drop (or more) to 1 liter of drinking water, adding 1 drop (or more) to 1 tablespoon of food, water misting with 4 drops (or more) added to 4 ounces (120 mL) of distilled water, application via Petting (diluted), direct application (neat or diluted), and even indirect diffusion with Frankincense on objects, cage papers, or other items in the environment. Frankincense remains an incredibly safe essential oil, that has been used in high amounts in these species. However, it is still advisable to start with lower amounts and gradually increase the amount of Frankincense that the animal is exposed to. While larger amounts and more aggressive routes of administration may be suggested, we have found clinically that they just are not necessary, and for some may carry adverse effects. For example, start with diffusing 3-4 drops in a water-based diffuser in an open room. If the exotic animal tolerates that, you can either increase the amounts of drops added, increase the length of exposure, or move towards a caging or tenting situation of diffusion. Likewise with a water spritzer, begin with 4 drops in a recipe, and you can gradually increase to 5-6 drops in the recipe if the condition warrants it.

Cats: All of the previous methods can be used with cats. The most common ways Frankincense is used with cats are: addition into the Feline Supportive Blend, via Petting (diluted), adding to litter box recipes, water-based diffusion including caging and tenting, mixing into foods, giving orally via capsule (diluted), giving directly in the mouth (they enjoy this less), direct application to tumors (neat or diluted), direct application to skin (neat or diluted), and ingestion via grooming after application. For oral use of Frankincense in cats, the best suggestion is to rely on the normal grooming practices of an applied diluted topical blend containing Frankincense. If further oral administration is desired, you will likely start with very small amounts of oil (toothpick dip) mixed into canned or moist foods. As the cat accepts the lesser amount, you can gradually increase how much is added to the food. Smaller empty gel capsules can be obtained from health food stores and pharmacies, and can be filled with Frankincense in carrier oil to be "pilled" into the cat. Directly dripping the Frankincense into the mouth of a cat has been done, however they often drool and salivate profusely, and quite honestly, unless a severe emergency with absolutely no other options available, this method is highly unnecessary. With most cats, the act of "pilling" or dripping an essential oil into their mouth, is not likely to be greeted with joy for long, and indeed we have seen over use of these routes, which have caused gastrointestinal "burn out". While I am still quite impressed at the safety level demonstrated, in light of the extreme administrations I have witnessed by well-meaning pet parents – we just do not have to do these things in order to help our companions.

For cats who need a more chronic and consistent exposure to Frankincense, my preference is to find many easy and small ways to layer their exposures to Frankincense, instead of trying to shove a pill down their throat. I like to find multiple methods that the individual finds acceptable, or you will soon have your cat continually hiding under the bed when they see you coming. In severe conditions, such as cancer, layering your methods of application can be the best way to ensure higher levels of "cat friendly" exposure. For example a cat experienced water-based diffusion on an almost continual basis, with a variety of blends containing Frankincense. Then, Frankincense can also be included in their daily exposure to a litter box recipe within their litter box. Applications of the Feline Supportive Blend with Frankincense could be completed daily, and in some cases even more frequently. Tolerated amounts could be mixed into foods.

That being said, if I truly felt a condition called for it, and there was ample evidence to show responses without harm, I will gladly force a capsule of Frankincense "down my cats throat" whether they like it or not. Yet, if I can achieve results with multiple cat friendly methods, eliminating the need to use more aggressive measures is in the cats' best interest.

If oral use of Frankincense is deemed necessary through work with your veterinarian, start with very low amounts ideally mixed into foods or carrier oils as a buffer. Gradually increase amounts as your cat tolerates it. When placing into a capsule or directly dripping into the mouth, start with 1 drop (we always recommend diluted in a carrier oil), once or twice a day. Depending on the severity of the situation, more Frankincense may be chosen to be given straightaway. Many cats enjoy eating raw organic coconut oil, and we have been successful in mixing some essential oils into this for direct ingestion or by mixing it into foods for consumption. Maximum levels for Frankincense use have not been established; and we have witnessed up to 10 drops (or more) per day of Frankincense given in severe cases of cancer. It is ideal to split the daily amount into 3-4 doses throughout the day. Administering these levels of oral Frankincense is most likely to be achieved only with capsule administration, and should always be considered carefully and with full cooperation and monitoring with a veterinarian.

Dogs & Larger: All of the previous methods discussed can be used for dogs, horses, and large animals. Favorite methods of exposure remain with water-based diffusion or diluted topical applications of Three Part Blends. In severe cases of cancer, air diffusion has been used in all methods including caging and tenting, although I strongly recommend starting with water-based diffusion. Dogs are much more likely to eat higher levels of Frankincense within their foods, and are much easier to give a capsule to. Horses can have their bottom lip pulled out, and the oil dumped into the little pocket that is created. Frankincense is well used when included in the Canine or Large Animal Support Blends. Direct neat application of the oil to tumors and skin is generally tolerated. Use within water-mists and shampoos is also an excellent way to use Frankincense.

With tumors, it is important to recognize that many will look much worse before they look better. Tumors such as Sarcoids in horses or Mast Cell Tumors in dogs may go through stages of death and irritation before they resolve. For the most part, I am comfortable with this happening, however it solely depends on if the animal itself is comfortable with the event. Tumors growing, itching, weeping, burning, or being chewed at may warrant a lighter approach until the body can catch up with the rejection of the cancer. Though, this decision is best made on an individual basis and with veterinary advice regarding the severity of the condition at hand.

For oral use of Frankincense, extremely large amounts have been consumed by dogs and larger animals. In the past, the amount of Frankincense that was ingested was based more on the owner's financial budget, and less on the actual maximum amount that could be consumed. However, with time, we have not noted an additional benefit that directly corresponds to the excessive amounts given orally. For example, we were no more likely to reverse a cancer situation in a dog getting two drops per day, versus 5mL per day. And in reality, we saw cases of gastrointestinal irritation and "burn out" occur from the high amounts of essential oils being given orally.

My preference now is to layer our exposures to Frankincense when we desire the use to be high. I heard one human aromatherapist call this "live embalming" – which made me absolutely giggle. But I think in a way this is how I view layering of application methods. I want the potentially beneficial essential oil to penetrate deeply and through many tissues throughout the body. I also want to optimize all routes of absorption – so having some avoid first pass metabolism by being inhaled, having some absorbed through the skin on a slower more consistent rate, and possibly having some rectally or orally administered, ensures that I have multiple areas and multiple differences in metabolism to benefit by. I would not want a cancer case to "only" rely on the use of Frankincense alone, but I also would not like a cancer case to rely on exposure to the Frankincense to be only by ingestion of a capsule. Therefore, exposures should be layered, with diffusion, topical applications, possible oral administrations or rectal administrations, etc.

When a veterinarian deems it beneficial to attempt administering higher levels of Frankincense orally, a general guideline would be to approach an end point ingestion of 10 drops per 20 pounds (9 kg) of body weight twice a day. Although, there have been many dogs who have easily consumed over 5 times this amount without toxicity. This sort of aggressive protocol is of course mainly used for severe cases of cancer. With more stable and less aggressive forms of cancer or tumors, starting with low amounts and gradually increasing the amounts given until effects are seen is suggested. Although very large volumes of Frankincense can be administered, some situations respond to quite low amounts, and it would be wasteful to use excessively more essential oil than is actually needed for an animal.

For oral use of Frankincense in large animals – there has been very large amounts given without apparent harm. Although, it also did not appear to carry with it the same large benefits as the dose. A general guideline would be to approach an end point ingestion of 10 drops per 100-200 pounds (45-90 kg) of body weight per day for severe cases of cancer. Thankfully, we see responses in animals with much less being administered, so please never feel that being able to give only one or two drops per day is not a worthwhile endeavor. I have been amazed at what only one drop of Frankincense can do for a huge animal such as a horse. Never underestimate the power of a drop of oil.

Frankincense (Boswellia frereana)

This Frankincense tends to carry higher levels of α-pinene than the other species. It can be commonly found on the essential oil market, and is regarded more so for skin care properties. This oil is not used for veterinary aromatic medicine, and Boswellia carterii is suggested.

Frankincense, Sacred (Boswellia sacra)

Sacred Frankincense is relatively new to the world of Frankincense oil, and has already met with a bit of controversy. Whether it is truly a novel species or not, this version of Frankincense seems to be a bit more powerful than "regular" Boswellia carterii and is sometimes reported to be much more emotionally and spiritually connecting. For some animals, it can be a bit overwhelming and my preference remains to use Boswellia carterii for work with veterinary aromatic medicine. Sacred Frankincense especially became popular through promotion through large essential oil companies, and now many suppliers have made a Boswellia sacra available for purchase. For the most part, it would appear that Boswellia sacra can be used similarly to Boswellia carterii, and may indeed be from the same plant. However, my preference is still to use Boswellia carterii with animals.

Frankincense (Boswellia serrata)

This Frankincense is from India, and may contain higher levels of α-thujone within its constituent profile than other species. While there is quite a lot of research to show that Boswellia serrata gum resin shows promise as an anti-inflammatory, analgesic, diuretic, and anti-cancer agent – the essential oil remains less researched and also less used within the world of Veterinary Aromatic Medicine. The use of Boswellia carterii is suggested.

Galangal (Alpinia galanga)
Also called Siamese Ginger, this oil is not currently recommended for use within Veterinary Aromatic Medicine. Galangal is also an essential oil with GRAS status.

Galbanum (Ferula gummosa)
This essential oil has not been used extensively with animals. While it may be appropriate for water-based diffusion, it is not currently recommended for use within Veterinary Aromatic Medicine.

Garlic (Allium sativum)
While garlic itself has a lot of health properties, the essential oil is incredibly strong. While there may be clear benefits to the oral administration of Garlic oil it is not recommended for use with animals at this time.

Geranium (Pelargonium graveolens)
Geranium is an oil which can be used for many purposes in the animal kingdom. Hepatitis, Fatty Liver Disease, skin conditions, ringworm, Herpes infections, hormone balancing, liver and pancreas stimulation, and dilation of bile ducts for liver detoxification. Emotionally it helps to release negative memories and eases nervous tension. Used less as a single it is widely used in blends and products for animals. Geranium has GRAS status.

You may note variations in the geranium oils available, most notably Rose Geranium (Pelargonium roseum), Reunion or Bourbon Geranium, etc... For the most part, these may often be used interchangeably. However, many companies may market their geranium incorrectly, listing different species without a true understanding of which oil is which. Many Rose Geranium products on the market, I find to be of poor quality. I purely source geranium based on the highest quality available, and typically prefer a Bourbon Geranium (Pelargonium graveolens) for work with Veterinary Aromatic Medicine.

Birds: In birds, Geranium by itself has not been used widely at this time, however in conditions such as Fatty Liver Disease, Geranium is likely to be of aid. Birds have been more consistently exposed to Geranium through the water-based diffusion of blends. The following methods are suggestions for use in birds, however, please note that these methods have not been used in high numbers of birds at this time. For birds water-based diffusion of Geranium (1-4 drops in a diffuser) or within Three Part Blends is suggested. The addition of 1 drop to 1 tablespoon of natural ointments for the application to feet would be appropriate. It is also likely that this oil can be used in drinking water (1 drop per liter) or mixed into foods. The use of Geranium within a water spritzer is likely to be very successful. Starting with only 1 drop of Geranium to 4 ounces (120 mL) of distilled water, or with adding 1 drop of Geranium to the Feather Spray Recipe would be recommended starting points. The addition of Geranium to the Small Animal Supportive Blend would also be appropriate. Before using Geranium in birds, it is first recommended to have explored the use of other more commonly administered oils.

Exotics: All of the previously mentioned methods could be used with exotic pets as well. Exotic pets have certainly been exposed to Geranium in much higher levels than birds, and have a wider range of options for its use. These methods are recommended: water-based diffusion, addition into Small Animal Supportive Blends, use in Three Part Blends via water-based diffusion or diluted topical applications, addition into drinking water (1 drop per liter), addition into foods, direct application (diluted – especially in cases of ringworm), water spritzers, and adding to aquariums and soaking water. Where oral ingestion is considered, dilute 1 drop of Geranium oil to 2 mL of Coconut Oil. Using the diluted solution, give 1 drop once to twice a day, starting with very low amounts, and gradually increasing to the recommended amount. This can be mixed into foods or given directly when possible.

Cats: All of the previously mentioned techniques could be used with cats. The most common ways Geranium would be used for a feline are: water-based diffusion via a Three Part Blend, topical applications of a Three Part Blend (diluted), addition into the Feline Supportive Blend, Petting (diluted), litter box blends, and direct application (neat or diluted) especially in cases of ringworm. Oral administration could be considered in severe cases of Fatty Liver Disease, and would begin with the same recommendations as stated above. Oral administration of Geranium has not been used widely in cats at this time, and careful monitoring with a veterinarian is recommended. It is most likely, that ingestion via grooming of diluted blends, is more than adequate use for cats. When possible, selection of more cat appropriate oils is suggested in place of Geranium.

Dogs & Larger: All of the previously mentioned methods can be used for these animals as well. Stronger concentrations of Geranium can easily be used for direct topical application, especially in cases of ringworm where neat application is recommended. Addition into the Canine or Large Animal Body Supportive Blends or use within Three Part Blends is especially recommended for Herpes infections. When oral use is considered for dogs – dilute 1 part Geranium with

10 parts carrier oil – use 1 drop or more of this solution twice a day, for each 20 pounds (9 kg) of body weight. For horses and others starting with 1 drop per 500 pounds (225 kg) of body weight, given orally twice a day is a good starting point. Monitor responses and adjust according to individual need.

Ginger (Zingiber officinale)

Ginger is most commonly used within blends for use with animals for all types of gastrointestinal issues, and has GRAS status. This oil is most commonly used for nausea (especially car sickness) in dogs, and may help reduce stomach ulcers, H. pylori infections, intestinal spasms, and inhibit Aspergillus (fungus). Ginger is well indicated in cases of abnormal GI motility, whether too much or too little. Ginger is also wonderful for warming and anti-inflammatory responses, as well as bronchodilation. It is important to note that Ginger also contains anti-coagulant properties. Care must be taken with Ginger oil in animals who are bleeding, have a tendency to bleed, or are on any sort of anti-coagulant therapy. The over use of essential oil(s) that have anti-coagulant actions, especially in oral administration, can produce a temporary and dose dependent increase in bleeding and reduction of clotting. Ginger is also wonderfully warming and helpful to muscular conditions, it should not be underestimated in contribution to animal athletes, and as a musculoskeletal aid.

Birds & Exotics: Ginger is mainly used within Three Part Blends for water-based diffusion or diluted topical applications. Use within the Small Animal Supportive Blend is suggested.

Cats: Ginger is mainly used within Three Part Blends for water-based diffusion, diluted applications topically, or within litter box recipes. Use within the Feline Supportive Blend is most suggested.

Dogs: Ginger is mainly used within blends for dogs, however Ginger as a single oil is used commonly for car sickness, and sometimes may have a stronger effect for this condition than a blend alone. While I still recommend trying a Three Part Blend first due to the synergy of other oils, it is not uncommon to use Ginger as a single for this situation. Ginger will mainly be used within Three Part Blends for water-based diffusion, or diluted topical applications. Petting onto the stomach (diluted), diffused directly or indirectly (for example placing a few drops on a cotton ball inside of the transport crate), or direct oral administration can be considered. Ginger is an excellent addition to the Canine Supportive Blend to provide routine health and function to the gastrointestinal system. Dripping the oil directly into the mouth (diluted) to achieve buccal absorption, seems to be the most effective method for severe nausea. For oral use with dogs – dilute 1 part Ginger with 4 parts carrier oil – use 1 drop or more of this solution, for each 20 pounds (9 kg) of body weight. For dogs who are approximately 50 pounds (23 kg) and larger, generally one neat drop is given orally in total – however dilution into a "serving" of carrier oil is still suggested. Oral administration can be repeated multiple times as needed for nausea, generally every 10-20 minutes. Due to the anti-coagulant potential of Ginger, a maximum dose of 3 neat drops per 20 pounds of dog should likely be followed. Needless to say, if you have approached this recommended maximum of drops, and your dog is still nauseated, a different oil is well indicated!

Horses & Larger: Ginger is most commonly used within blends for these animals, however can be used as a single when desired. Ginger would most commonly be used by addition to drinking water, addition to foods, used within the Large Animal Supportive Blend, applied via Petting (diluted), or used within Three Part Blends. For ingestion, 1 drop per 500 pounds (225 kg) of body weight, given orally twice a day is a good starting point. Monitor responses and adjust according to individual need.

Goldenrod (Solidago Canadensis)

Goldenrod is not commonly used for animals at this time. However, its properties indicate it may be helpful for Fatty Liver Disease, liver conditions, urinary tract and bladder conditions, hypertension, and as a diuretic. Although the use of other more commonly used oils would be recommended first, Goldenrod is an oil that could be called upon for difficult or non-responsive cases. Working closely with a veterinarian to monitor blood work and responses, when using uncharted essential oils is wise.

Birds & Exotics: Goldenrod has not been used extensively in these species at this time. In cases where other essential oils have not yielded sufficient results, or where the severity of the case calls for the addition of this essential oil, the following methods would be appropriate to use: water-based diffusion within Three Part Blends.

Cats: The same comments as noted for Birds & Exotics is true for cats as well. The following methods would be most suitable for use in cats when needed: adding to the Feline Supportive Blend, water-based diffusion within Three Part Blends, and addition into litter box recipes. Oral administration would be achieved through grooming of the Feline Supportive Blend, it is unlikely that further oral administration would be advised.

Dogs & Larger: Although Goldenrod has not commonly been used in these animals, dogs and larger animals can often easily be transitioned into the use of more novel oils, by scaling their usage to match human recommendations. Addition into the Canine or Large Animal Supportive Blends or use within Three Part Blends for water-based diffusion or diluted topical applications is suggested.

Grapefruit (Citrus paradisi)

Grapefruit oil is indicated for use with animals for conditions such as tumors, fatty tumors (lipomas), cancer, obesity, detoxification, diuresis, fluid retention, liver conditions, cognitive dysfunction, senility, and anxiety. Grapefruit is a photosensitizing oil, so application is recommended to sites that will not be exposed to direct sunlight or full spectrum UV lights within 12 hours. For example with horses, the use of Grapefruit oil can be designated to the underside of the belly. Because of fur and feathers, we have yet to witness a photosensitive side effect with the use of these oils, but that is not to say it cannot happen. We are better off to heed the warning, than to regret it later.

Another common question regarding Grapefruit oil is if it interacts with medications. Many people are told to avoid drinking grapefruit juice or eating grapefruit while they are on prescription medications. It does appear that the Grapefruit Essential Oil is different in action than the meat or juice of the fruit itself, and I have known many humans and animals who use the oil right alongside of other medications with no ill effects. In veterinary medicine, it is actually a recommended practice to strategically use grapefruit juice to effectively reduce the amounts of prescription drugs that are needed for a patient. Many other resources now support this evidence as well such as *Medicinal Essential Oils* (Johnson, 2017) and *Essential Oil Safety* (Tisserand and Young, 2nd Edition 2014). I have no reservations using Grapefruit oil together with prescription medications. Grapefruit oil has GRAS status.

Birds & Exotics: Grapefruit oil is used in the following ways: water-based diffusion, addition to drinking water (1 drop or more per liter), addition to foods, addition into Small Animal Supportive Blend, used within Three Part Blends for water-based diffusion or diluted topical applications, adding to aquarium or soaking water, water misting (4 drops or more in 4 ounces (120 mL) of distilled water, application to perches (avian), Petting (diluted, non-avian), direct application (diluted, especially to fatty tumors), and direct ingestion when desired (rodents, ferrets, and such licking the oil off of our hands). For oral ingestion, there really has not been a maximum amount witnessed. For most animals, the strong taste of the essential oil will be the limiting factor on how much we add to food or water. Starting with small amounts (toothpick dips) and gradually increasing the amount based on taste preference and response is recommended.

Cats: All of the methods mentioned for Birds & Exotics can be used for cats, and some cats may drink or ingest Grapefruit oil as well. Cat friendly methods for the use of Grapefruit oil include: water-based diffusion within Three Part Blends, addition to the Feline Supportive Blend, and addition to litter box recipes. Keep in mind that with topical applications, cats will ingest certain levels of the essential oil when they groom.

Dogs & Larger: All of the methods discussed can be used as well. The most common methods of use will be water-based diffusion within Three Part Blends, diluted topical applications within Three Part Blends, addition to the Canine or Large Animal Supportive Blends, as a direct application (diluted), and oral administration. For large barns or arenas, air style diffusion may be considered. When oral use is considered, higher concentrations of Grapefruit oil are likely to be tolerated, and generally can easily be given in foods. For oral use in dogs – 1 drop or more can be given twice a day, for each 20 pounds (9 kg) of body weight. Start with a smaller amount, dilute within food or carrier oil, and gradually increase as needed. For horses and others starting with 1 drop per 100-200 pounds (45-90 kg) of body weight, given orally twice a day is a good starting point. Monitor responses and adjust according to individual need.

Helichrysum (Helichrysum italicum)
Also called Immortelle, Everlasting, or Helichrysum angustifolium (synonym), Helichrysum is surely one of my favorite oils. It truly is miraculous and worthy of use in almost every condition, and has obtained GRAS status. You will never be wrong selecting Helichrysum, and it has been used in many ways, in all forms of animals. Helichrysum is indicated in cases of blood clots as an anticoagulant, but is also used in cases of hemorrhage, bleeding, and bruising. This is the interesting thing with many natural remedies, is that they tend to bring the body to a point of homeostasis. Whatever is needed within the body appears to be honored. Much like eating food that nourishes certain aspects of health, we are merely providing the body with the tools it needs for health, and the body mainly decides on what to do with those tools, and when.

In animals, Helichrysum is especially indicated for nerve regeneration and neurologic conditions, hearing impairment, circulatory and blood vessel disorders, heart disease, blood clots, liver disease, hypertension, chelation of chemicals, toxin exposure, poisoning, vaccination detoxification, healing of lacerations and wounds, for control of pain, and as a topical anesthetic. There is not much that Helichrysum does not contribute to, and it falls into a category of "must have" oils in my opinion.

Helichrysum is often included within pain recipes intended for oral use in animals. Within blends with Copaiba and/or Myrrh, there seems to be an enormous synergistic effect for pain management, and is well tolerated by many species.

Diffusing Helichrysum in situations of lung bruising or trauma (pulmonary contusions), such as in animals who have been hit by a car, has proved incredibly helpful in recovery. Caging or Tenting with water-based diffusion to gain penetration of the lung tissues, works wonderfully. Combining this diffusion with oils that also aid in oxygenation, reduction of inflammation, and healing (Cedarwood, Copaiba, Frankincense) provides nothing short of near miraculous results in our veterinary hospital. I have witnessed severe lung trauma reverse in 12 hours, where typically bruising of the lungs would continue to worsen for the first 24 hours.

Birds & Exotics: Helichrysum has been used in many ways in all species. Water-based diffusion (with caging or tenting), addition to Small Animal Supportive Blends, inclusion in Three Part Blends for diffusion or dilute topical applications, in drinking water (1 drop or more per liter), in foods, direct oral use, in water spritzers (starting with 1 drop per 4 ounces (120 mL) of distilled water and working up to 4 or more drops), mixed into natural ointments (1 or more drops in 1 tablespoon), adding 1-4 drops into the Feather Spray Recipe, adding 1-5 drops into 2 mL of carrier oil and using for topical application, via Petting (diluted for non-avian species), via Perches and indirect exposure, in soaking water and aquariums, added to shampoos or rinses, and directly topical (neat or diluted). For oral consumption, often 2 drops is added to 2 mL of carrier oil, and 1 drop or more of this diluted solution is given orally, usually 2-3 times a day. This diluted solution can also be mixed into foods as well. The animal is monitored for response, and given repeated doses as needed. The concentration of the solution can be increased as needed as well. Many respond to this initial dilution, and maximum limits of Helichrysum ingestion have not been determined. It does appear that there is an extremely wide range of safety with this oil.

Case Example: A bird with a broken wing was given a solution of 2 drops of Helichrysum, 1 drop of Copaiba, and 1 drop of Myrrh in 2 mL of carrier oil for pain management. Approximately 1 drop of this solution was administered by syringe, directly into its mouth, 2-3 times a day. The bird experienced so much comfort from this remedy, that traditional pain medications were not needed, and the little bird was difficult to keep quiet and rested! Please also see the Myrrh essential oil description for more information on this Pain Recipe.

Cats: All of the previously mentioned techniques can be used with cats as well. Helichrysum does appear to be best tolerated when added to the Feline Supportive Blend for topical use in cats, this also provides for adequate oral exposure and ingestions for most situations and needs. Addition into litter box recipes is well tolerated. Inclusion into Three Part Blends for water-based diffusion or diluted topical applications work very well.

When pain management or clinical support is needed for a severe condition in cats, often 1 full drop can be given orally for an average sized cat at one time. Dilution of this drop is suggested in carrier oil prior to administration, however, neat drops have been given for buccal absorption. Even kittens weighing less than 1 pound (0.5 kg) have received a maximal dose of 3 drops of neat Helichrysum (diluted) orally at one time, with no ill effects. Cats will generally salivate in response to the oral administration of the oil. This is fairly expected, although not all cats do this. While these recommendations describe maximum use that could be considered, it should be in cooperation and with monitoring by your veterinarian. Oral consumption due to normal grooming, is often more than adequate for most cases.

Dogs & Larger: Helichrysum can be used in all of the ways mentioned previously as well as included within Canine and Large Animal Supportive Blends, direct topical application (neat or diluted), and oral administration. Use within Three Part Blends is preferred. For oral use in dogs – 1 drop or more can be given twice a day, for each 50 pounds (22 kg) of body weight. Start with a smaller amount, and gradually increase as needed. For horses and others starting with 1 drop per 200 pounds (90 kg) of body weight, given orally twice a day is a good starting point. Monitor responses and adjust according to individual need.

Helichrysum splendidum
Also called Peta, this oil has made its debut in the aromatherapy world, likely marketed by some to obtain sales through the name "Helichrysum". It is not used with animals, nor is it recommended for use with animals at this time.

Hemp (Cannabis sativa)
Do not confuse the essential oil of Hemp with the cold pressed or carrier oil of hemp seed, nor with "CBD" oil. These are all different. Hemp essential oil contains basically no THC levels (the part of Cannabis that is psychoactive), and does not contain CBD either. Hemp essential oil does contain respectable levels of β-caryophyllene and sometimes Myrcene making it anti-inflammatory. However, Copaiba is likely a much better oil to select when these properties are desired. CBD oil (which is not Hemp essential oil) should be collected by CO_2 extraction, so that it contains these heavier weight plant extracts.

Hinoki (Chamaecyparis obtusa)
While I did name my cat after this oil, it is not commonly used with animals at this time. While water-based diffusion is likely to be of no concern, it is not recommended for use in Veterinary Aromatic Medicine at this time.

Holy Basil (Ocimum sanctum)
As an oil rather high in Eugenol, it may be prone to causing sensitization. Research has shown potential effects on Leishmaniasis, blood pressure and platelet aggregation, decreasing cholesterol, and possesses anti-inflammatory properties. Holy Basil is not widely used with animals, and is not suggested for use with Veterinary Aromatic Medicine at this time.

Hops (Humulus lupulus)
Research shows that Hops essential oil may have anti-inflammatory and analgesic properties, and would be quite beneficial for allergies. This oil is not used commonly with animals at this time, and is not suggested for use with Veterinary Aromatic Medicine at this time. Hops essential oil contains β-caryophyllene and has GRAS status. Copaiba is an excellent oil to consider for replacement.

Hyssop (Hyssopus officinalis)

Hyssop has many indications for use in animals, and is generally regarded as a purging oil. It is reported to be a decongestant and diuretic, as well antimicrobial. Hyssop tends to be a mild oil topically, but when taken internally can be quite aggressive.

Hyssop is indicated whenever you would like to "expel" something from the body – whether it is a toxin, poison, respiratory mucus, parasites, viruses, or bacteria. Common conditions that would call for the single oil of Hyssop include snake bites, tick paralysis, poisoning, parasites, and viral infections. There is a cautionary statement in some references to avoid the use of Hyssop with epilepsy. Most reported cases of convulsions came from excessive oral use of this oil, and we have not witnessed any problems with the use of Hyssop within blends and when used appropriately. Hyssop is not recommended for oral use beyond light exposure through grooming. In animals with seizures, and who may excessively consume applied oils, you may wish to exercise increased caution. I prefer the use of Hyssop within blends, to further "dilute" the total exposure to this oil.

Birds & Exotics: Hyssop as a single has not been used commonly in these species. The most recommended uses of Hyssop would be to include the oil within the Small Animal Supportive Blend, or within Three Part Blends for water-based diffusion. In cases of severe need, water misting (1 drop to 4 ounces) could be considered – however it is important to recognize that these techniques have not been used commonly for these animals at this time, and close veterinary monitoring would be important.

Cats: The most common ways to use Hyssop with cats is by addition to the Feline Supportive Blend. Inclusion in Three Part Blends for water-based diffusion or diluted topical applications, as well as within litter box recipes can be considered.

Dogs & Larger: The most common ways to use Hyssop in these animals is by inclusion into the Canine or Large Animal Supportive Blends, within Three Part Blends for water-based diffusion or diluted topical applications. If oral use of an oil is desired for poisoning or toxin situations (snake bite), Helichrysum is the suggested oil.

Jasmine (Jasminum officinale)

Jasmine is an absolute and not a true essential oil, and is also frequently adulterated. Due to the fact that absolutes may contain traces of solvents, they are not recommended for use with Veterinary Aromatic Medicine or with animals (even if just with diffusion). Oddly enough however, Jasmine obtains GRAS status.

Juniper Berry (Juniperus communis)

Juniper is indicated as a digestive cleanser and stimulant, for liver conditions, kidney conditions, to promote the excretion of toxins, promote nerve regeneration, for fluid retention, and for urinary infections. Juniper Berry oil has GRAS status. Many of the reports for adverse issues with Juniper essential oil may be related to its oxidized, and therefore more harmful form. It is imperative that fresh and well stored Juniper is used with animals.

Birds: Juniper has not been used widely with birds at this time. Water-based diffusion within Three Part Blends in an open or small room is the recommended method of exposure.

Exotics: Juniper is recommended within Three Part Blends for water-based diffusion or diluted topical applications. It can also be added to the Small Animal Supportive Blend, or for ferrets used within the Feline Supportive Blend. Oral use of Juniper has not been established in exotic animals at this time except for normal grooming exposure.

Cats: Juniper is recommended within Three Part Blends for water-based diffusion or diluted topical applications. It can also be added to the Feline Supportive Blend. Oral use of Juniper has not been established in felines at this time beyond normal grooming exposure.

Dogs & Larger: Juniper is recommended within Three Part Blends for water-based diffusion or diluted topical applications. Addition into the Canine or Large Animal Supportive Blends is an excellent suggestion. If oral use is considered for these animals, it is reserved for when topical applications have failed to yield sufficient results. For oral use in dogs – 1 drop of Juniper is diluted in 5 drops of carrier oil. 1 drop or more of this dilution can be given twice a day, for each 50 pounds (22 kg) of body weight. Start with a smaller amount, and gradually increase as needed. For horses and others, starting with 1 drop per 500 pounds (225 kg) of body weight, given orally twice a day is a good starting point. Monitor responses and adjust according to individual need.

Labdanum (See Cistus)

Laurus Nobilis (L. nobilis)

Laurus nobilis is also known as Bay Laurel. Laurus nobilis is indicated for nerve regeneration, nerve pain, loss of appetite, gingivitis, viral infections, as an anticonvulsant, for respiratory infections, to stimulate lymph flow, expel excess mucus, and especially for bacterial infections with Staphylococcus, Streptococcus, E. Coli, and Pseudomonas. Emotionally Laurus nobilis is said to enhance confidence and aid in focus and concentration.

Research indicates that Laurus nobilis should be looked into further for cases of myasthenia gravis, dementia and cognitive disorders, herpes virus, analgesia, and cancer.

Birds & Exotics: Laurus nobilis has not been used extensively with birds or exotic animals at this time, however it has been used within diluted topical blends in low concentrations, as well as within Three Part Blends used for water-based diffusion. When creating blends with Laurus nobilis, it is suggested to be used at a lower total addition than the other parts of the blend.

Cats: Most commonly Laurus nobilis is used via addition to the Feline Supportive Blend, or via water-based diffusion of a Three Part Blend. Less common methods of feline use include addition to the litter box and addition to Coconut Oil to rub gums affected with gingivitis. The most cat friendly methods are likely to be addition to the Feline Supportive Blend, with oral exposure and subsequent ingestion through normal grooming practices. While Laurus nobilis has been used orally as an antibiotic for cats with urinary tract infections and has been applied to abscesses directly (neat or diluted); further oral use and aggressive topical use of this oil should only be considered for difficult and critical cases, and would be started very slowly, with less than one drop given per day, and gradually increasing in amount. Veterinary monitoring with blood work and other laboratory tests (urinalysis) is advised before, during, and after administration.

Dogs & Larger: The use of Laurus nobilis can generally be much more widely used for these animals. The most common uses are within Three Part Blends for water-based diffusion and diluted topical applications, addition into the Canine or Large Animal Supportive Blends, and direct topical application (diluted).

If oral use for dogs is considered, 1 drop of Laurus nobilis can be diluted with 10 drops of carrier oil. 1 drop or more of this dilution can be given twice a day, for each 50 pounds (22 kg) of body weight. Start with a smaller amount, and gradually increase as needed. For horses and others, starting with 1 drop per 200 pounds (90 kg) of body weight, given orally twice a day is a good starting point. Monitor responses and adjust according to individual need.

For severe infections and conditions, Laurus nobilis has historically been given at a rate of 3 drops orally, 6 times per day, for animals 50 pounds (22 kg) and larger – although this is likely to be excessive in nature.

Lavandin (Lavandula x intermedia)
Lavandin is a hybrid of Lavender, and has obtained GRAS status. It generally will contain camphor, and is not recommended for use with animals.

Lavender (Lavandula angustifolia)
Lavender is one of the most adulterated and synthetically created essential oils on the market today. Very few available Lavender oils are pure enough to be called medical grade, or qualify for use in animals. Lavender is incredibly mild and well suited for use with all species of animal. It has been used extensively in even the most fragile of creatures. Lavender is especially indicated for skin conditions, wound healing, ringworm and other fungal skin infections, for muscular concerns, for calming effects, for burns and frostbite, and high blood pressure. Lavender has GRAS status.

Lavender also has significant research with dementia, and is highly indicated for use with Cognitive Dysfunction, anxiety, post-traumatic stress, poor sleeping, and other emotional concerns.

Oddly enough, I often hear reports of people who say that Lavender should not be used around asthmatics, while research clearly shows that Lavender suppresses respiratory inflammation, and is well indicated for allergy, respiratory irritations, and asthmatics. My theory on this mindset is purely that the cautions have been equated to poor, adulterated, extended, synthetic, or fragrance grade Lavender oils. In clinical use of Lavender, when screened appropriately for animal and veterinary use, water-based diffusion of this oil has been quite helpful for asthma, collapsing trachea irritation, kennel cough, and all sorts of upper respiratory and sinus irritations and infections.

Birds & Exotics: Lavender can be used in many ways including; water-based diffusion (including caging and tenting), use within Small Animal Supportive Blend, in water spritzers (up to 20 drops per 4 ounces of distilled water), in soaking waters, pools, and aquariums, Petting (dilute or neat in non-avian species), applied to perches (avian), added to drinking water (1 drop or more per liter of water), added to foods (1 drop or more per tablespoon), applied by direct topical application (dilute or neat), added to natural ointments or shampoos (1 drop or more per tablespoon), and by indirect diffusion on cotton balls and cage papers. Lavender is exceptionally suited for use within Three Part Blends both for water-based diffusion or diluted topical applications. The Feather Spray Recipe is by far the most common way to apply Lavender to birds, and is often used as the first line exposure technique for Lavender oil.

Cats: All of the mentioned methods can be used for cats. The most cat friendly methods include use of the Feline Supportive Blend, water-based diffusion alone or within Three Part Blends, and addition to litter box recipes. Petting (neat or diluted) and addition into shampoos and ointments can also be considered. While some cats may or may not enjoy a water-mist, preparations for conditions such as Ringworm, may be water-misted onto the cat for a dispersed coverage of oils if the cat is so willing.

Dogs & Larger: Lavender can be used in any method, and has also been used by air diffusion and direct oral administration. The amounts of Lavender that can be applied safely to these animals are much higher, however usually unnecessary. The most recommended methods of Lavender exposure are water-based diffusion as a single or within a Three Part Blend, diluted topical applications as a single or within a Three Part Blend, use within the Canine or Large Animal Supportive Blends, via a water-misting application, and by addition into shampoos, washes, rinses, or ointments. Often, solutions and preparations created with Lavender, can utilize Lavender in higher total percentages of the blend when desired, and can then create a functional dilution of "hotter" oils for topical use. For example, if one drop of Oregano is added to 30 drops of Lavender, we can still have some benefits of antifungal properties of both oils for spot treatment of Ringworm on a horse, however, the Oregano will not be as strong as if it were applied directly. Starting with smaller amounts, and pre-diluted oil, is always recommended as many animals respond to lesser amounts. However, if needed, much larger quantities can be applied safely.

If oral use is considered for dogs – 1 drop of Lavender can be diluted with 10 drops of carrier oil. A maximum of 1 drop or more of this dilution can be given twice a day, for each 20 pounds (9 kg) of body weight – is suggested. Start with a smaller amount, and gradually increase as needed. For horses and others, starting with 1 drop per 200 pounds (90 kg) of body weight, given orally twice a day is a good starting point. Monitor responses and adjust according to individual need.

Lavender, Spike (Lavandula latifolia)
Spike Lavender is often adulterated, and also contains camphor. While it has obtained GRAS status, it is not recommended for use with animals.

Ledum (Ledum groenlandicum)
Also called Labrador Tea, Greenland Moss, and Rhododendron groenlandicum; Ledum is often used in animals for its benefits to the liver. Conditions such as hepatitis, elevated liver enzymes, fatty liver disease, vaccinosis, ascites, liver cancer, and fluid retention are benefited by Ledum.

Birds & Exotics: Ledum has not been used extensively with birds or exotic animals at this time. The recommended initial method of use would be water-based diffusion within a Three Part Blend (3-4 drops added to a diffuser, in an open room). The addition of Ledum to the Small Animal Supportive Blend would also be suggested when topical use is desired. Ledum has been used in animal research, and if oral use was considered the addition to foods would be most appropriate to start with – adding a toothpick dip or more into 1 tablespoon of food or 1 drop per liter of drinking water. Ledum is likely to be helpful in many forms of liver disease. Monitor cases closely with a veterinarian. It is advisable to only move towards other methods in which to use Ledum, only after water-based diffusion or diluted topical use has not yielded adequate results.

Cats: Cats can use Ledum in all of the ways mentioned for Birds & Exotics. The most cat friendly methods of use include addition into Three Part Blends for water-based diffusion or diluted topical applications, by addition into the Feline Supportive Blend, and by addition into litter box recipes. Oral use should mainly be achieved through normal grooming processes. In severe cases, additional oral use can be considered. Some cats may ingest Ledum in food or water, and monitoring liver values with a veterinarian is important to evaluate how much essential oil is needed. Start with a very small amount, and work your way up to a maximum of 1-2 drops per day. Adjust the amount according to the individual needs and responses. Oral administration beyond grooming, is only recommended when all else has failed, and you are working directly with a veterinarian.

Dogs & Larger: Ledum would most commonly be used through water-based diffusion or diluted topical application of a Three Part Blend, by addition into the Canine or Large Animal Supportive Blends, Petting (diluted), direct topical application (diluted), addition to foods, addition to water, and direct oral administration. Again, oral administration is only deemed necessary if diffusion and topical use has not been adequate. If oral use is considered with dogs – 1 drop of Ledum can be diluted with 10 drops of carrier. 1 drop or more of this dilution can be given two or more times a day, for each 20 pounds (9 kg) of body weight. Start with a smaller amount, and gradually increase as needed. For horses and others, starting with 1 drop per 200 pounds (90 kg) of body weight, given orally twice a day is a good starting point. Monitor responses and adjust according to individual need.

Lemon (Citrus limon)

Lemon oil is widely used in all species, and in many routes. It has a very wide safety margin and has GRAS status. Lemon is particularly used with animals for anti-tumoral properties, immune stimulation, to increase white blood cells, for obesity and lipomas (fatty tumors), for gentle cleansing and detoxification, for anti-bacterial properties, to cleanse the air and reduce disease transmission, for urinary tract infections, hypertension, digestive issues, and anxiety.

Lemon oil is also used to remove sticky substances from animals such as tree sap, medical adhesive tape, or chewing gum. I have found that by applying Lemon oil diluted in Fractionated Coconut Oil to these items, they are easily removed from an animal. Lemon oil can be quite irritating to skin if not diluted, make sure to always dilute for topical use, even if removing adhesive (see more information under Dogs & Larger). Lemon is a photosensitizing oil; avoid applying to skin that will be exposed to sunlight or full spectrum UV light within 12 hours. This oil is used commonly in the Feather Spray for birds, and we have not noted a photosensitizing issue for fully feathered birds at this time. However, I would still advise caution, as many birds using the Feather Spray Recipe are missing feathers and have fully exposed skin. Caution with full and natural sunlight is more likely needed, than with the full spectrum indoor lighting commonly used for birds and reptiles.

Birds & Exotics: Lemon oil has been used in many, many ways: water-based diffusion (including caging and tenting), addition to the Small Animal Supportive Blend, within the Feather Spray Recipe, added to drinking water (1 or more drops per liter), added to foods (generally up to 1 drop per tablespoon), addition to natural ointments and to carrier oils, water spritzers (up to 20 drops per 4 ounces), Petting (diluted non-avian), and allowed to be directly ingested when animals chose to lick the oil off of hands and other items. Lemon is an excellent addition to Three Part Blends for water-based diffusion or diluted topical applications.

Cats: Lemon oil has been used for cats, and without the related concern you will find online and expressed by the media. Please see the chapters discussing cats, oils, and research for more details. The most cat friendly methods for the use of Lemon is water-based diffusion within a Three Part Blend. The addition of Lemon can be considered to the Feline Supportive Blend as well. For sticky substances, diluted topical use would be appropriate – usually in a 1-5% concentration range. Addition to litter box recipes, and other Three Part Blends for diluted topical applications can also be considered. Some cats may ingest Lemon oil in foods or water as described for Birds & Exotics, however ingestion via the normal grooming process is likely to be more than adequate for our needs. We have not noted photosensitivity issues for cats who are fully furred, however the recommendation to apply the oil where the sun will not contact the skin (stomach), is a wise recommendation for cats with outdoor exposure, as well as for use with hairless breeds exposed to direct sunlight.

Dogs & Larger: Lemon is most commonly used in water-based diffusion alone or within Three Part Blends, and is often used within diluted massage recipes for Fatty Tumors (lipomas). Lemon can be included within the Canine and Large Animal Supportive Blends, applied diluted within Three Part Blends, added to shampoos, ointments, or water-mists, and may be considered for addition into foods, direct topical application (diluted), Petting (diluted), and oral administration. Air diffusion has been used in larger barns or areas as well.

Lemon oil applied directly to the skin, should almost always be diluted in a carrier oil, or in the case of a water-mist dispersed heavily. Follow dilution recommendations for your species, however, a 5-10% concentration is common, especially in cases of adhesive removal. Starting with smaller amounts or more diluted oil, is still recommended as many animals respond to lesser amounts. However, if needed, much larger quantities can be applied safely.

For topical applications, blends containing Lemon oil could be applied to the underside of the belly of Goats, Horses, and other Large Animals who may be exposed to the sun. Photosensitivity has not been noted in furred areas, but caution is still a wise idea.

When oral use is considered for dogs – 1 drop of Lemon can be diluted with 10 drops of Coconut Oil. 1 drop or more of this dilution can be given twice a day, for each 20 pounds (9 kg) of body weight. Start with a smaller amount, and gradually increase as needed. For some dogs, approximately 1-2 full drops of Lemon oil will be consumed twice a day in foods, when determined by a veterinarian to be necessary. For horses and others, starting with 1 drop per 200 pounds (90 kg) of body weight, given orally twice a day is a good starting point. Monitor responses and adjust according to individual need.

Lemon Balm (see Melissa)

Lemon Catnip (see Catnip, Lemon)

Lemon Eucalyptus (see Eucalyptus citriodora)

Lemon Myrtle (Backhousia citriodora)
An Australian oil which is commonly used in perfumery and cooking. Caution should be used with topical applications, as it is a strong oil, and can cause irritations. Reports show this oil carries antifungal and antimicrobial properties, and is excellent for freshening, deodorizing, and cleansing the air. Use within Three Part Blends with water-based diffusion is the suggested use of this oil. It has a powerful odor profile, so it is likely to be needed in much lower concentrations within blends. This oil may commonly be adulterated with synthetic citral, so caution with sourcing is advised.

Lemon-Scented Ironbark (Eucalyptus staigeriana)
This lesser-known oil is from Australia, and carries a fresh lemon-type scent. This oil is being used within blends for water-based diffusion most commonly. Use within Three Part Blends for water-based diffusion is suggested use for this oil at this time. This oil is reported to have anti-oxidant, antifungal, and antimicrobial properties, and it is quite pleasant for room freshening, cleansing,

and deodorizing. Apparently, this essential oil was the flavoring ingredient for the "lemon cordial" in Australia for many years, which likely would gain it some sort of ingestion status.

Lemon-Scented Tea Tree (Leptospermum petersonii)

Also called Lemon Tea Tree, this tea tree is not within the Melaleuca family. High in geranial, this Australian essential oil has some research supporting that it lowers plasma insulin and increased glucose tolerance in rats. This oil is most commonly recommended to be used within Three Part Blends for water-based diffusion at this time. There is current use including topical applications within blends to animals as well.

Lemongrass (Cymbopogon flexuosus)

Lemongrass is used with animals for a variety of conditions. It has powerful antifungal action, regenerates connective tissue and ligaments, improves circulation, promotes lymph flow, is anti-inflammatory, antibacterial, and anti-parasitic. It is specifically useful for bladder infections, respiratory and sinus infections, cruciate injuries, muscle injuries, Salmonella, MRSA (Methicillin Resistant Staphylococcus Aureus), fluid retention and edema, digestive issues, and parasites. Lemongrass is a rather "hot" oil when applied to animals topically, and is generally used diluted. Lemongrass is yellow in color, and will stain light and white colored animals temporarily. Lemongrass has GRAS status.

Birds: Lemongrass can be used via water-based diffusion (starting with 2 drops added to the diffuser), including caging and tenting techniques. Most commonly, Lemongrass should be used within Three Part Blends for water-based diffusion or when appropriate, diluted topical applications. Lemongrass can be considered for ingestion, and is generally added to foods, with one or more toothpick dips of oil being added into 1 tablespoon of soft foods. Starting with a small amount, and gradually increasing is recommended. Careful monitoring with a veterinarian, with blood work and laboratory monitoring is wise. Oral use of Lemongrass could kill normal flora of the gastrointestinal tract, so caution is recommended. In very small percentages, Lemongrass has been included within blends that are water-misted onto birds, including parrots and finches. However, I would suggest use of regular Feather Spray Recipes first, only resorting to the addition of Lemongrass in extreme and unresponsive situations.

Exotics: All of the methods in which we use Lemongrass for birds, can also be used for other exotics. With most non-avian exotic animals, Lemongrass can be used in many more ways. Caution is used with exotics who are "hind-gut fermenters" – as the powerful antibacterial action of Lemongrass may overwhelm their natural intestinal flora. Use of gentler essential oils is recommended for Rabbits, Guinea Pigs, and Chinchillas. The addition of 1 drop of Lemongrass to the Small Animal Supportive Blend can be considered, when the use of Lemongrass is deemed necessary. The same methods used for birds, should be used when diluting and adding Lemongrass to foods for exotic animals.

Cats: Lemongrass would most commonly be used within Three Part Blends for water-based diffusion or diluted topical applications. Use of Lemongrass as a single, can include water-based diffusion, Petting (diluted), and direct topical applications (diluted). In general, the addition of 2 drops Lemongrass to the Feline Supportive Blend is suggested for topical use, or to gain oral administration through grooming. Addition to litter box recipes, shampoos, and ointments is also suggested. Oral administrations have been used, but usually as a last resort. Amounts ingested via grooming of diluted blends, are likely to be more than adequate. For additional oral administration 1 drop of Lemongrass is diluted in 10 drops of carrier oil. Give 1 drop of the diluted solution, further diluted into foods, twice a day. Monitor responses and increase the amount given as needed for the individual. Oral administration of Lemongrass as a single oil is generally reserved for when other oils have not been effective.

Dogs & Larger: Lemongrass is more commonly used for these animal species. The most common methods of use include water-based diffusion and diluted topical applications within Three Part Blends, addition into the Canine or Large Animal Supportive Blends, direct topical application (most often diluted), Petting (most often diluted), water and oil misting, addition into ointments, shampoos, and by oral ingestion. When oral use is considered for dogs – 1 drop of Lemongrass can be diluted with 3 drops of carrier oil. 1 drop or more of this dilution is further diluted into foods, and given twice a day, for each 20 pounds (9 kg) of body weight. Start with a smaller amount, and gradually increase as needed. For horses and others, starting with 1 drop per 200 pounds (90 kg) of body weight, given orally twice a day is a good starting point. Monitor responses and adjust according to individual need.

Lime (Citrus aurantifolia)

There are two versions of lime oil that are readily available on the market. Steam Distilled and Cold Pressed. Steam Distilled lime oil is more reminiscent of candy, and does not contain photosensitizing properties. Both are used within Veterinary Aromatic Medicine, however when therapeutic properties of lime are desired, the cold pressed oil is more often selected. However, if humans plan to use the oil for fragrance, lime scented diffusion, or their own topical applications, then the steam distilled version may be more desirable. Both lime oils have GRAS status, and the Cold Pressed oil should adhere to the caution of not exposing skin to sunlight within 12 hours of topical applications.

Not only does lime have one of the best fragrance profiles on earth, it is also reported to be antiseptic, antiviral, antibacterial, anti-inflammatory, an appetite stimulant (don't worry it won't make you eat if you don't need to!), anti-spasmodic, immune supportive, helpful for weight management, reduces anxiety, depression, is uplifting, regenerative, and a circulatory aid! Whew – I knew I loved lime for a reason!

Lime is most commonly used in Three Part Blends, and mainly within water-based diffusion for animals at this time. However, it can be considered for use in all of the ways described for Lemon and other citrus oils.

Mandarin (Citrus reticulata)

Mandarin oil has GRAS status, and can be found listed as Red, Yellow, and Green Mandarinl. Red Mandarin is generally cold pressed from the ripe fruit, while Green Mandarin is expressed from the green unripe fruit, and naturally Yellow is somewhere in between. Although a citrus oil, it is usually not considered photo-toxic as it contains low levels of furanocoumarins. The petitgrain, or leaf distillation of Mandarin, is photosensitizing, however we do not use the petitgrain in veterinary aromatic medicine at this time. Most commonly, I select Red Mandarin for use with animals. Mandarin should be used as described for other citrus oils such as Lemon and Tangerine when desired. Mandarin oil is reported to have great properties for emotional support and is uplifting, while soothing, and would be indicated for sleeplessness, anxiety, and nervous conditions.

Physically Mandarin is reported to be antiseptic, antispasmodic, aids circulation, blood purification, lymph flow, digestion, may be gastroprotective and aid in healing of ulcers, supports the liver and neurologic systems, and may be indicated for use with seizures and epilepsy.

Manuka (Leptospermum scoparium)

Manuka essential oil is of course different from Manuka Honey which is quite a popular natural remedy. The essential oil is created from the New Zealand Tea Tree plant, and is reported to have many of the similar properties as Tea Tree (Melaleuca alternifolia) while being more mild in nature. At this time, Manuka is not commonly used with animals, but it does appear to be of low concern.

Marjoram (Origanum majorana)

Also called Sweet Marjoram, this oil is well known as one of the "muscle" essential oils, but is also indicated for body and joint discomfort, arthritis, respiratory conditions (expectorant and mucolytic), ringworm, muscle spasms, muscle conditions, increasing motility of the gastrointestinal tract (promotes intestinal peristalsis), fluid retention, lowering blood pressure, vasodilation, circulatory disorders, and nerve pain. Marjoram carries effects for menstrual problems and PMS in humans, which likely carries over into other hormonal issues in animals, such as excessive sexual drive. Marjoram has GRAS status.

Birds: Marjoram is most commonly used within Three Part Blends for water-based diffusion (including caging and tenting) or for diluted topical applications, within the Small Animal Supportive Blend, by addition to foods (1 toothpick dip to 1 drop added per tablespoon of food), addition to drinking water (1 drop per Liter of water), Perch applications (diluted), indirect diffusion, and by mixing 1 drop into 1 tablespoon of natural ointments applied to non-feathered areas. Marjoram is especially helpful for crop infections, crop stasis, respiratory conditions, excessive egg laying, excessive sexual drive, and hormonal issues in birds. Starting with diffusion alone is often enough to give benefits. Advancing to more intensive exposure is generally used after diffusion has not proven to be effective enough. Marjoram has not been added to a water spritzer at this time.

Exotics: Marjoram can be used in all of the methods discussed for birds, and is most commonly used within Three Part Blends for water-diffusion or diluted topical applications, or within the Small Animal or Feline Supportive Blends (ferrets). It can also be considered for application via Petting (diluted), and direct topical application (generally diluted, except for ringworm where neat application is more likely). It is likely that Marjoram could be added to the soaking water of reptiles, turtles, and other zoo animals for muscular concerns, fungal infections, and to promote intestinal activity. Starting with very small amounts (a toothpick dip) of Marjoram added to the water would be advisable, then gradually increasing the amount of exposure.

Cats: Marjoram is most commonly used within the Feline Supportive Blend. Other cat friendly methods of use include water-based diffusion of Three Part Blends, Petting (diluted), addition to natural ointments, addition to litter box recipes, and direct topical application (generally used diluted first, but may increase to neat application with difficult cases of ringworm).

It is likely unnecessary to administer Marjoram orally beyond basic grooming behavior.

Dogs & Larger: Marjoram will most commonly be used within Three Part Blends for water-based diffusion or diluted topical applications. In dog and larger animals, Marjoram is most commonly used within the Canine or Large Animal Supportive Blends. Application by Petting (diluted), by direct topical application (neat or diluted), by adding into natural ointments or shampoos, adding into soaking or swimming water, and by oral administration when other methods have not been adequate or it is deemed necessary – may be considered. For oral use in dogs – 1 drop of Marjoram can be diluted with 6 drops of coconut oil. 1 drop or more of this dilution can be given twice a day, for each 20 pounds (9 kg) of body weight. Start with a smaller amount, and gradually increase as needed. For horses and others, starting with 1 drop per 200 pounds (90 kg) of body weight, given orally twice a day is a good starting point. Monitor responses and adjust according to individual need.

May Chang (Litsea cubeba)
May Chang is reported to have antibacterial, anti-inflammatory, and antifungal properties as well as often being indicated for the support of the cardiovascular system. Research indicates it may have actions against cancer cells, reduces anxiety, repels insects, and has been effective against Microsporum canis and other dermatophytes (ringworm). The most common ways to use May Chang include within Three Part Blends for water-based diffusion or diluted topical applications. Addition into the species specific Supportive Blends can also be considered for all species.

Melaleuca alternifolia (Melaleuca alternifolia)

Also called Tea Tree, Melaleuca alternifolia is likely to be the most controversial essential oil used in animals. This oil became popular quickly, which spurred an abundance of poor quality, contaminated, and synthetically created "oils" to flood the consumer market very quickly. It is true that use of poor quality Melaleuca "essential oil" has indeed killed cats. Cases of toxicity that have enough data to trace and research the events at hand, have always revealed very poor grade and synthetic essential oils or their gross misuse and over-dosage. In one case, a bottle of essential oil was spilled, and a cat came into contact with the spillage. The cat seizured the next day and died. The brand was a basic "over-the-counter" variety that can be purchased in most health food stores.

Research quoted most often in regards to the concern about Melaleuca with cats, indeed had 60mL of the essential oil applied to three cats. This is an insane overdose, and we should be reluctant to claim toxicity as a rule, when clear poisoning is occurring.

In contrast, as a veterinarian, I have witnessed extreme uses of essential oils, and am always quite impressed by the relative safety demonstrated. A feline patient presented to our veterinary clinic for evaluation prior to an essential oil protocol being started. Blood work was obtained, and this cat proceeded to receive 4 drops of Melaleuca alternifolia, directly into its mouth, twice a day. Blood work was re-evaluated after one week of administration and was completely normal. This is not to say that cats should have oils administered to them in this manner, quite the opposite. I rarely use Melaleuca alternifolia with cats in general. However, when you are exposed to what the general public may do, and the actual medical details of it, it is quite enlightening. I for one, do not think we should ignore the data that even excessive use of oils provides us.

Melaleuca alternifolia is antibacterial, antifungal, antiviral, antiparasitic, and anti-inflammatory. It is indicated for yeast and bacterial infections of the skin, ringworm, candida, sinus and lung infections, hypertension, and skin conditions. Research shows that Melaleuca can reduce oral bacteria, improve gum health, reduce stomatitis and inflammation in the mouth, reduce histamine-induced allergic skin reactions, kills lice, inhibits sarcoptic mites, reduces warts, and has effects against resistant bacterial strains such as MRSA.

Quite honestly, the hullabaloo about Tea Tree (Melaleuca alternifolia) is best summarized by Tisserand and Young within the 2nd Edition of *Essential Oil Safety* stating, "Much nonsense has been written about tea tree oil safety." I encourage everyone to read this important reference, for accurate information on safety and known data for all essential oils.

Birds: Melaleuca oil of any species must be of the utmost quality for use in birds. Methods of use include water-based diffusion via a Three Part Blend (generally 3-4 drops added to a diffuser – caging and tenting can be used), use within natural ointments, and by addition into the Small Animal Supportive Blend. The topical use of Melaleuca may be considered in severe cases through addition to Feather Spray Recipes, often starting with one drop added to 4 ounces and applied via water-misting applications. This again is only in severe cases of need, and with direct monitoring and instruction by a qualified veterinarian.

Exotics: Melaleuca can be used for exotic animals similarly to as described for birds. The most common methods of use include water-based diffusion within a Three Part Blend, addition to the Small Animal Supportive Blend, and diluted topical applications of a Three Part Blend. Addition into shampoos and ointments can also be utilized.

Cats: Some people will feel more comfortable taking a cautious approach to the use of Melaleuca for felines, and this is completely fine. There are so many other essential oils to choose from, that the use of Melaleuca in cats is likely unnecessary. However, it is nice to know that if a case seems to be completely unresponsive to other remedies, or if Melaleuca seems like the perfect oil to use – this is still a viable option to consider. Veterinary monitoring and pre-exposure blood work is always recommended, and especially so that the documentation of the safe use of Melaleuca in cats can be further demonstrated. The use of Melaleuca within blends is highly recommended, as it further dilutes the effective exposure to Melaleuca, while still providing its synergistic actions. It should be recognized that Melaleuca is actually used within many pet products, including those for cats, and has been found to be safe when used properly.

The most cat friendly methods of use of Melaleuca alternifolia include; addition into the Feline Supportive Blend (starting with 1 drop added), water-based diffusion of Three Part Blends, addition into natural ointments or shampoo, applications of diluted Three Part Blends, and direct topical application (diluted). Oral administration beyond grooming, is likely unnecessary, and would be reserved for only the most severe of conditions, and only under strict veterinary monitoring. It is highly likely that other essential oils could be used instead of Melaleuca.

Dogs & Larger: Melaleuca alternifolia can be used with many methods of application, with the most common forms being water-based diffusion within Three Part Blends, addition into the Canine or Large Animal Supportive Blends, diluted topical application within Three Part Blends, direct topical application (diluted or neat), addition into various carriers, ointments, or shampoo, and when deemed necessary by the oral route. It may be less likely for Melaleuca to be consumed in water or food due to its strong flavor, however some animals seem to enjoy it. We have seen dogs who self-select to lick Melaleuca oil off of human hands, treated areas, or even other animals. When ingestion via licking and grooming occurs, we have no concern, and have usually found it beneficial.

If oral use in dogs is considered – 1 drop of Melaleuca Alternifolia can be diluted with 10 drops of carrier oil. 1 drop or more of this dilution can be given twice a day, for each 20 pounds (9 kg) of body weight. Start with a smaller amount, and gradually increase as needed. Most often, the diluted oil should be added additionally to foods. For horses and others, starting with 1 drop per 300 pounds (135 kg) of body weight, given orally twice a day is a good starting point. Monitor responses and adjust according to individual need.

Melaleuca Ericifolia (Melaleuca ericifolia)
Also called Rosalina or Lavender Tea Tree, Melaleuca ericifolia is a slightly milder form when compared to alternifolia. Its properties include antibacterial, antifungal, antiviral, anti-parasitic, and anti-inflammatory actions. It is indicated specifically for Herpes Virus and respiratory and sinus infections. Melaleuca ericifolia can be used in all of the ways mentioned for Melaleuca alternifolia – however ericifolia has been used much less commonly with animals. In cats, exotics, and birds the use of Melaleuca ericifolia should start cautiously as the use of this oil has not been widely documented.

Melaleuca Quinquenervia – chemotype C (Melaleuca quinquenervia)
This essential oil is also known as MQV, Broad-leaf Paperbark, and Niaouli – this particular chemotype is cineole rich. This oil is most commonly used within blends, and extensive use as a single has not been well documented. Properties suggest this oil would be indicated for respiratory and sinus infections, allergies, insect bites, parasites, and wound healing. Suggested uses of MQV include water-based diffusion within Three Part Blends, diluted topical applications within Three Part Blends or species specific Supportive Blends. Addition into natural ointments and shampoos is likely a wonderful method of use to consider. Water-based diffusion is generally the method selected when use of an

"un-documented" essential oil is initiated in animals. Careful monitoring and gradual increases in exposure intensity is recommended.

Melaleuca Quinquenervia – chemotype LN (Melaleuca quinquenervia)

Also called Nerolina, this is a chemotype rich in linalool and nerolidol. It is reported to be antifungal, antimicrobial, miticidal, calming and relaxing, as well as helpful to freshen and deodorize rooms. It likely can be used in all of the ways mentioned for MQV above.

Melissa (Melissa officinalis)

Melissa is also known as Lemon Balm. Melissa essential oil falls into the category of a "must-have" oil for me. Although it can be considered expensive, the massive benefits from very small amounts of this oil make the investment well worthwhile. Melissa is a powerful oil with a very high vibrational energy. Melissa is most likely one of the highest regarded oils in terms of anti-viral properties, and it is especially indicated with Herpes Viruses and Avian Influenza. Melissa also has very high anti-histamine type actions. Melissa is used for many conditions including depression, grief, anxiety, cognitive dysfunction, viral infections, pruitis (itching), hives, seizures, nerve pain, vertigo, diabetes, as a replacement for anti-histamines, and for anaphylaxis. Melissa oil is one to try when you have tried everything else without results. I am continually amazed at reports of what Melissa oil has helped with, and the possibilities seem quite endless.

Research indicates that Melissa may have actions against cancer cells, induces apoptosis (cancer cell death), improves dementia, may help neurodegenerative disease, and may reduce blood triglycerides when given orally.

Birds: The most common use of Melissa has been by addition to drinking water (1 drop per liter). This is widely accepted, and when needed 2 drops per liter can be used. Other common methods of use include water-based diffusion alone or within Three Part Blends, and by addition into foods (starting with a toothpick dip per tablespoon). 1 drop could be added to the Small Animal Supportive Blend for topical use with severe viral situations, where other methods have not yielded results. Melissa is generally not used within Feather Spray Recipes or as a water-mist in these species.

Exotics: All of the methods for birds can be used for exotics. Other methods of use include addition of 1 drop of Melissa into the Small Animal Supportive Blend, addition into Three Part Blends for diluted topical applications, and via Petting (diluted). In severe viral situations addition into soaking waters and aquariums can also be used, starting with adding a toothpick dip, and gradually increasing the amount used. Melissa is quite a powerful and intense oil, and many times portions of the drinking water solution (1 drop per liter) will be added to aquariums, soaking water, and foods to reduce the intensity.

Cats: All of the methods listed for birds and exotics can be used in cats. The most cat friendly methods include the addition of 1 drop of Melissa to the Feline Supportive Blend, water-based diffusion of Three Part Blends, addition to litter box recipes (often only 1 drop), and via diluted topical applications of Three Part Blends. Petting (diluted) can be considered, but generally at a 1% concentration – use within blends is preferred. Ingestion of this oil should mainly be achieved via normal grooming behavior of topically applied diluted blends. If a cat will ingest the oil in foods or in drinking water, it can be considered, especially in severe viral situations, allergic reactions, or anaphylaxis. Melissa is especially indicated for Feline Leukemia, FIP, Feline Corona Virus, FIV, Feline Herpes Virus, Feline Distemper, other viral conditions. Melissa has also been used successfully for seizures.

If more extensive oral use is considered for cats, diluting 1 drop in 1 liter of water, and mixing 3-5mL of this solution with foods is recommended. No maximum amount has been reached with this method, and even up to 3-5 mL of "Melissa water" could be administered, 2-6 times a day. Alternately, 1 drop of Melissa can also be diluted in 30 drops of carrier oil, and 1 or more drops of this dilution can be given directly in the mouth or via capsule. This dilution can be given twice a day or more, as needed for the severity of the condition. For chronic viral infections, a much slower introduction to the oil can be followed.

It is important to note that exposure via topical applications and subsequent grooming, along with the layers of water-based diffusion and use within the litter box, is often adequate to obtain therapeutic levels of Melissa use. With some cats, daily to twice a day applications of oil blends containing Melissa may be needed for a duration of time. Adjust according to response, and be willing to give it some time prior to jumping to extremely aggressive methods of administration.

Dogs & Larger: Melissa is most commonly used by addition into the Canine or Large Animal Supportive Blends. Water-based diffusion or diluted topical applications within Three Part Blends is well accepted. Application as a single via Petting (diluted) and direct topical application (diluted) is less commonly used. Addition into water-mists, shampoos, and ointments can be considered. One or more drops of Copaiba and/or Frankincense can also be added to blends containing Melissa oil, helping to magnify and providing synergistic effects in order to enable less Melissa oil to be used, especially if expense is a concern.

If oral use for dogs is considered, 1 drop of Melissa can be diluted with 20 drops of carrier oil. 1 drop or more of this dilution can be given twice a day, for each 20 pounds (9 kg) of body weight. Start with a smaller amount, and gradually increase as needed. For horses and others, starting with 1 drop per 500 pounds (225 kg) of body weight, given orally twice a day is a good starting point. Monitor responses and adjust according to individual need.

Monarda (Monarda fistulosa)

Also called Bee Balm; Monarda is an up and coming oil to the marketplace I am sure. It is being reported to have levels of Thymoquinone, a constituent with huge amounts of beneficial research, however the levels of this component seem to vary widely with the type of plant and location of growth. One farm is selectively re-distilling Monarda, to achieve high levels of almost pure TQ (Thymoquinone) – however this should definitely be treated more as a pharmaceutical by nature than an essential oil. Most likely, if we want an all-natural source of TQ – it should be obtained through Black Cumin oil at this time, instead of through manipulated essential oils. Monarda as an essential oil in its own right, is reported to have many beneficial properties, however it is not commonly used with animals at this time.

Mountain Savory (Satureja montana)

Also called Winter Savory, this essential oil is often considered as a gentler version of Oregano. Summer Savory is the cultivated version of this oil, while Winter (Mountain) Savory is wild grown. Its actions are similar to oregano and include strong antibacterial, antifungal, antiviral, anti-parasitic, anti-inflammatory, and immune stimulating properties. It is especially indicated for MRSA, mastitis, spinal and back conditions, as well as viral infections (such as Herpes and FIV.) Mountain Savory has GRAS status.

Birds & Exotics: Mountain Savory has not been used extensively at this time, however it seems likely that it can be used similarly to Oregano, and may be a more mild selection to utilize. Please see Oregano for a description of methods of application.

Cats: Mountain Savory has not been used extensively with cats at this time, however it seems likely that it can be used similarly to Oregano. It would be most indicated in cases of Feline Herpes Virus and FIV (Feline Immunodeficiency Virus.) Please see Oregano for a description of methods of application.

Dogs & Larger: Mountain Savory can be used in all of the ways that Oregano is used and recommended. Please see Oregano for a description of methods of application. Mountain Savory would be especially indicated for use with viral infections, Equine Herpes Virus, spondylosis, and other back conditions.

Mugwort (Artemisia vulgaris)
Also called Wormwood, this essential oil is not recommended for use with animals.

Mustard (Brassica nigra)
Mustard is not recommended for use within Veterinary Aromatic Medicine.

Myrrh (Commiphora myrrha)
Myrrh is used in many ways with animals. Its medical properties make it well indicated for use with diabetes, cancer, hepatitis, fungal infections, tooth and gum infections, skin conditions, and as an analgesic. Myrrh is also supportive for many endocrine and hormonal conditions including support of the thyroid, growth hormone production, pituitary gland function, and hypothalamus function.

One of the more common uses of Myrrh in animals is for pain management. Myrrh is often given in combination with Copaiba and Helichrysum in an oral form, with very effective results. We have seen this combination replace the use of many traditional pain medications in the veterinary hospital. Topically, Myrrh has also been helpful in controlling pain and aiding in the healing of post-surgical sites.

Birds: Myrrh is most commonly used within natural ointments, which are not applied to feathered areas. For pain management 1 drop of Myrrh, 2 drops of Helichrysum, and 1 drop of Copaiba are added to 2 mL of fractionated coconut oil. Approximately 1 drop (or 0.05 mL) of this solution is given orally, to a bird up to 100 grams in weight. For larger birds, starting with one drop is still advisable; however it is likely that increased amounts could be used if needed. The dose was repeated every 8 hours for a particular individual, however the judgment on when to re-dose should be placed more on response than on a specific time frame. This blend was very effective in controlling the discomfort associated with a broken wing in our veterinary hospital, and the bird required no further pain medications or injections.

Myrrh can also be considered for addition into the Small Animal Supportive Blend, or within natural salves and ointments (1 or more drops per tablespoon). Due to its resinous and sticky nature, caution is used with Myrrh in regards to application and possible adherence to feathered areas. Water-based diffusion of Three Part Blends containing Myrrh is highly suggested. Diluted topical applications of Three Part Blends, or use within Feather Spray Recipes can be considered if skin healing and regeneration is needed as in cases of mutilation. However, careful care should be used, and with direct aid from an experienced avian veterinarian.

Exotics: Myrrh can be used in all of the ways mentioned for birds. Oral use of Myrrh would follow the same recipes to start with, however it is likely that the concentration of the Pain Recipe could be increased to 2 drops of each oil added into 2 mL of fractionated coconut oil. This solution would be given orally or mixed with foods at a rate of 1 or more drops per 5 pounds (2 kg) of body weight. For most exotics, starting with one drop and judging response and duration of the response, is the best way to establish a dosing regimen.

Myrrh would most commonly be used via water-based diffusion or diluted topical applications of Three Part Blends. Myrrh can also be used by addition to soaking water (starting with 1 toothpick dip into 1 liter of water), and by addition into the Small Animal Supportive Blend. Considerations can also be made for use in water-mists, especially for skin conditions.

Cats: Myrrh is especially indicated for hyperthyroidism, pain management, ringworm, use after surgeries, hepatitis, diabetes, and skin conditions. Cat friendly methods of use include addition into the Feline Supportive Blend, addition to litter box recipes, water-based diffusion and diluted topical applications within Three Part Blends, or addition to shampoos and ointments.

For pain control with cats, it has been quite adequate for blends containing Myrrh, Copaiba, and Helichrysum to be ingested via grooming practices alone.

In the past, the cat Pain Recipe started with 5 drops each of Myrrh, Helichrysum, and Copaiba per 2 mL of fractionated coconut oil. This solution was given orally directly, by capsule, or within foods if the cat is willing. 5 drops or more of this dilution could be given, 3 or more times per day. Cats often salivate when given any essential oil orally, and this was an expected event. However, cats rejoiced everywhere (as well as their owners), when we recognized that simple topical applications, topical absorption, inhalation absorption, and grooming actions resulted in comfort without all the hassle. While we can still consider use of the oral Pain Recipe for cats in severe need, it should be used mainly as a last resort.

The Pain Recipe described above, or diluted Three Part Blends, can also be used to apply near surgical incisions. Direct application to a surgical incision is rarely necessary, and application directly next to the incision works well. For most surgical areas, I prefer a mild water-mist, often containing Myrrh which can be misted lightly over the area after shaking well. This distributes a very fine layer of the beneficial essential oils, without being irritating or greasy. A Three Part Blend of Lavender, Copaiba, and Myrrh could be used in a water-mist for incisions. Often times, Myrrh may be used in lesser amounts than the other oils within the water-mist due to its resinous nature. Approximately 10 drops of this blend, can be added to 30mL (1oz) of distilled water. Mist onto location 2-3 times a day or as needed, noting that cats are not necessarily fond of sprays.

Dogs & Larger: All of the methods discussed for other species, can be considered for Dogs & Larger Animals. The most common methods include addition into the Canine or Large Animal Supportive Blends, water-based diffusion or diluted topical applications of Three Part Blends, Petting (diluted, especially over the neck or thyroid gland area), direct topical application (neat or diluted), addition into natural ointments, salves, or shampoo, and by oral administration. See the instructions above for Cats – on preparing a water-mist for incisions and surgical sites.

If oral use is considered for dogs, 1 drop of Myrrh can be diluted with 10 drops of fractionated coconut oil. 1 drop or more of this dilution can be given twice a day, for each 20 pounds (9 kg) of body weight. Start with a smaller amount, and gradually increase as needed. For horses and others, starting with 1 drop per 500 pounds (225 kg) of body weight, given orally twice a day is a good starting point. Monitor responses and adjust according to individual need.

An effective Pain Recipe for dogs is 1 drop of Helichrysum, 1 drop of Myrrh, 1 drop of Copaiba, within 10 drops of carrier oil. This is placed within a gel capsule and given orally, and is reserved for more severe situations. This amount is generally used for dogs approximately 50 pounds (23 kg) in weight, and can be dosed 2-3 times a day. Adjustments should be made accordingly for other weights. This blend is generally used for more severe pain situations such as an injury, trauma, or surgery. The patient should be monitored closely, ideally in cooperation with a veterinarian, and amounts and dosing frequency adjusted based on the individual.

Myrtle (Myrtus communis)

Myrtle is used mainly in animals for liver, prostate, thyroid, and respiratory concerns. It may be listed as Green or Red Myrtle, with the Green most commonly being of the α-pinene chemotype, and the Red being of the 1,8-cineole chemotype. Most commonly Green Myrtle is selected for use with Veterinary Aromatic Medicine. Myrtle is also reported to be a bronchodilator, eases coughs, is an expectorant and decongestant, supports urinary tract health, and encourages restful sleep. Research shows that Myrtle may be effective in lowering blood glucose levels, reduces spasm of intestine, and creates vasodilation and increased circulation which may be helpful in circulatory disorders such as ear margin vasculitis, laminitis, or for human Raynaud's Syndrome.

Birds: Myrtle is not commonly used as a single with birds. Water-based diffusion within Three Part Blends is appropriate. Topical application of Myrtle would most likely be accomplished through addition to the Small Animal Supportive Blend. Use of Myrtle should be in full cooperation and monitoring with an avian veterinarian.

Exotics: Myrtle has also not been commonly used as a single for exotic animals, but has been used within blends on a more extensive basis. Myrtle is most commonly used with water-based diffusion of a Three Part Blend. For topical applications, addition into the Small Animal Supportive Blend or Feline Supportive Blend (ferrets) is suggested. Diluted topical applications of Three Part Blends may also be considered.

Cats: Cat friendly methods in which to use Myrtle include water-based diffusion within Three Part Blends, addition into the Feline Supportive Blend, and by addition into litter box recipes.

Dogs & Larger: Myrtle is often indicated for dogs with hypothyroidism, liver disease, and prostate disease. Myrtle can be used in all of the application methods for these animals and is most commonly used via addition into the Canine or Large Animal Supportive Blends. Water-based diffusion within Three Part Blends is also widely used, and greatly accepted. Petting (diluted – especially over the thyroid or neck area) can be considered for Myrtle as a single oil as well. Rectal Instillation of Myrtle has been used for cases of prostatic disease (see that chapter for more details). Oral administration can also be considered, although is not commonly used.

When oral use is considered for dogs – 1 drop of Myrtle can be diluted with 10 drops of carrier oil. 1 drop or more of this dilution can be given twice a day, for each 20 pounds (9 kg) of body weight. Start with a smaller amount, and gradually increase as needed. For horses and others, starting with 1 drop per 500 pounds (225 kg) of body weight, given orally twice a day is a good starting point. Monitor responses and adjust according to individual need.

Myrtle, Lemon (see Lemon Myrtle)

Neroli (Citrus sinensis, Citrus aurantium)

Also called Orange Blossom oil, Neroli is often found as a solvent extracted absolute and not a true essential oil. While there are steam distilled essential oils available, Neroli has not been used as a single oil extensively in animals at this time. It has mainly been used within blends for water-based diffusion, and this would appear to be a safe and effective route of use for all animals as long as a proper quality and confirmed steam distilled oil is used. Diluted topical applications within Species Specific Supportive Blends would be appropriate, as long as quality, steam distilled oil is confirmed. Neroli is very expensive, and often adulterated, regardless of claims of quality. Reported properties indicate it may be useful for anxiety, depression, hypertension, heart disease, and may have anti-convulsant properties. Neroli has GRAS status.

Nerolina (see Melaleuca quinquenervia chemotype LN)

Niaouli (see Melaleuca quinquenervia chemotype C)

Nutmeg (Myristica fragrans)

Nutmeg is a magnificent oil with many supportive properties including anti-inflammatory, anticoagulant, antiparasitic, analgesic, liver protecting, stomach protecting against ulcers, circulatory stimulation, adrenal support and stimulation, muscle relaxation, and the increase of growth hormone and melatonin production. Conditions in animals that are aided by Nutmeg include; arthritis, heart disease, hypertension, liver disease, gastric ulcers, digestive disorders, parasites, nerve pain and neuropathy, adrenal stress and fatigue, and Addison's Disease. Nutmeg has GRAS status.

Care must be taken with Nutmeg oil in animals who are bleeding, have a tendency to bleed, or are on any sort of anti-coagulant therapy. The over use of essential oil(s) that have anti-coagulant actions, especially in oral administration, can produce a temporary and dose dependent increase in bleeding and reduction of clotting.

Birds: Nutmeg is mainly used within blends for birds, and is not commonly selected as a single. In birds the most common method of exposure would be within addition to the Small Animal Supportive Blend, by water-based diffusion within Three Part Blends, or by adding into foods (starting with 1 toothpick dip per tablespoon).

Exotics: Nutmeg is most commonly used to support the adrenal glands in ferrets, and is most commonly used via addition into the Small Animal or Feline Supportive Blend (ferrets). Other recommended methods of exposure include water-based diffusion within Three Part Blends, and even addition into routine shampoos or litter box recipes can be considered for appropriate species. Oral use is generally only moved towards when other methods of use have failed to be effective. If oral use is considered, 1 drop of Nutmeg is diluted in 2 mL of carrier oil, and 1 drop or more of this dilution can be added to foods or given orally, twice a day. Monitor for responses and adjust according to individual need.

Cats: Cats can also use Nutmeg as described for exotics and birds. Cat friendly and recommended methods of using Nutmeg include addition into Feline Supportive Blend, water-based diffusion within Three Part Blends, and addition into litter box recipes. Consumption of nutmeg through regular grooming process is of no concern, and the only way we generally expose cats to ingestion of nutmeg oil.

Dogs & Larger: Nutmeg will most commonly be used through addition into the Canine or Large Animal Supportive Blends. Water-based diffusion or diluted topical applications within Three Part Blends is also appropriate. Petting (diluted, especially over the adrenal gland area), addition to foods, and direct oral administration can be considered.

If oral use in dogs is considered, 1 drop of Nutmeg can be diluted with 30 drops of carrier oil. 1 drop or more of this dilution can be given twice a day, for each 20 pounds (9 kg) of body weight. Start with a smaller amount, and gradually increase as needed. For horses and others, starting with 1 drop per 500 pounds (225 kg) of body weight, given orally twice a day is a good starting point. Monitor responses and adjust according to individual need. See the cautionary statement regarding bleeding and anticoagulant activity.

Ocotea (Ocotea quixos)

Also called Ishpingo, Ocotea has been made popular mainly through one large essential oil company. It is not widely available on the essential oil market, although the tree itself has been used for over 500 years. Ocotea's claim to fame is as a choice for Diabetes and pancreatic disorders, antihistamine-type actions, and is often mentioned for undocumented actions against internal parasites. Research reveals that Ocotea may be useful for high blood pressure, clotting disorders, gastro-protective properties, fungal infections, and inflammation.

For similar actions and properties, more animal-safe and more commonly used oils are available for Veterinary Aromatic Medicine. Cinnamon and Copaiba are highly suggested for use when these properties are desired for animals.

Caution and careful monitoring with a veterinarian is recommended whenever Ocotea is used with animals receiving Insulin or oral hypoglycemic medications. Ocotea (or any essential oil intended to lower blood sugar) may lower the need for these medications, so much so, that continued administration of prescribed insulin dosages, may prove dangerous. When working with a veterinarian, it is helpful to describe that you will be using a natural remedy that may reduce the required levels of Insulin or other diabetic medications. Most veterinarians are familiar with the careful monitoring and adjusting of Insulin doses in diabetic animals – especially when we are first introducing the therapy. In the case of essential oil use with diabetes, we basically monitor "in reverse," slowly exposing the animal to the natural remedy, while performing the same careful monitoring and blood glucose curves, at intervals determined by the veterinarian. Over time, Insulin and medication requirements may lessen, and a reduction in dosage can be made with your veterinarian.

Due to the limited availability, and often questionable quality, Ocotea is not recommended for use with animals at this time.

Opoponax (Commiphora guidotti)
Also called Sweet Myrrh, this essential oil has not been used commonly with animals at this time. It is not recommended for use within Veterinary Aromatic Medicine, and if similar properties are desired, oils with much more data and records of use with animals are suggested. Myrrh and Frankincense would be most commonly suggested as alternatives.

Orange, Bitter – see Bitter Orange

Orange, Sweet (Citrus sinensis)
Orange oil has been used extensively in all species of animals, and in almost every way imaginable. With a high Limonene content, Orange oil is often recommended for antitumoral benefits. Orange oil is commonly indicated for cancer, depression and anxiety, support of the liver and glutathione production, support of lymph drainage, as a diuretic, and for health in general. Orange has GRAS status.

Orange is a photosensitizing oil; avoid applying to skin that will be exposed to sunlight or full spectrum UV light within 12 hours. This oil is used commonly in the Feather Spray Recipes for birds, and we have not noted a photosensitizing issue for fully feathered birds at this time. However, I would still advise caution, as many birds using the Feather Spray Recipe are missing feathers and have fully exposed skin. Caution with full and natural sunlight is more likely needed than with the full spectrum indoor lighting, commonly used for birds and reptiles.

Birds & Exotics: Orange oil has been used in many, many ways: as a single via water-based diffusion (including caging and tenting), within Three Part Blends for water-based diffusion or diluted topical applications, added to Small Animal or Feline Supportive Blends (ferrets), within the Feather Spray Recipes, added to drinking water (1 or more drops per liter), added to foods (1 or more drops per tablespoon), addition to natural ointments, salves, and shampoos, within water spritzers (up to 20 drops per 4 ounces), via Petting (diluted non-avian), and allowed to be directly ingested when animals chose to lick the oil off of hands and other items.

Cats: Orange oil is most commonly used via water-based diffusion within Three Part Blends, and by addition into the Feline Supportive Blend for topical applications. Addition into the Small Animal Supportive Blend can also be utilized for feline topical applications. Addition into litter box recipes can also be considered, although would generally not be selected as the most cat friendly exposure route. Some cats may ingest Orange oil in foods or water as described for Birds & Exotics, but regular grooming from topical applications is likely to be more than adequate when internal use is desired. We have not noted photosensitivity issues for cats who are fully furred, however the recommendation to apply the oil where the sun will not contact the skin (stomach), keep the cat indoors, or avoid use in hairless cats exposed to sun is wise. Also see the chapters on Metabolism Theory for more information on cats and citrus oils.

Dogs & Larger: Orange oil is most commonly used as a single via water-based diffusion (including caging and tenting), within Three Part Blends for water-based diffusion or diluted topical applications, added to the Canine or Large Animal Supportive Blends, added to ointments, salves, or shampoos, used within water mists or oil mists for diffuse application to larger areas, added into foods, and for direct topical application (generally diluted).

Orange oil applied directly to the skin, should always be diluted to the amounts recommended for your species of interest. Starting with smaller amounts or more diluted oil is still recommended as many animals respond to lesser amounts. However, if needed, larger quantities can often be applied safely.

Applications containing Orange oil could be applied to the underside of the belly of Goats, Horses, and other Large Animals who may be exposed to the sun. Photosensitivity has not been noted in furred areas, but caution is still a wise idea.

If oral use is considered for dogs, 1 drop of Orange oil can be diluted with 10 drops of carrier oil. 1 drop or more of this dilution can be given twice a day, for each 20 pounds (9 kg) of body weight, generally combined with food. Start with a smaller amount, and gradually increase as needed. For horses and others, starting with 1 drop per 200 pounds (90 kg) of body weight, given orally twice a day is a good starting point. Monitor responses and adjust according to individual need.

Oregano (Origanum vulgare)

Oregano is often included within many Body Supportive Blends. High in phenols, it is a powerful oil. Properties of Oregano include antioxidant, antiviral, antibacterial, antifungal, antiparasitic, anti-inflammatory, anti-allergenic, wart removing, anticancer, bronchodilation, expectorant, diuretic, and immune stimulation. Oregano can almost be indicated for every condition, and when used properly is an oil renowned for health benefits worldwide. Unfortunately, Oregano is commonly adulterated with synthetic carvacrol, and poor grade, altered, diluted, and manipulated Oregano is often widely presented in today's market. Oregano is known as a "hot" oil, and care must be taken to properly dilute, and monitor the skin of animals exposed to it. In general, Oregano is not selected for diffusion applications due to its hot nature. Oregano has GRAS status.

Research has shown Oregano to be effective for a variety of cancers, elimination of internal parasites, inhibition of many strains of antibiotic resistant bacteria (MRSA), and reducing stomatitis among other things.

Birds: Oregano has mainly been mixed into foods and used within the stronger Avian Drip & Rub Technique recipe. With addition into foods, 1 toothpick dip is mixed into 1 tablespoon of food, and gradually increased to even 1 drop per tablespoon of food. This can be used as a powerful natural antibacterial agent, but has also been used to contact papillomas (warts) within the digestive tract. Within the Avian Drip & Rub Technique, Oregano is likely to benefit any condition, however, this technique is not always easy to administer to every bird and is reserved mainly for severe cases and conditions. Water-based diffusion of this oil could be considered in extremely low amounts within a blend, but mainly as a last resort when other less irritating oils have been tried without adequate results, and for severe conditions such as Aspergillosis, air sac infections or tumors, or unresponsive sinusitis.

Exotics: Oregano is mainly used with less sensitive species, through addition into the Small Animal Supportive Blend or within the Feline Supportive Blend. Addition into foods has also been used, with the same protocols as described for birds. Care must be taken with Rabbits, Guinea Pigs, and Chinchillas as they are considered "hind-gut fermenters" – therefore the aggressive use of a powerful antibacterial agent like Oregano, could damage their delicate intestinal flora. Please make sure to see the sections for these animals specifically, for more information on their individual needs and recommendations. Water-based diffusion of Oregano could also be considered as described for birds, but again, only as a last resort. For cases of severe warts, stronger solutions of Oregano can be considered for topical application directly to the wart. Rabbits are the most likely exotic species to get warts, so caution must be used if Oregano is considered for them. Please see the Rabbit section for specific recommendations for this species.

Cats: Oregano is most commonly used within the Feline Supportive Blend. Addition to natural ointments (1 drop per tablespoon), or diluted topical applications of Three Part Blends directly to areas of fungal infection (ringworm) can also be considered. Most commonly, when use of Oregano is desired, it should be accomplished through use of the Feline Supportive Blend, including for ingestion, which will generally be adequate through normal grooming behaviors. More aggressive oral use of Oregano is not suggested for cats at this time, without distinct and direct monitoring and administration through an experienced veterinarian. Please see comments in Birds and Exotics for information on water based diffusion of Oregano.

Dogs & Larger: Oregano is most commonly used through the Canine and Large Animal Supportive Blends. Direct application (neat or diluted), addition into natural ointments, salves, and shampoos, addition into bug sprays and bug repellent recipes, addition into massage oils and bases, addition into soaking solutions for Large Animals), addition into foods, and direct oral administration can be considered for oregano. Care should always be taken to use the most benign methods of exposure first with such an aggressive oil; only increasing your level of exposure when other methods have not yielded enough results.

In horses, the bottom lip has been "squeezed out" to create a little pocket, and even neat Oregano has been very well tolerated in this manner. However, dilution of the Oregano is still advised, and at least a 50:50 dilution is suggested. Cattle and other large animals will often ingest Oregano in grain, hay, or feeds. Oregano can be mixed with many liquids or food items including Honey, Maple Syrup, Agave, Apple Sauce, or other items and can then even be delivered orally with a syringe.

Oregano is most commonly used orally for antibacterial properties and is often used in cases of bacterial infection (urinary infections, mastitis, tendon infections, bacterial diarrhea, etc...). The carvacrol content of Oregano is especially suited for the urinary system, as carvacrol is excreted rapidly in the urine, concentrating its properties there. Topical application of Oregano is useful for warts, sarcoids, mastitis, canker, abscesses, and fungal infections.

If oral use is considered for dogs – 1 drop of Oregano oil can be diluted with 10 drops of carrier oil. 1 drop or more of this dilution can be given twice a day, for each 20 pounds (9 kg) of body weight. Start with a smaller amount, and gradually increase as needed. Some dogs will lick a diluted Oregano solution off of your hand, or greatly enjoy the flavor mixed with foods. We often find this licking and ingesting behavior when the Canine Supportive Blend is used, and we allow it fully, along with the benefits it may impart. For Oregano delivered orally by capsule, Oregano should always be diluted with a carrier oil. Special consideration should be made of the gut flora of dogs receiving oral Oregano, and probiotics during and after administration may be warranted.

For horses and others, starting with 1 drop of Oregano per 200 pounds (90 kg) of body weight, given orally twice a day is a good starting point. After figuring the total amount of Oregano that will be given, it is still suggested to dilute or add to foods for use. Monitor responses and adjust according to individual need. In cases of mastitis and more severe infections – even 10 total drops of Oregano have been given orally twice a day. Special care should be considered of the gastrointestinal flora, and it is a good idea to follow the use of oral Oregano with probiotics.

Oregano, Onites (Origanum onites)
This version of Oregano is not widely available, but has made its debut on the aromatherapy market and is often quoted in research. It is not recommended for use with animals at this time.

Palmarosa (Cymbopogon martinii)
Palmarosa has not been used extensively as a single oil in animals at this time, and is most commonly used within blends. Palmarosa has GRAS status, and properties suggest its use to be excellent for conditions such as fungal infections (ringworm and dermatophytes), sebaceous cysts, cardiovascular disease (especially arrhythmias), oily skin conditions (seborrhea oleosa), wound healing, skin cell regeneration, and nervous system support. Palmarosa may be especially indicated for cases of Aspergillosis as some research has shown it to reduce spread, growth, and production of fungal mycotoxins. Research has also shown Palmarosa as effective in killing sarcoptic mites both topically and as a fumigant (diffusion), and may also have effects against ticks. Emotionally Palmarosa helps with stress and anxiety, as well as feelings of jealousy and possession. Over protective or possessive animals may find benefit with this oil.

Birds: Use of Palmarosa is most commonly through water-based diffusion of Three Part Blends. Addition to the Small Animal Supportive Blend or to Feather Spray Recipes can also be considered. When indicated diluted topical use of Three Part Blends or addition into natural ointments or salves could be considered. Ingestion beyond normal exposure, is not suggested.

Exotics: Use of Palmarosa is most commonly through water-based diffusion of Three Part Blends. Addition to the Small Animal Supportive Blend or to the Feline Supportive Blend (ferrets) can also be considered. Addition into water-misting recipes is also appropriate. When indicated diluted topical use of Three Part Blends or addition into natural ointments, shampoos, or salves can be considered. Ingestion is not suggested beyond normal grooming or licking behaviors.

Cats: Use of Palmarosa is most commonly through water-based diffusion of Three Part Blends. Addition into the Feline Supportive Blend is the most suggested route for any topical use. Addition into water-misting recipes can be considered, but many cats do not enjoy water-mists. When indicated diluted topical use of Three Part Blends or addition into natural ointments, shampoos, or salves can be considered. Addition into litter box recipes is also appropriate. Ingestion is not suggested beyond normal grooming activities.

Dogs & Larger: Palmarosa can be used in a variety of ways. Most commonly Palmarosa will be added to the Canine or Large Animal Supportive Blends or used via water-based diffusion or diluted topical applications of Three Part Blends. Addition into water-mists, natural ointments, salves, and shampoos is an excellent route for exposure. Direct topical applications can be considered (dilute or neat). Ingestion beyond normal grooming or licking behaviors is not suggested, however if a dog seems very intent on licking your hands with Palmarosa, you should not be concerned.

Palo Santo (Bursera graveolens)

Palo Santo is sometimes referred to as the "South American Frankincense" and is also called Holy Wood or Sacred Wood. Highly regarded as a spiritual oil, it is no mistake that these oils often carry many powerful medical benefits with them. This essential oil became very popular due to the promotion of sales by large essential oil companies. Sadly, Palo Santo (a wild-growing small tree) is regarded as a critically endangered species in Peru. While the essential oil is mainly produced in Ecuador, this appears to be only due to the fact that the plant is not officially recognized in this country as endangered. The extinction of a plant is never worth obtaining an essential oil, nor the medical properties it is reported to have. Palo Santo is reported to be useful for conditions such as cancer (especially lung and breast), cartilage repair, joint conditions, tendon and ligament repair and health, as an insect repellant, for skin tags, depression, emotional cleansing, warding off negative energy, pain control, healing, fungal infections, skin conditions, immune stimulation, and even antibacterial and antiviral actions. It is fairly mild in scent, and with skin application. Palo Santo is high in limonene, and so many other oils can contribute this constituent. Frankincense is an excellent replacement for this oil.

There are some cautionary statements regarding use during pregnancy and with children under 18 months of age, as well as cautions with oral use. While evidence to support these cautions has not been noted clinically, Palo Santo is not recommended for use with animals at this time.

Patchouli (Pogostemon cablin)

Patchouli is a wonderful oil that has been used widely with humans and animals. It is especially indicated for nausea, vomiting, hypertension, any form of skin condition, and for general calming effects. It is a great oil to consider for incredibly itchy skin, horses with summer itch, or other weepy or oozing sores. It is quite a strong oil in scent, and a very little amount added to a blend, is often all that is needed. Patchouli is incredibly mild to the skin, and neat use has often been used without concern. However, for animals, neat use results in overwhelming scent concerns, more than dermal irritation. Less is more, in regards to this oil's use.

Patchouli is mainly used within blends for animals, however often in lesser amounts than the other oils contained within that blend. When a blend may call for equal parts of oils, I may actually use 10% of that amount or less when considering Patchouli. As many humans will consider this fragrance for their own use, in general animals are fine being exposed to Patchouli on their humans.

Birds & Exotics: Patchouli is most commonly used within blends for water-based diffusion or diluted topical applications. Again, much lower percentages of Patchouli are generally required within animal blends. Addition into natural ointments, shampoos, and salves can also be considered. Addition into the Small Animal or Feline Supportive Blends can also be considered when appropriate. Adding 1 drop into the Feather Spray Recipe, water misting (1 drop or less per 4 ounces (120 mL), and application via Perches and Hands (diluted) could be considered. Although it has not been used extensively in an oral manner, routine ingestion through licking or grooming behaviors is of no concern, and is likely to be beneficial, especially for cases of regurgitation and nausea.

Cats: The most cat friendly methods of use for Patchouli will be within blends for water-based diffusion. Addition into the Feline Supportive Blend, or within blends intended for diluted topical applications can also be used. However, much lower percentages and additions of Patchouli are generally required within animal blends. Addition into natural ointments, salves, and shampoos, as well as inclusion into litter box recipes can also be considered. The oral use of Patchouli has been used for situations of severe nausea and vomiting, and exposure to routine grooming is often adequate for any oral need.

Dogs & Larger: Patchouli is most commonly used through water-based diffusion and diluted topical applications of Three Part Blends, or within the Canine or Large Animal Supportive Blends. Again, much lower percentages of Patchouli are generally required within animal blends. Direct application (diluted), addition into natural ointments, shampoos, massage oils, addition to wading pools and soaking water, and application via Petting (diluted) can also be considered. Oral use beyond normal licking or grooming behavior is unlikely to be necessary, however it does not cause concern if a dog or other animal appears quite attracted to ingesting this oil.

Pennyroyal (multiple spp.)

Basically this is one of those oils that we say, "Don't, just don't." There are just no indications that make me feel that the use of this essential oil would be worthwhile. With all of the cautionary tales involving Pennyroyal, it is just not an oil to be found in any collection.

Pepper, Black (Piper nigrum)

Black Pepper is more commonly used with animals now, than it was previously. Used most commonly in the "Flea Bomb Recipe", Black Pepper is also indicated for obesity, stimulating metabolism, for digestive problems, increasing circulation, as an analgesic and anti-inflammatory, for nerve and muscle pain, arthritis, and fungal infections. Black Pepper is also often indicated to help humans stop smoking. Black Pepper has GRAS status.

Steam distilled Black Pepper is prone to oxidation, and should be carefully stored to prevent spoilage. CO_2 extracts are becoming more widely desired and available, as more of the plant materials are present within them, and they also appear more resistant to oxidation damage. Black Pepper is certainly a CO_2 extract to consider the use of. Only in the CO_2 extract, do we find the beneficial compound piperine, which is often used to enhance the absorption of curcumin found in Turmeric. This is one situation, for which the CO_2 extract may become a more valuable player than the essential oil. The CO_2 extract is known to be more stable, and have a longer shelf life than the essential oil.

Flea Bomb Recipe: This recipe is so powerful, that it is recommended that humans, animals, and fish tanks be removed from the home or room while administering this treatment. If the area to be treated can be confined, some people have been successful in treating one room at a time, moving their diffuser from room to room, and evacuating to a distant part of the home. If you have fragile animals, it is likely best to have them leave the home completely. Diffusion with an air-style diffuser is mandatory for this application to penetrate more fully, and aid in potential elimination of insects and pests within the home. While a water-based diffuser can be used, the goal is to permeate the area with oils that might degrade and repel insects, which makes the concentrations available through water-based diffusion, less likely to accomplish.

- In a 15 mL glass essential oil bottle:
- Add approximately 70 drops each of Black Pepper, Peppermint, Oregano, and Orange essential oils.
- Set the dials on the air diffuser to full strength, and non-stop diffusion.
- Diffuse for at least 2 to 4 hours.
- The more severe the flea problem, the more you should desire to penetrate the room with these oils.
- Moving furniture and bedding, and vacuuming thoroughly is important. The entire home must be treated.

Birds & Exotics: Black Pepper is mainly used within blends or in diluted topical applications. Diffusion of this oil is less commonly selected for delicate animals, however inclusion into blends in small percentages for water-based diffusion is fine. Addition into the Small Animal Supportive Blend, into natural ointments, salves, or shampoos, or within Three Part Blends for diluted topical applications can be considered. Ingestion through regular grooming or licking is of no concern, however direct oral administration is generally not used.

Cats: Black Pepper is mainly used within blends or in diluted topical applications. Diffusion of this oil is less commonly selected for delicate animals, however inclusion into blends in small percentages for water-based diffusion is fine. Addition into the Feline Supportive Blend, into natural ointments, salves, or shampoos, within Three Part Blends for diluted topical applications, or addition into litter box recipes can be considered. Ingestion through regular grooming practices is likely all that would be necessary when oral use is considered, and is of no concern.

Dogs & Larger: Black Pepper is mainly used within blends or in diluted topical applications for severe obesity, arthritis, nerve and muscle pain, circulation disorders, or fungal infections (especially in Large Animals). Addition into the Canine or Large Animal Supportive Blends is suggested. Use within Three Part Blends can also be considered, and when considered for water-based diffusion, often just lower total percentages of Black Pepper will be added to a blend. Oral administration is very possible, and exploration especially with the CO_2 extracts is likely. If oral use in dogs is considered – 1 drop of Black Pepper can be diluted with 20 drops of carrier oil. 1 drop or more of this dilution can be given twice a day, for each 20 pounds (9 kg) of body weight. Start with a smaller amount, and gradually increase as needed.

For horses and others, topical use of Black Pepper as a single is much more likely to be tolerated, and would be indicated generally if blends or other essential oils have failed. Situations that would warrant the use of Black Pepper as a single or in much stronger concentrations would include severe and unresponsive nerve and muscle pain, obesity, metabolic syndrome, and fungal infections. Dilution for oral use should likely start at 1 drop Black Pepper in at least 5 drops of carrier oil; then giving 1 drop per 500 pounds (225 kg) of body weight, orally twice a day would be a recommended starting point. Monitor responses and adjust according to individual need.

Peppermint (Mentha piperita)

Peppermint is an interesting oil. For one so common, it can be found on many extremes of the quality spectrum. One must truly know distillation practices, to obtain a very high quality and aesthetically pleasing peppermint oil. In the past, it has been used last in the sequence of oil applications as it is a "driving" oil, which means that it appears to enhance the penetration of other oils. Often Peppermint will be applied after layering several other oils in a topical application. Peppermint's medical properties include anti-inflammatory, antitumoral, antiparasitic for worms, antibacterial, antiviral, antifungal, gall bladder and digestive stimulation, pain relief, and abnormal appetite suppression. It is indicated for conditions such as arthritis, obesity, Herpes infections, papilloma (warts), candida, diarrhea, nausea, vomiting, and colic. As part of Drip & Rub Recipes, it is likely to add enhancement to every situation.

Young children have had respiratory reactions to the Menthol in Peppermint, and so its use in high concentrations is not recommended for human children under 18 months of age. This condition has not been witnessed in animals, but it would be wise to be cautious with the use of neat Peppermint oil in very small puppies or kittens. Many foals and calves have been exposed to even neat peppermint, as early as 1 day of age, and it does not appear that large animals have this tendency for respiratory sensitivity. With diluted solutions as suggested in this book, we have not noted any concerns for animals, or humans applying them, in regards to issues with intensity.

Birds & Exotics: Peppermint is used less often as a single in these animals. With birds the most common use is by mixing into foods, starting with a toothpick dip and increasing up to 1 drop within 1 tablespoon. Adding to water can be considered, however for birds that bathe in their water, this may not be a good choice, as it could feel very "cold" and sting the eyes. It can be considered for use within the Small Animal Supportive Blend and is included within the stronger Avian Drip & Rub Recipe. While Peppermint can be water diffused – it should generally be combined with other oils, within blends, and often at a lower ratio than other oils. Peppermint is most commonly used within digestive Three Part Blends, and has been diffused quite often for digestive purposes. Peppermint could also be added to natural ointments, salves, and shampoos when desired, for topical application to non-feathered areas (1 drop or less to 1 tablespoon.)

With other exotics, Peppermint is also most commonly through addition to the Small Animal Supportive Blend or the Feline Supportive Blend. Addition to foods has also been commonly utilized for many exotics. Naturally, consider if Peppermint is a taste that would be appropriate for the animal you wish to use ingestion with, as use of items such as Copaiba or Ginger, may be far more accepted. The methods described for birds can also be used for most exotic species. It is likely that large amounts of diluted Peppermint can be consumed safely, however the intense flavor is more likely to limit the amounts that can be mixed into foods, and clinically, it appears an unnecessary route of administration in most situations.

Cats: There are opinions that cats and Peppermint oil should not be combined. In practice, I have found this issue to be more of a "how" the Peppermint oil is used, and not a function of Peppermint oil in itself. Peppermint is a strong oil, and with cats I often think of applying oils to them as if I would apply them to my own face, or to the face of my child. If you consider applying neat Peppermint oil to your face, I am sure you would agree it will be an intense experience. Even diluted, Peppermint can pack quite a bit of zing to a topical application. With a cat's very opinionated view on the world, an application of Peppermint that would be too intense, is likely to be remembered. Within the Feline Supportive Blend, Peppermint is used for some cats even twice a day. There are some cats who truly enjoy Peppermint and seek it out when their humans use it. This makes great sense actually, as both Catnip and Peppermint are within the mint family. The majority of cats absolutely love the Feline Supportive Blend applications, and in decades we have not witnessed any issue with Peppermint being in the solution. However, it is important to remember that there is quite a low percentage of Peppermint within the blend. Only 4 drops of Peppermint is contained within 30 mL (1 ounce), making it quite a dilute solution of both Peppermint, and the final total concentration of essential oils as a whole.

The most cat friendly way to use Peppermint is within the Feline Supportive Blend or within Three Part Blends intended for digestive concerns or for just amazing scents. Three Part Blends containing small amounts of Peppermint (Citrus and Peppermint for example) are often water diffused in animal homes for pure human enjoyment, and we have not witnessed reason for concern. While I would avoid diffusion of Peppermint as a single, it does have its place within diffusion, and retains its decongestant, anti-inflammatory, and sinus opening properties to impart. Addition into natural ointments (1 drop per tablespoon), salves, or shampoos can also be considered. When ingestion is desired, you should not have to look beyond normal grooming practices of diluted blends for adequate exposure.

Dogs & Larger: The most common methods of use include within the Canine and Large Animal Supportive Blends, within Three Part Blends for water-based diffusion or diluted topical applications, direct application (diluted), addition into natural ointments, salves, shampoo, massage oils, adding to wading pools and soaking water, addition into foods, addition into drinking water, and by direct oral administration.

When oral use for dogs is considered – 1 drop of Peppermint can be diluted with 10 drops (or more) of carrier oil. The dilution of Peppermint in this situation is important for the lowering of the intense flavor of the oil, and increased dilution should be considered for most animals prior to administration. Up to 5 drops or more of this diluted solution (basically an entire drop of Peppermint oil per day) can be given twice a day, for each 20 pounds (9 kg) of body weight. Start with a smaller amount, and gradually increase as needed, as most animals likely do not need that much in actuality.

For horses and others, starting with 1 drop per 200 pounds (90 kg) of body weight, given orally twice a day is a good starting point. Monitor responses and adjust according to individual need. Certainly much larger amounts of Peppermint are administered to these animals orally in certain cases. With colic in horses, 20 drops of Peppermint is commonly administered orally, and 20 drops of Peppermint is applied topically every 20 minutes, often for multiple doses. Please see Colic within the Equine Conditions for more information on this protocol. While dilution of oral Peppermint for large animals has not been necessary, it is still recommended. For most large animals, we are relying on the absorption through mucous membranes in the mouth (buccal absorption) than through a swallowing type of ingestion.

Peru Balsam (Myroxylon balsamum)
There is little information on this oil, but it is cautioned as a source of skin sensitization. It is not recommended for use with animals at this time, however high quality oil may be able to be used within blends via water-based diffusion.

Petitgrain (Citrus sinensis, Citrus aurantium)
Also called Orange Leaf, bitter orange leaf, sour orange leaf - Petitgrain has not been used extensively as a single oil in animals at this time. Medical properties indicate its use for conditions such as nystagmus and vestibular disease, anxiety, and muscle spasms. There are different forms of Petitgrain, which are all distilled from the leaf of the citrus plant. So one might find a Petitgrain of Mandarin, Orange, Lemon, Bergamot, or Lime etc. While Petitgrain is not commonly used with animals at this time, it is likely that inclusion within blends for water-based diffusion will be of no concern.

Pine (Pinus sylvestris)
Also called Scotch pine, Pine oil is useful with animals for conditions such as lice, fleas, mange and skin parasites, lung infections, arthritis, urinary tract infections, lymphatic stimulation, anxiety, and sinus infections. It may show

great value for hormone and cortisone-like activity as well as anti-diabetic properties. Pine is often used within blends in small amounts. Pine oil is not recommended for oral use (which eliminates its purposes with animals distinctly). While there are many types of pine essential oil (dwarf, grey or Jack, black, white, red or Norway, etc...), Scotch Pine remains the one most consistently available and in use with animals.

Birds & Exotics: The main use of Pine is through water-based diffusion (including caging and tenting.) Other appropriate uses of Pine would be through addition of 1 drop to the Small Animal Supportive Blend, addition to natural ointments (1 drop per tablespoon), Perch and Hand applications (generally diluted), and diluted topical applications of Three Part Blends (non-avian species mainly). For birds and exotics with skin parasites, it is likely that a water-based diffusion in a tented situation may be sufficient to permeate the skin with the oil. Starting with 1 drop in a diffuser, and with careful monitoring, the amount diffused could gradually be increased in concentration (adding more drops the diffuser.) As the animal tolerates it, 4 drops or more could be water diffused in a tenting situation, for 20 minutes, 2-4 times a day. This technique would be especially useful for skin mites in hedgehogs. However, it is important to recognize that other essential oils have a wider safety margin, have been used much more commonly, and can be considered consumable by animals, making Pine a far less recommended option.

Cats: Pine would most commonly be considered for water-based diffusion within Three Part Blends. While it is likely that Pine could be added successfully (and has) to the Feline Supportive Blend, litter box recipes, shampoos, ointments, and salves, the avoidance of oils with ingestion concerns is the best recommendation for species such as cats, who are almost continually grooming.

Dogs & Larger: Pine would most commonly be considered for water-based diffusion within Three Part Blends. Pine can safely be added to the Canine or Large Animal Supportive Blends, or to Three Part Blends for diluted topical applications, however consideration should be made for dogs who may ingest larger amounts of the oil through ointments or salves. The addition of Pine to shampoos, wading pools and soaking water, and other massage oil recipes for large animals has been well accepted and effective. Air diffusion for larger barns or arenas can be considered when needed, generally within Three Part Blends.

Plai (Zingiber montanum)
A wonderful up and coming oil in Veterinary Aromatic Medicine, Plai is a member of the ginger family. Known mainly for its antioxidant and anti-inflammatory actions, Plai is thought to be quite safe. However, more data is needed at this time for wide spread use in animals to be recommended.

Ravensara (Agathophyllum aromatica, Ravensara aromatica)
The leaf derived oil of Ravensara is the most commonly found in the aromatherapy market. Much confusion has been placed between Ravensara and Ravintsara – however even between "known" species there appears to be quite a wide array of chemical analysis. In general, Ravensara or Ravintsara oils are not widely used with animals at this time. See more information within the Ravintsara description for how to use Ravensara.

Ravintsara (Cinnamomum camphora)
Ravintsara is regarded for antiviral properties in animals, especially for Herpes virus. Ravintsara may also be useful for hepatitis, lung infections and pneumonia, and cancer. It has been part of the confusion between Ravintsara and Ravensara – and in general it is not widely used with animals at this time. The camphor chemotype of this oil is not recommended for use with animals.

Birds & Exotics: Ravintsara has been used in small concentrations within blends. Water-based diffusion can be considered for both Ravintsara and Ravensara. More extensive use of Ravintsara is not suggested at this time.

Cats: Ravintsara is also more commonly used within blends in small concentrations, and most often with water-based diffusion. Addition in small amounts into the Feline Supportive Blend and litter box recipes has been utilized.

Dogs & Larger: Ravintsara is also more commonly used within blends in small concentrations, and most often with water-based diffusion. Ravintsara can be considered for addition into the Canine or Large Animal Supportive Blends, air diffusion in large barns or areas, diluted topical applications within Three Part Blends, addition to natural ointments, salves, and shampoos. Ravintsara is not recommended for oral use beyond normal licking or grooming behaviors.

Roman Chamomile (see Chamomile, Roman)

Rosalina (see Melaleuca ericifolia)

Rose (Rosa damascene)

Rose oil (also called Rose Otto) for use with animals, should only be obtained by steam distillation and never its cheaper absolute counterpart. High quality steam distilled oil is quite expensive, and often carries some level of crystallization at room temperatures and colder. Often this oil has to be warmed gently (by hugging close to the body is great) to get it fully mobile and flowing.

In terms of properties, Rose has no equal. It is of the highest vibrational energy reported for essential oils. This makes this oil one of the "Life Force Oils," which we routinely use in our veterinary clinic for animals who are very weak, and who are close to death. When the situation is correct, Rose can elevate an animal's energy and seemingly ability to live, simply by smelling the open bottle. If it truly is the animal's time to pass, this event is not prevented, however we see a more serene and peaceful transition. Owners and animal friends experience great relief and acceptance of the passing, with the combined use of Rose and Frankincense.

Rose has research and properties that suggest it is useful for conditions such as anxiety, conflict between animals, releasing traumatic memories, hypertension, seizures, Herpes infections, skin conditions, and ulcers. Since Rose is also a more expensive oil, it is often used within blends and at lesser concentrations. It is quite a powerful oil, and its scent within a blend can become overpowering. A small bottle of Rose is well worth the investment, and you are likely to only need very small amounts. Ingestion of Rose beyond normal exposure through grooming or licking behaviors is not suggested.

Birds & Exotics: Rose oil is most commonly used within blends in low amounts. Water-based diffusion of blends containing Rose oil, is the most common and recommended method of use. The indirect diffusion of a human wearing the oils, wafting an open bottle near-by, or placing a drop (can be diluted) on a cotton ball or tissue is also used commonly.

Cats: The same statement that was made for birds and exotics also holds true for cats. In some situations, we have applied Rose oil to cats via the Petting technique (diluted), and 1 drop can be added to the Feline Supportive Blend when desired. The vast majority of the use of Rose remains in the use of the blends for water-based diffusion, although addition in small amounts to litter box recipes can also be considered.

Dogs & Larger: Rose oil will most commonly be used in small amounts within blends for water-based diffusion. For larger animals, water-spritzers containing Rose may be useful to obtain exposure and responses. Humans can also wear Rose or blends containing Rose for additional actions. Rose most certainly can be included in Three Part Blends, Canine or Large Animal Supportive Blends, and within natural ointments, salves, or shampoos. Due to the expense of this oil, it is most likely to be reserved for emotional work, and less likely to be utilized in treatment of physical conditions or topical applications.

Rosemary (Rosmarinus officinalis – Cineole Chemotype)

Rosemary oil has many benefits in the world of animals. It has GRAS status, and has been used in French hospitals to disinfect the air, and as part of the blends we used for this purpose in our veterinary hospital. We see vast reduction in transmission of upper respiratory infections and kennel cough when blends containing this oil are diffused on a regular basis in shelters, hospitals, grooming facilities, boarding facilities, or any other location where multiple animals will be in contact.

Rosemary as a single oil has been noted to have bug repelling properties, and seems especially good at repelling Asian Beetles and Box Elder Bugs that invade our homes. Through the diffusion Rosemary itself, we have noted continually less of these bugs entering our home and clinic. Rosemary's medical benefits include liver protection, stimulation of hair growth, reduction of blemishes, antitumoral, antifungal, antibacterial, and antiparasitic actions as well as the enhancement of mental clarity. Conditions benefiting from Rosemary would include infectious diseases (especially air borne), liver conditions, lung infections, hair loss, cognitive dysfunction, dementia, and fungal infections.

There is a lot of interesting research regarding Rosemary, and even studies that show that tracheal muscle contractions due to inflammation and irritants, were lessened through exposure to the essential oil. This confirms what we have seen clinically; that coughs and conditions such as collapsing trachea, greatly improve through the presence of water-based diffusion of essential oils, and especially of blends containing Rosemary.

There are cautionary statements in regards to the use of Rosemary with children under 4 years of age. This appears to be due to the high 1,8-cineole content of this chemotype, and not fully to Rosemary itself. While Rosemary as a single oil is not used extensively with animals, and certainly not with very young animals, it has been used within blends quite commonly, even in the presence of day old animals. The use of Rosemary as a single oil, is likely best avoided in animals less than 6 months of age as a precaution, but the use within blends and within proper dilutions and ratios, has shown no clinical concern. Water-based diffusion is likely to remain fine for all ages and conditions.

There is also a caution regarding the use of Rosemary in those with high blood pressure. This has basically been dispelled in Tisserand & Young's well respected book - *Essential Oil Safety*; 2nd Edition. There are just so many cautions that become "urban legend" and they are difficult to shake in the essential oil world, especially with the online buzz that can be created and perpetuated.

The last "urban legend" that arises with Rosemary are the many reports to be cautious regarding seizures or epilepsy with Rosemary exposure or use. I even see humans wishing to avoid Rosemary Extract (a natural preservative) within foods and shampoos. The link to Rosemary and seizures, comes from the possible high Camphor content, especially related to the Camphor chemotype of Rosemary. 1,8-cineole is also often incriminated for seizure potential. It is the over-exposure to these constituents, and often by themselves, that we should be concerned with, not the Rosemary as a whole. The levels required to be "neurotoxic" are quite high, and should not be related necessarily to Rosemary by itself, and especially not when used with proper methods.

Birds & Exotics: The use of Rosemary has mainly been limited through its use within blends. Water-based diffusion (starting with 1 drop, and gradually increasing to 4 drops in a diffuser) is the recommended use for Rosemary as a single. Rosemary can be considered for addition into the Small Animal or Feline Supportive Blends, Three Part Blends for water-based diffusion or diluted topical applications, and added to natural ointments, salves, and shampoos. In severe situations, oral use of Rosemary can be considered starting with a toothpick dip added into 1 tablespoon of food. The addition into drinking water is also a likely method of ingestion (1 drop or less per liter.)

Cats: The use of Rosemary is mainly through use within blends, and most commonly through water-based diffusion. Addition of 1 drop into the Feline Supportive Blend, addition to litter box recipes, and diluted topical use of Three Part Blends can be considered. Ingestion of Rosemary beyond normal grooming practices is not suggested.

Dogs & Larger: Rosemary can be used in many application methods for these animals. The most common methods of use include water-diffusion within Three Part Blends, addition into the Canine or Large Animal Supportive Blends, use within Three Part Blends for water-misting or diluted topical applications, direct application (diluted), or by addition into natural ointments, salves, and shampoos. Addition to wading pools and soaking water, application via Petting (diluted), air diffusion in large areas, addition into foods, addition into drinking water, and direct oral administration can be considered. In general, ingestion beyond normal licking or grooming behaviors is not suggested.

If oral use is considered for dogs – 1 drop of Rosemary can be diluted with 20 drops (or more) of carrier oil. Increased dilution of Rosemary may be necessary for some dogs. 1 drop or more of this diluted solution can be given twice a day, for each 20 pounds (9 kg) of body weight. Start with a smaller amount, and gradually increase as needed, as most animals likely do not need that much in actuality.

For horses and others, starting with 1 drop per 500 pounds (225 kg) of body weight, given orally twice a day is a good starting point. Monitor responses and adjust according to individual need.

Rosemary (Rosmarinus officinalis – Verbenone Chemotype)

Another chemotype of Rosemary that is also used within the animal kingdom. The main directions of the Cineole chemotype also apply here. Verbenone has been shown to have synergistic effects with the antibiotics erythromycin and ampicillin in research, and increased their concentrations in the lung. There is also evidence that Verbenone may act on platelets, inhibiting aggregation.

Rosewood (Aniba rosaeodora)

Also called Bois de rose, this essential oil is listed on the CITES protection list. It has been used sparingly within the animal kingdom, however due to high rates of synthetic and adulterated oil on the market, I do not recommend its use with animals.

Rue (Ruta graveolens)

Rue is a bit of a controversial oil, and while some fear it, others have used it quite successfully. Its odor however, is one that often limits its use to very small amounts. It contains potential phototoxic properties, and so applications to the skin should not be exposed to direct and intense sunlight for 12 hours. However, we have yet to note photosensitivity reactions in animals to date. Rue is considered safe for human consumption by the FDA and is used in food flavorings at low levels. Emotionally, Rue seems to have a very grounding effect, and is often used is very small amounts in emotionally based blends.

Sage (Salvia officinalis)

Also called Dalmatian Sage, this is the most common version of Sage used with animals, however it has mainly been used in small concentrations within blends. Due to its camphor content, Sage is less selected for use within Veterinary Aromatic Medicine. As a single oil, Sage is indicated for hormonal issues, cognitive dysfunction, cancers, prostate problems and urinary tract infections, conditions in need of bone remodeling, diabetes, gall bladder conditions, and liver disease. There are cautionary statements within references to avoid the use of Sage with epileptics (seizures) and with high blood pressure. It is likely wise to avoid Sage in animals with these conditions. In general, the use of Sage in the animal kingdom is not widely recommended.

Birds & Exotics: The use of Sage has mainly been limited to its use within blends. Water-based diffusion (starting with 1 drop, and gradually increasing to 4 drops in a diffuser) is the recommended route for desired exposure to Sage. It is likely that Sage may be helpful to ferrets, who are commonly affected with prostatic disease. Addition into the Small Animal Supportive Blend can likely be considered. Ingestion beyond normal grooming or licking behaviors is not suggested at this time.

Cats: The use of Sage should mainly be considered through water-based diffusion within blends. The addition of 1 drop to the Feline Supportive Blend or inclusion within litter box recipes can be considered.

Dogs & Larger: Sage will mainly be used within blends, with the most common exposure through water-based diffusion. Addition into the Canine or Large Animal Supportive Blends, Three Part Blends, natural ointments, salves, and shampoos, can be considered. Ingestion beyond normal licking and grooming behaviors is not suggested. For prostate disorders, Rectal Instillation can also be considered – please see that chapter for more information.

St. John's Wort (Hypericum perforatum)
This essential oil is not recommended for use with animals.

Sandalwood (Santalum album)
Also referred to as Indian, East Indian, White, Yellow, or Mysore Sandalwood. This plant currently protected from over-harvest – however Santanol (a company located in Western Australia) is currently cultivating and harvesting true Santalum album. This should be the source desired for this oil. True Sandalwood is a lovely oil indicated for conditions such as Herpes Virus infections, Papilloma (warts), cancer, as an immune stimulant, and for urinary and cystitis cases as santalols are eliminated via the urine. It is used both as a single and is also commonly used within blends. The use of Sandalwood in cancer cases has been powerful emotionally and physically. Emotional benefits of Sandalwood include grounding, acceptance, reduction of stress, guilt, and aggressive behavior, reduction of irritability and despondence, sleep improvement, and improvement of memory and brain function.

Birds & Exotics: Sandalwood is most commonly used within blends. Water-based diffusion, addition into the Small Animal Supportive Blend, addition of 1 drop to the Feather Spray Recipes, water misting (1 drop in 4 ounces (120 mL) of distilled water), addition to natural ointments (1 drop per tablespoon), salves, or shampoos, diluted topical applications of Three Part Blends, direct topical application (diluted 1 drop in 20 drops of carrier oil), Perch and Hand applications (generally diluted), and indirect diffusion on humans and cotton balls can be considered.

Cats: The most cat friendly methods of use include addition into the Feline Supportive Blend, addition into Three Part Blends for water-based diffusion or diluted topical applications, addition into litter box recipes, and direct application (generally diluted.) Oral administration beyond routine grooming behaviors is not suggested. In cases of cancer and severe Herpes infection, further ingestion could be investigated in strict cooperation with veterinary monitoring. If oral use is considered for cats, addition into foods is suggested. Start with a toothpick dip within a Tablespoon of food, and gradually increase the amount. A maximum oral amount is generally obtained by 1 drop of Sandalwood being diluted with 10 drops of carrier oil. One or more drops of this solution can be given twice a day, generally added to foods. Since this has not been used widely in cats at this time, using other methods of application is recommended first, along with careful monitoring with a veterinarian.

Dogs & Larger: The most common methods of use include addition into topical blends and through water-based diffusion. Addition into the Canine or Large Animal Supportive Blends, Three Part Blends for water-based diffusion or diluted topical applications, direct application (neat or diluted), application via Petting (diluted), addition into natural ointments, salves, and shampoos is most commonly utilized. Ingestion beyond normal grooming or licking actions is generally not suggested.

If oral use for dogs is considered – 1 drop of Sandalwood can be diluted with 3 drops (or more) of carrier oil. 1 drop or more of this diluted solution can be given twice a day, for each 20 pounds (9 kg) of body weight. Start with a smaller amount, and gradually increase as needed, as most animals likely do not need that much in actuality.

For horses and others, starting with 1 drop per 300 pounds (135 kg) of body weight, given orally twice a day is a good starting point. Monitor responses and adjust according to individual need.

Sandalwood (Santalum spicatum)
Also called Australian Sandalwood, it is often used as a replacement for Indian Sandalwood. It is not as rich in santalol, and now with viable and responsible harvests of Santalum album in Australia – album is likely to remain the preferred species of use. It can be used in the ways described for Santalum album.

Saro (Cinnamosma fragrans)
From Madagascar, this essential oil is high in 1,8-cineole. It is not widely used with animals at this time, although most profiles indicate it is likely safe.

Sassafras (many species)
This essential oil is not recommended for use with animal species.

Savory (see Mountain Savory)

Spearmint (Mentha spicata)

Spearmint oil is used with animals for a variety of conditions including increasing metabolism, for obesity, as a mucolytic (breaks up mucus), as a gall bladder stimulant, for liver disorders, and as a digestive aid. Research indicates Spearmint would be beneficial for nausea and vomiting, reduction of intestinal spasms, high blood pressure, fungal infections, COPD and inflammatory lung conditions, to increase athletic performance, and as an anti-inflammatory and antinociceptive agent. Spearmint is most commonly used within blends for animals, however may be desired at lower amounts than the rest of the blends ingredients. Spearmint has GRAS status.

Birds & Exotics: Spearmint would most commonly be used through addition to the Small Animal Supportive Blend, to Three Part Blends for water-based diffusion or diluted topical applications, and may be considered for use by addition to drinking water (1 drop per liter), or addition to foods (up to 1 drop per tablespoon).

Cats: The same comments for birds and exotics apply to the use of Spearmint with cats. The most cat friendly methods of use include water-based diffusion within blends, addition into the Feline Supportive Blend, and addition to litter box recipes (usually in a lower amounts than other ingredients within the blend). It greatly depends on the cat if they will ingest Spearmint within foods or water. Ingestion of Spearmint beyond normal grooming practices is likely to be unnecessary. When further ingestion is desired, starting with a toothpick dip into 1 liter of water, and gradually increasing to 1 drop per liter, is a good method to get cats used to the flavor. For oral administration, addition into foods is most likely to be successful. Start with 1 drop of Spearmint diluted in 20 drops (or more) of carrier oil. 1 drop or more of this dilution can be given, twice a day or as needed. Oral use is generally reserved for more severe issues, and is not used commonly for cats.

Dogs & Larger: Spearmint is most commonly used within blends, and can be added to the Canine and Large Animal Supportive Blends, Three Part Blends for water-based diffusion or diluted topical applications, addition into natural ointments, salves, and shampoos. While ingestion beyond normal licking and grooming is usually not needed; addition into foods, addition into drinking water, and direct oral administration can be considered.

If oral use is considered for dogs – 1 drop of Spearmint can be diluted with 10 drops (or more) of carrier oil. Increased dilution of Spearmint may be necessary for some dogs. 1 drop or more of this diluted solution can be given twice a day, for each 20 pounds (9 kg) of body weight, generally mixed into foods. Start with a smaller amount, and gradually increase as needed, as most animals likely do not need that much in actuality.

For horses and others, starting with 1 drop per 300 pounds (135 kg) of body weight, given orally twice a day is a good starting point. Monitor responses and adjust according to individual need.

Spike Lavender (see Lavender, Spike)

Spikenard (Nardostachys jatamansi)

Spikenard is listed on the CITES protection list, and careful regard should be considered in the purchase and use of this oil. Often referred to as "Jesus' Oil" as it was said to be used to anoint the feet of Jesus before the Last Supper. It has been a precious oil throughout history, even before biblical times, and its health benefits are often powerful. Conditions that may benefit from the use of Spikenard include severe bacterial or viral disease, breast cancer, heart arrhythmias, migraines, skin conditions, wounds requiring the regeneration of skin, lymph circulation, allergies, constipation, nervous tension, and when stimulation of the immune system is needed.

Birds & Exotics: Spikenard is most commonly used by water-based diffusion within blends for these species. Addition into the Small Animal Supportive Blend, Three Part Blends for water-based diffusion or diluted topical applications, addition of 1 drop to the Feather Spray Recipes, water misting (1 drop per 4 ounces (120 mL) of distilled water), Perch or Hand application (diluted), indirect diffusion (onto objects within diluted Three Part Blends), and addition into natural ointments (1 drop per tablespoon), salves, or shampoos can also be considered. Oral use of Spikenard is not recommended beyond normal diluted topical exposure and licking and grooming behaviors.

Cats: Cat friendly methods of use include water-based diffusion within Three Part Blends, addition into the Feline Supportive Blend, and addition into litter box recipes. Oral ingestion of Spikenard is only suggested through normal grooming behaviors of diluted topical blends containing Spikenard. Addition into natural ointments, salves, water-mists, or shampoos can also be considered.

Dogs & Larger: Spikenard can be used by addition into the Canine or Large Animal Supportive Blends, Three Part Blends for water-based diffusion or diluted topical applications, direct application (diluted), application via Petting (diluted), and by additions into natural ointments, salves, water-mists, or shampoos. Ingestion beyond normal grooming and licking behaviors is not suggested at this time.

Spruce, Black (Picea mariana)

Spruce is a very special oil, rich in spiritual connection and is often indicated for arthritis and bone conditions, sinus and respiratory infections, nerve and back pain, immune stimulation, spasms, inflammation, hormonal concerns, thyroid and adrenal support, fungal infections, and parasites. Spruce is helpful to release emotional blocks and is a very balancing and grounding oil. It is helpful in many behavioral conditions and is often linked to confidence, acceptance, forgiveness, and security. Research has also shown Black Spruce to have effects against MRSA.

Birds & Exotics: Spruce is most commonly used within Three Part Blends for water-based diffusion (including caging and tenting). Addition into the Small Animal Supportive blend, addition of 1 drop into the Feather Spray Recipes, water misting (1 drop added to 4 ounces (120 mL) of distilled water), addition to natural ointments, salves, or shampoos, addition to soaking water and aquariums (starting with a toothpick dip), Perch applications, and indirect diffusion can be considered. Ingestion beyond normal grooming and licking behaviors is not suggested.

Cats: The most cat friendly methods to use Spruce include the addition into the Feline Supportive Blends and water-based diffusion within Three Part Blends. Diluted topical applications of Three Part Blends, use in litter box recipes, addition into natural ointments, salves, or shampoos, and indirect diffusion (often a diluted drop of a blend placed on a cotton ball, and placed inside a cat carrier), can also be considered. Oral use of Spruce in cats is generally limited to ingestion via normal grooming behaviors.

Dogs & Larger: Spruce is most commonly used through addition into the Canine and Large Animal Supportive Blends, addition into Three Part Blends for water-based diffusion or diluted topical applications, direct application (diluted), application via Petting (diluted), addition into natural ointments, salves, or shampoos, addition to wading pools and soaking water, addition into bathing or soaking solutions, addition into foods, addition into drinking water, and by direct oral administration. In general, the oral use of Spruce beyond normal grooming and licking behaviors, is widely unnecessary.

If oral use is considered for dogs – 1 drop of Spruce can be diluted with 10 drops of edible carrier oil (coconut oil). 1 drop or more of this diluted solution can be given twice a day, for each 20 pounds (9 kg) of body weight, generally mixed with foods. Start with a smaller amount, and gradually increase as needed.

For horses and others, starting with 1 drop per 100-200 pounds (45-90 kg) of body weight, given orally twice a day is a good starting point. Monitor responses and adjust according to individual need.

Spruce, Other Varieties

Other varieties of Spruce include Hemlock, Red, White, Norway, etc... However, these species of Spruce should not be considered interchangeable with Black Spruce. The use of these Spruce species is not well documented with animals at this time, and their use is not recommended.

Star Anise (see Anise, Star)

Tagetes (Tagetes minuta)

Also known as Wild Marigold, this oil is not widely used nor suggested for use with animals at this time.

Tangerine (Citrus tangerina)

There is some confusion between Mandarin and Tangerine oils. Citrus reticulata is used to describe both, however they are quite different. Tangerine is easily used in all animals and in many routes, and is an essential oil with GRAS status. Its use is indicated for cases of spasm, tumors and cancer, digestive problems, liver problems, parasites, fluid retention, edema, sleeplessness, anxiety, obesity, circulation disorders, and depression.

Tangerine is not actually considered to be photosensitizing; however there could still be issues for sensitive people when strong concentrations are applied. Avoid applying in concentrations higher than 30% to skin that will be exposed to sunlight or full spectrum UV light within 12 hours. Due to proper use of oils and dilution rates suggested for animals, concern is likely not needed where animals are concerned.

Birds & Exotics: Tangerine oil has been used in many ways: via water-based diffusion (including caging and tenting), within the Small Animal Supportive Blend, added to topical recipes, within the Feather Spray Recipe (replacing either Lemon or Orange, drop for drop), added to drinking water (1 or more drops per liter), added to foods (1 or more drops per tablespoon), addition into natural ointments, water spritzers (up to 20 drops per 4 ounces), Petting (diluted non-avian), and allowed to be directly ingested when animals chose to lick the oil off of hands and other items.

Cats: The most cat friendly methods of use include water-based diffusion within Three Part Blends, addition into the Feline Supportive Blend, and by use within litter box recipes. Some cats will ingest Tangerine oil in foods or water as described for Birds & Exotics, however ingestion beyond normal grooming habits is likely unnecessary.

Dogs & Larger: Common methods of use include addition into the Canine and Large Animal Supportive Blends, Three Part Blends for water-based diffusion or diluted topical applications, addition into foods, addition into drinking water (1 drop or more per liter for dogs), direct topical application (generally diluted), air diffusion, and direct oral administration. Follow the basic directions for Orange oil for ingestion.

Tangerine oil applied directly to the skin, is usually best diluted in a carrier oil such as Fractionated Coconut Oil. Starting with smaller amounts or a more diluted oil, is still recommended as many animals respond to lesser amounts. However, if needed, much larger quantities can be applied safely.

Tansy, Blue (Tanacetum annuum)
Blue Tansy (also called Moroccan Blue Chamomile) has not been used extensively as a single in animals at this time. It has been used within some proprietary human blends, without much consequence. Medical properties of Blue Tansy indicate its use for inflammation, analgesia, pain control, reduction in itching, hormone-like activity, and as a relaxant. At this time, Blue Tansy is not recommended routinely for use with animals. I suggest the use of German Chamomile instead, when this oil is being considered.

Tansy (Tanacetum vulgare)

Common Tansy (from Idaho specifically) was made especially popular by one specific essential oil company. While it was reported to have a great many uses by those within that company, it is not an oil which I use widely, nor recommend routinely. It is well known for its insect repelling action, and also has actions of analgesia and immune stimulation. Although it is listed as an anticoagulant, many people have placed this essential oil onto the wounds of large animals, and have not only found it to stop the bleeding, but at the same time repel flies and other insects from attacking the wound. Tansy has been a common ingredient in many bug repellant recipes.

There are cautionary statements against using Tansy while pregnant or nursing. It is a wise recommendation to heed this warning for animals as well, however many pregnant horses, cows, goats, and dogs have been exposed to Tansy within bug repelling recipes, with no ill effects. Due to its constituent profile (especially camphor and thujone content), Tansy is not recommended for use with animals at this time.

Tarragon (Artemisia dracunculus)

Tarragon is used with animals primarily for gastrointestinal concerns and internal parasites. Medical properties indicate its use with intestinal disorders, urinary tract infections, for nausea and vomiting, behavioral hormonal issues, for seizures, and as an antispasmodic. Its use as a single is common in the deworming practices of large animals.

There is a cautionary statement in some references to avoid the use of Tarragon with epilepsy. I have not witnessed any problems with the use of Tarragon containing blends and products with animals known to have seizures, and current research and safety textbooks do not indicate Tarragon as a seizure risk. In fact, there is one research article which claims anticonvulsant properties associated with certain chemotypes of Tarragon (Sayyah et al, *J. Ethnopharmacol.* 2004 Oct;94(2-3):283-7).

Birds & Exotics: Tarragon is most commonly used within blends created to support the digestive tract. Addition to the Small Animal Supportive Blend, to Three Part Blends for water-based diffusion or diluted topical applications, and addition into foods can be considered. Oral consumption is reserved for when other methods have not been effective, or in cases of dire need under supervision of a veterinarian. Starting points for food administration would be with a toothpick dip into 1 tablespoon of food.

Cats: The most cat friendly uses of Tarragon include addition into the Feline Supportive Blend, addition into Three Part Blends for water-based diffusion or diluted topical applications, and addition into litter box recipes. Ingestion of Tarragon beyond normal grooming practices of diluted topical blends, is likely unnecessary.

Dogs & Larger: Tarragon is most commonly used by addition into the Canine or Large Animal Supportive Blends, addition to Three Part Blends for water-based diffusion or diluted topical applications, direct topical application (diluted), Petting (diluted), addition into foods, and direct oral administration. Oral administration is unlikely to be necessary, and topical and diffusion applications are often sufficient.

If oral use is considered for dogs, 1 drop of Tarragon can be diluted with 10 drops of carrier oil. 1 drop or more of this diluted solution can be given twice a day, for each 20 pounds (9 kg) of body weight, generally adding into foods. Start with a smaller amount, and gradually increase as needed.

For horses and others, starting with 1 drop per 200 pounds (45-90 kg) of body weight, given orally twice a day is a good starting point. Monitor responses and adjust according to individual need.

Deworming protocols have been used in horses, with 6 drops of Tarragon given to an average sized horse, in the lip, twice a day for one week. This was recommended to start on a full moon, and repeated monthly or as needed. While some people did note apparent results, the outcome is inconsistent at best. Working with a veterinarian to monitor fecal egg counts, and responses to any natural deworming regimen is important. Please see Deworming in Equine Conditions for more information.

Tea Tree (see Melaleuca alternifolia)

Thyme (Thymus vulgaris)

Thyme essential oil has several chemotypes available. Of the more common is Thymol and Linalool. Each have their own properties that make them attractive to use. Thyme (thymol) has very powerful effects. Medical properties show that Thyme is anti-aging, liver protective, anti-inflammatory, highly antimicrobial (effective against MRSA), antifungal (Aspergillus, yeast, others), antiviral

(Herpes), antiparasitic (giardia, protozoa, lice, stomach worm), eases coughs, and may encourage bone remodeling. It is especially indicated for use as an overall immune supportive oil. Emotionally and mentally, Thyme may contribute to better concentration, confidence, and assurance. Thyme is a "hot" oil, and care must be taken to monitor the skin of animals exposed to it, and to also use caution if diffusing.

Thyme (linalool) is a milder version, however due to the high levels of linalool, may be more prone to oxidation damage. Most commonly the thymol chemotype is used within Veterinary Aromatic Medicine.

The repeated use of Thyme, or the use of Thyme that is overly concentrated, has resulted in hair loss in some animals at the site of application. This occurrence is most common in animals receiving repeated, frequent, or overly concentrated applications, even if the area never became red or irritated. Mostly what is seen is a flakey scab, which peels off with the hair. To date, all hair loss has grown back. There may be other oils that contribute to this hair loss phenomena, however Thyme seems to be a prominent component in the event, as often the hair loss was located where a drop of Thyme fell on the skin. With proper use of this oil, and especially within the blends and concentrations recommended in this book, it is very unlikely to see this occur. However, if beginning signs are noted, take action to reduce the total amount of Thyme within your blend, or to dilute the blend further as a whole. Lessening the frequency of application may also be effective to reduce hair loss.

Water-based diffusion of this oil could be considered in extremely low amounts, and especially combined with other oils to further dilute the entire recipe. This would be reserved for only the most severe of cases, especially fungal infections, when other oils have not yielded enough results. Strict veterinary monitoring is suggested.

Birds & Exotics: Thyme has mainly been used within the stronger Avian Drip & Rub Recipe or within the Feline Supportive Blend for selected species (ferrets). In severe situations, addition into foods can be considered and would begin with 1 toothpick dip of Thyme mixed into 1 tablespoon of food, and would then be gradually increased. This can be used as a powerful antibacterial, antifungal, antiviral, and antiparasitic agent in resistant cases. Moving towards the oral use of Thyme, is generally reserved for when other methods of use have failed.

Care must be taken with Rabbits, Guinea Pigs, and Chinchillas as they are considered "hind-gut fermenters." The aggressive use of a powerful antibacterial agent like Thyme, could damage their delicate intestinal flora.

Please make sure to see the sections for these animals specifically, for more information on their individual needs and recommendations. However, it is interesting to note new research indicating that Thyme oil added to the foods of rabbits, actually strengthened their intestinal integrity while maintaining a balanced gut microbiome (Placha et al, *Effect of thyme oil on small intestine integrity and antioxidant status, phagocytic activity and gastrointestinal microbiota in rabbits.* Acta Vet Hung. 2013 Jun;61(2);197-208).

Cats: Thyme is most commonly used within the Feline Supportive Blend. Addition to natural ointments (1 drop per tablespoon), salves, or shampoos, or diluted topical applications of Three Part Blends directly to areas of fungal infection (ringworm) can also be considered. Most commonly, when use of Thyme is desired, it should be accomplished through use of the Feline Supportive Blend, including for ingestion, which will generally be adequate through normal grooming behaviors. More aggressive oral use of Thyme is not suggested for cats at this time, without distinct and direct monitoring and administration through an experienced veterinarian.

Dogs & Larger: Thyme may be used a bit more aggressively in these animals, than in cats and smaller. The most common method of application is within the Canine and Large Animal Supportive Blends. Addition to Three Part Blends for diluted topical applications, direct application (neat or diluted), addition into natural ointments, salves, and shampoos, addition into massage oils and bases, addition to soaking water for Large Animals, addition into foods, and direct oral administration (diluted) have been utilized. Many dogs and even some horses and livestock, will lick the supportive blends and dilutions off of your hands or themselves after application. This is of no concern, and actually may be quite beneficial. It is often honored when an animal craves ingestion of these blends, and they are allowed to consume it at their discretion.

When oral use in horses is considered, the bottom lip can be "squeezed out" to create a little pocket, and diluted Thyme can be dripped right in. Often, oral Oregano is used as a first choice, as it has been used a more extensively via the oral route, but Thyme is easily an option for stubborn cases. Cattle and other large animals will often ingest diluted Thyme in grain, hay, or feeds. Thyme can be mixed with a variety of foods including Honey, Maple Syrup, Agave, Apple Sauce, or other items and can be delivered orally with a syringe. Thyme is most commonly used orally in cases of severe bacterial, fungal, or parasitic infection.

When oral use of Thyme is considered for dogs – 1 drop of Thyme oil can be diluted with 10 drops of carrier oil. 1 drop or more of this dilution can be given twice a day, for each 20 pounds (9 kg) of body weight, generally added to foods.

Start with a smaller amount, and gradually increase as needed. Some dogs will lick a more diluted Thyme solution or a blend containing Thyme off of your hands, or greatly enjoy the flavor mixed with foods. When this occurs, it is of no concern. When mixing into foods, further dilution may be required due to the strong flavor of the Thyme.

On average, approximately ½ drop of Thyme per 20 pounds (9 kg) of dog body weight is given per day. Some dogs may need less, and some dogs may need more, careful monitoring and adjusting for the individual dog is important. For Thyme delivered orally by capsule, generally the desired amount of Thyme is added to the empty capsule (and other oils if indicated), and the capsule is filled the rest of the way with a carrier oil prior to administration. Special consideration should be made of the gut flora of dogs receiving oral Thyme, and probiotics may be indicated after any oral administration of powerful antibacterial essential oils.

For horses and others, starting with 1 drop per 500 pounds (90 kg) of body weight, given orally twice a day is a good starting point. Thyme oil should be diluted in a carrier oil, Applesauce, or other foods for oral administration. Monitor responses and adjust according to individual need. In cases of severe infections – it is likely that more Thyme can certainly be given. It is more common to use oral Oregano in large animals, so we often rely on this oil as a first choice. Special care should be considered of the gastrointestinal flora, and it is a good idea to follow the use of oral Thyme with probiotics.

Tsuga (Tsuga canadensis)
Also known as Hemlock Spruce or Eastern Hemlock, Tsuga is most commonly recommended for use as a blood purifier and for detoxification and vaccinosis. It is "related" to the popular Homeopathic remedy Thuja, which is widely used for vaccination detoxification. Medical properties also suggest the use of Tsuga for analgesia, arthritis, respiratory conditions, kidney and urinary infections, skin conditions, and venereal diseases. Its use within Veterinary Aromatic Medicine is not widely recommended at this time.

Tulsi (See Holy Basil)

Turmeric (Curcuma longa)

The CO_2 extract of Turmeric rhizome is likely to be of the most benefit in Veterinary Aromatic Medicine. Curcumin, which is the main beneficial compound we are often looking for from Turmeric, is not found within the classic steam distilled essential oil of this plant. However, the CO_2 extract does contain Curcumin. It is likely that the CO_2 extract has a bright future in Veterinary Medicine, however the essential oil is not recommended for use with animals at this time.

Valerian (Valeriana officinalis)

Valerian has been extensively utilized for tranquilizer type effects in the medical community. It generally has a very calming effect on the central nervous system. It is well indicated for sleep disturbances and cognitive dysfunction, restlessness, anxiety, and emotional concerns in animals. Mention has been made several times about the herbal preparation of Valerian "building up" within a system, and that caution needed to be taken with the use of Valerian herb. Further research revealed descriptions of the actual need for buildup of the herb to be effective, and no data could be found on actual reports of the herb or essential oil causing issues. The oral use of Valerian has been quite extensively used in humans and animals, and no concern has been noted.

The use of Valerian within several human recipes indicated for pain management has been used in animals.

Birds & Exotics: Valerian has not been used extensively with these species. The use of Valerian is suggested within Three Part Blends for water-based diffusion or diluted topical applications. Addition to the Small Animal Supportive Blend or Feline Supportive Blend (for ferrets) is suggested when use of Valerian is desired. Research has shown that Valerian has been ingested in quite high amounts without harm.

Cats: If the use of Valerian is desired, the most cat friendly methods of use include addition to Three Part Blends for water-based diffusion, addition to the Feline Supportive Blend, and addition into litter box recipes. The oral consumption of Valerian is likely more than adequate through regular grooming behaviors of diluted topical applications.

Dogs & Larger: Common methods of use include addition into the Canine or Large Animal Supportive Blends, addition into Three Part Blends for water-based diffusion or diluted topical applications, addition into foods, Petting (diluted), and direct oral administration.

If oral use is considered for dogs – 1 drop of Valerian can be diluted with 10 drops of carrier oil. 1 drop or more of this diluted solution can be given twice a day, for each 20 pounds (9 kg) of body weight, generally mixed with foods. Start with a smaller amount, and gradually increase as needed.

For horses and others, starting with 1 drop per 500 pounds (225 kg) of body weight, given orally twice a day is a good starting point. Monitor responses and adjust according to individual need.

Vanilla (Vanilla planifora)

Vanilla, as it is currently available on the market, is for the most part not appropriate for use with animals. Being either within an alcohol extraction, or as an absolute, the possible benefits do not outweigh the quality issues or alcohol exposure. CO_2 extracted vanilla is likely to be an option for high quality availability of vanilla essential oil, however it is hard to come by, a bit hard to work with, and is very expensive. At this time, I recommend not using vanilla for animals.

Vetiver (Vetiveria zizanioides)

Vetiver is well known for anti-inflammatory properties, and is indicated for conditions such as anxiety and behavioral concerns, to reduce anger and fear, encourage focus, provide grounding, for arthritis, circulatory stimulation, oily skin, and as an antispasmodic.

Given orally, Vetiver has been reported to have wonderful anti-histamine actions, and reduces itching very well. Oral use has mainly been within dogs and larger animals.

Birds & Exotics: Vetiver has most commonly been used within blends, with the most common use being water-based diffusion within Three Part Blends. Addition into the Small Animal or Feline Supportive Blend can also be considered. Ingestion beyond normal grooming or licking behaviors is not suggested at this time.

Cats: Vetiver is recommended for use with cats by addition into Three Part Blends for water-based diffusion or diluted topical applications, addition into the Feline Supportive Blend, and by addition to litter box recipes. The oral consumption of Vetiver beyond normal grooming behavior is not suggested at this time.

Dogs & Larger: Vetiver would most commonly be used within Three Part Blends for water-based diffusion or diluted topical applications, by addition into Canine or Large Animal Supportive Blends, and can be considered for addition into natural ointments, salves, or shampoo. Water-mists can also be created for emotional work – to coat bedding or the area in which the dog resides.

If oral use for dogs is considered – 1 drop of Vetiver can be diluted with 10 drops of carrier oil. 1 drop or more of this diluted solution can be given twice a day, for each 50 pounds (23 kg) of body weight, generally mixed with foods. Start with a smaller amount, and gradually increase as needed.

For horses and others, starting with 1 drop per 500 pounds (225 kg) of body weight, given orally twice a day is a good starting point. Monitor responses and adjust according to individual need.

In some deworming protocols, Vetiver may be included as an antispasmodic (decreasing intestinal cramping from the passing of worms.)

Vitex (Vitex agnus castus)
Also known as Chaste Tree or Chaste Berry, Vitex has been heralded for neurologic health issues, even though some references state concerns with its use with epilepsy or seizures. Vitex has been found to be a nervine, with relaxing properties, and quite helpful for shaking and neurologic concerns. Vitex is also reported to help balance hormones and the endocrine system, especially the thyroid. While it is not widely used with animals at this time, its use can be considered in water-based diffusion, diluted within Three Part Blends, and added to Body Supportive Blends.

Western Red Cedar (Thuja plicata)
This essential oil seems to have some wonderful properties in certain cases of Post-Traumatic Stress Disorder (PTSD). In general, water-based diffusion within blends would be utilized in the animal kingdom, however, it remains a lesser utilized oil for animals.

White Cypress (Callitris glaucophylla)
This essential oil from Australia is wonderful in a fixative nature. As a thick and "heavy" oil, it tends to make other oils last a bit longer. A gentle fragrance, it is reported to carry anti-inflammatory and antifungal actions. It is not widely used within the animal kingdom at this time, but its use in small proportions within blends is proving useful.

Winter Savory (see Mountain Savory)

Wintergreen (Gaultheria procumbens)
Wintergreen certainly carries a bit of controversy with its use within the animal kingdom, and especially in cats. Wintergreen is likely one of the most synthetically created essential oils on the market today, and I believe that this is the primary reason for all of the negative reports and issues related to its use. At this time, I do not feel that there is high enough quality Wintergreen available on the market, to warrant its use with animals. Especially when we consider that there are so many other "ultra-safe" oils available to use, that are highly animal friendly, and just as anti-inflammatory, if not more so. When pure Wintergreen oil has been used properly in the past, many animals (even cats) have actually benefited, and we witnessed no harm. Even with that, there simply does not appear to be a good enough reason that we "have to" use Wintergreen in the animal kingdom.

Care must be taken with Wintergreen oil in animals who are bleeding, have a tendency to bleed, or are on any sort of anti-coagulant therapy. The over use of essential oil(s) that have anti-coagulant actions, especially in oral administration, can produce a temporary and dose dependent, increase in bleeding and reduction of clotting. Wintergreen is one of very few essential oils that I feel carries a possibility of being substantially over-dosed when given orally, and could cause significant concern.

Wintergreen is often especially used for conditions such as blood clots, spasms, inflammation, to dilate blood vessels and increase circulation, for analgesia, to reduce blood pressure, arthritis, pain, fatty liver disease, and muscle and nerve pain.

A note on performance and competition animals: Methyl Salicylate, a main constituent of Wintergreen oil, is often contained within the listings of banned substances for horses and other animals entered in competitions such as racing and endurance events. To date, and to my knowledge, there has never been a positive testing result from the use of a truly natural Wintergreen. More studies are being completed to understand the blood levels, metabolism, and clearing of essential oils, however at this time, you may choose to avoid the use of oils such as Peppermint, Ginger, or Wintergreen at least 3 days before an event, or just replace their use with oils that carry no controversy at all, such as Copaiba.

Wormwood (Artemesia sp.)
This essential oil gets great press for being toxic and causing so many problems. In my opinion, it is an oil that is hardly ever used anymore – and just shouldn't be used. Then, problem solved.

Yarrow (Achilles millefolium)
Yarrow essential oil comes in several versions, and is a very polymorphic species. While not widely used with the animal kingdom, the Blue or Chamazulene chemotype of Yarrow is the more commonly used version with animals. Yarrow is reported to have inhibited convulsions, and is likely to be of benefit in neurologic conditions and epilepsy.

Ylang Ylang (Cananga odorata)
Ylang Ylang is used with animals for antispasmodic effects, vaso-dilation, antidiabetic effects, antiparasitic properties, to regulate heartbeat, for heart arrhythmias, hypertension, anxiety, depression, hair loss, and intestinal problems. It is often thought of as a "Yin and Yang" oil, balancing male and female or positive and negative energies. Emotionally it combats low self-esteem, increases focus of thoughts, filters out negative energy, and restores confidence and peace.

Ylang Ylang is available in several forms, and many essential oil companies will not designate which version you are purchasing. Ylang Ylang "Complete" is the most appropriate form for animal use, however many suppliers will supply Ylang Ylang from different countries, as well as different distillation types known as 1st, 2nd, 3rd, Complete, or Extra. There is a different chemical profile for each of these versions, which are fractional distillations of Ylang Ylang. The Complete version is a combination of all of the fractions, and is considered more close to the actual whole essential oil. Ylang Ylang Complete is the preferred oil for Veterinary Aromatic Medicine.

While I have noted a few cautionary statements to avoid the use of Ylang Ylang if blood pressure is too low – I have not found this to be accurate clinically nor in further research. Ylang Ylang has GRAS status, and is generally considered non-toxic.

Birds & Exotics: Ylang Ylang has most commonly been used within blends for these species. The use of Ylang Ylang should start with water-based diffusion within Three Part Blends when desired. The addition of 1 drop into the Small Animal Supportive Blend is also likely to be well tolerated. Consideration can be made for the addition of 1 drop into the Feather Spray Recipe, Perch and Hand applications, indirect diffusion, and by Petting (diluted) in non-avian species. It is important to have careful monitoring, in cooperation with a veterinarian, when you use protocols that have not been widely used in your species before.

Cats: The use of Ylang Ylang for cats is recommended through water-based diffusion of Three Part Blends, or through addition to the Feline Supportive Blend or to Litter Box recipes. The oral consumption of Ylang Ylang should be accomplished through grooming after diluted topical applications. There is little need for further oral use in cats, however with careful pre-exposure monitoring with a veterinarian, as well as monitoring of responses, more aggressive use could be considered. The direct oral use of Ylang Ylang has not been well documented in cats at this time.

Dogs & Larger: Ylang Ylang oil can be used in many methods of application for these animals. The most common methods of use include water-based diffusion via Three Part Blends, diluted topical applications of Three Part Blends, addition into Canine or Large Animal Supportive Blends, direct topical application (diluted), Petting (diluted). Direct oral administration in animals is likely not necessary, while it has been considered in the past.

Yuzu (Citrus junos)
While this citrus oil is common in the human flavoring world, it has not been used widely with animals at this time. It is likely to be appropriate for water based diffusion, however topical or oral administrations have not been explored adequately to warrant use.

Zdravetz (Geranium macrorrhizum)

This oil is not commonly used within the animal kingdom. It is not recommended for use at this time, however may hold hepatoprotective properties. High levels of Germacrone are present in this oil, and this constituent has reports of anti-cancer activity.

Zinziba (Lippia javanica)

A very interesting oil from Africa, also called Wild Verbena. This oil has not been used commonly within the animal kingdom. It is not recommended for use at this time.

ESSENTIAL OIL BLENDS

Here are some examples of oils you could combine within Three Part Blends for your needs. You may find that certain blends are more appropriate for dogs, while less appropriate for cats. If you intend to use a blend for a cat, please review each individual oil contained within the blend, and read the feline notes regarding the use of the oil. If it is mainly recommended for diffusion, and not topical application – please use the blend appropriately for your species. These are merely suggestions for Three Part Blends you could use.

Calming Recipes
There are many oils which will have calming effects whether you select them for diffusion or topical applications. Review oils for your individual species to dilute to the proper concentrations, or to select the route of administration you will use for your particular species.

- Lavender, Bergamot, Ylang Ylang
- Lavender, Frankincense, Orange
- Roman Chamomile, Bergamot, Ylang Ylang
- Frankincense, Rose, Roman Chamomile
- Valerian, Frankincense, Vetiver

Balancing Recipes
These recipes may be more balancing or grounding in nature.

- Myrrh, Frankincense, Spikenard
- Ylang Ylang, Clary Sage, Roman Chamomile
- German Chamomile, Copaiba, Ylang Ylang
- Melissa, Black Spruce, Balsam Fir
- Grapefruit, Ginger, Nutmeg
- Vetiver, Geranium, Patchouli

Nerve, Brain, Nervous System Recipes
- Helichrysum, Frankincense, Copaiba
- Geranium, German Chamomile, Frankincense
- Helichrysum, Balsam Fir, Vitex
- Melissa, Nutmeg, Black Pepper
- Spikenard, Black Spruce, Frankincense

Respiratory
- Cinnamon, Tangerine, Rosemary
- Eucalyptus globulus, Black Spruce, Copaiba
- Rosemary, Lemon, Eucalyptus radiata
- Balsam Fir, Black Spruce, Copaiba
- Marjoram, Lemon, Eucalyptus globulus

Air Freshening
- Cilantro, Lime, Black Spruce
- Lemon, Orange, Lavender
- Tea Tree, Lemon, Cypress
- Lemongrass, Citronella, Lemon
- Eucalyptus citriodora, Lemon, Catnip

Cleaning Recipes
- Black Spruce, Tea Tree, Lemon
- Lemongrass, Tea Tree, Eucalyptus radiata
- Cinnamon, Lemon, Rosemary
- Cilantro, Tea Tree, Lemon
- Lemongrass, Lemon, Tea Tree

Cognitive Function
- Helichrysum, Frankincense, Cypress
- Vetiver, Vitex, Frankincense
- Geranium, German Chamomile, Black Pepper
- Black Pepper, Frankincense, Copaiba
- Melissa, Frankincense, Black Spruce

Physical Pain
- Copaiba, Helichrysum, Frankincense
- Peppermint, Copaiba, Marjoram
- Copaiba, Marjoram, Lemongrass
- Lavender, Black Spruce, Frankincense
- Balsam Fir, Copaiba, Frankincense

Digestive (GI) Recipes
- Tarragon, Ginger, Peppermint
- Anise, Ginger, Peppermint
- Copaiba, Ginger, Peppermint
- Fennel, Copaiba, Ginger
- Marjoram, Copaiba, Peppermint

Digestive recipes are some of the most commonly used essential oil blends in all forms of animals. They have been used extensively via the oral route, and dosages can become quite high with no reported ill effects, especially in horses and large animals. Take note that some oils such as ginger and peppermint carry with them a bit of an intense property - and could be a bit uncomfortable for topical application to cats and smaller. Most cats should start with the Feline Supportive Blend to see if their digestive needs are met with this blend. Then any of the single oils could also be additionally added when more support of the digestive system is needed. These blends could also be added to litter box recipes.

Digestive Recipes are most often used for intestinal concerns, diarrhea, vomiting, indigestion, colic, nausea, and motion or car sickness. Use for intestinal parasites remains inconsistent, and careful monitoring with your veterinarian is necessary to determine success.

Birds & Exotics: Digestive blends for these species can sometimes be used via water-based diffusion – however, you may wish to reduce the total amount of Peppermint within a blend when diffusion is desired. Oral administrations can also be considered. Addition to drinking water (1 drop per liter), addition to foods (1 drop per tablespoon), and Petting (non-avian species, diluted) are the most common methods of use. Using less quantity within foods may be necessary due to the strong flavors of some oils.

Cats: Most cats should start with the Feline Supportive Blend to see if their digestive needs are met. Then any of the single oils could also be additionally added when more support of the digestive system is needed. These blends could also be added to litter box recipes. Use of the Three Part Blends via water-based diffusion or diluted topical applications can be considered. Ingestion of the oils will occur from normal grooming, and is often enough for response.

If oral use is indicated, some cats may eat small amounts of the diluted Three Part Blends within their foods. Starting with a toothpick dip is recommended, then gradually increasing the amount to allow your cat to get used to the flavor.

Dogs & Larger: Use the Three Part Blends as described in all methods. Diffusion during car rides or topical applications may be helpful for car sickness. When oral use is desired in dogs – dilution of the blend is suggested to a 30% concentration or less, within a carrier oil such as Fractionated Coconut Oil. Raw Coconut Oil can also be considered, as long as your dog should not be avoiding excess fats due to its digestive concern.

On average, 10 drops of diluted digestive recipes have been given per 20 pounds (9kg) of body weight, twice daily or more frequently. Many dogs will respond to less, and it is advised to start with only 1 drop per 20 pounds initially and monitor for response. Start with a smaller amount, and gradually increase as needed. Many dogs respond to topical applications quite well, and you should always try those first. Diffusion has also been incredibly helpful.

For horses and others, digestive blends have been used more extensively, especially in cases of colic. Starting with 1 neat drop of the blend per 100 pounds (45 kg) of body weight, given orally twice a day is a good starting point. For many large animals, the digestive blend is dripped into the lip area, and absorbed buccally. Monitor responses and adjust and increase according to individual needs. There have been many cases of horses consuming upwards of 200 drops of some digestive blends in a day during severe situations. While this is likely an excessive situation, it is reassuring to know that we can re-administer in cases of colic as needed.

With colic protocols in horses, 20 drops of a digestive blend is often given to an average sized horse, in the lip, every 20 minutes. It is also commonly applied topically, and sometimes rectally, at the same time as oral administration is being given.

Hormonal Recipes
- Marjoram, Orange, Clary Sage
- Clary Sage, Ylang Ylang, Bergamot
- Lavender, Lemon, Orange
- Geranium, Bergamot, Ylang Ylang
- Copaiba, Frankincense, Clary Sage

Strong Antimicrobial Recipes
Situations for use of these sorts of blends include abscesses, mold situations, fungal and bacterial respiratory infections, etc. Please select oils that are indicated for use with your particular species of interest, and also the proper routes of administration for your species.

- Cinnamon, Clove, Rosemary
- Lemongrass, Tea Tree, Eucalyptus globulus
- Frankincense, Oregano, Thyme
- Lemon, Melaleuca alternifolia, Lemongrass

Endocrine Supporting Recipes
- Spearmint, Geranium, Nutmeg
- Myrtle, Myrrh, Nutmeg
- German Chamomile, Nutmeg, Black Cumin

Emotional Cleansing
- Rose, Melissa, Frankincense
- Geranium, Lemon, Ylang Ylang
- Spikenard, Frankincense, Black Spruce

New Animal Introductions
- Frankincense, Roman Chamomile, Ylang Ylang
- Lavender, Orange, Lemon
- Ylang Ylang, Black Spruce, Lavender
- Rose, Roman Chamomile, Frankincense

Birth & Delivery
- Geranium, Lavender, Roman Chamomile
- Bergamot, Frankincense, Ylang Ylang
- Palmarosa, Rose, Frankincense

Liver Support
- Grapefruit, Helichrysum, Celery Seed
- Ledum, Helichrysum, Copaiba
- Frankincense, Helichrysum, Ledum

Anti-Inflammatory Blends
- Copaiba, Helichrysum, Myrrh
- Marjoram, Peppermint, Copaiba
- Lavender, Copaiba, Frankincense
- Frankincense, Copaiba, Helichrysum
- Black Spruce, Copaiba, Helichrysum

Skin Blends
- Palmarosa, Helichrysum, Myrrh
- Melaleuca alternifolia, Rosemary, Copaiba
- Lavender, Copaiba, Frankincense
- Frankincense, Copaiba, Myrrh
- Lavender, Myrrh, Palmarosa

Odor Elimination
- Citronella, Lemongrass, Melaleuca alternifolia
- Rosemary, Lavender, Lemon
- Melaleuca alternifolia, Eucalyptus citriodora, Citronella

ESSENTIAL OILS: AVIAN

Birds (especially parrots) are a more specialized arena in veterinary aromatic medicine. Just as not every vet is an "avian vet" based on the fact that they are willing to examine a bird; it takes very special knowledge to properly screen essential oils for this delicate species. Pet birds are extremely sensitive to household toxins, and it is well known by bird owners that even the spray of an air freshener or the burning of a candle can be dangerous to a bird. Since many household fragrances are created with poor grade, adulterated, or synthetic essential oils, it was thought that all essential oils were toxic to birds. This has been found to be untrue. While birds have a distinct way that they should be exposed to essential oils, it is being found that they not only benefit, but thrive, with the addition of essential oils into their lives.

Prior to the use of any essential oil or essential oil based product with a bird, a thorough veterinary examination, by an avian veterinarian, is recommended. It is ideal if blood work (CBC and Chemistry Profile) can be performed prior to any start of natural remedies. Many avian patients initially present with pre-existing blood work abnormalities in my practice. So it is important to be able to document either the improvement of these values, or at least the stability of them while using essential oils. Clinicians have made misinterpretations of abnormal blood values in sick animals, due to the fact that they never obtained "pre-exposure" blood work. If we are using essential oils or other natural remedies for a bird, it is usually because they are already ill. Then if their condition degrades, it becomes a common thought to blame the natural remedy that was given. When in fact, if blood work would be available to compare with prior to the exposure, we would likely not see any deterioration in the values.

It is an important note, that although some essential oils may be listed for possible use, that not every essential oil has been used extensively for birds at this time. Read the individual description for a particular item, and if it states that it has not been used commonly in animals, then it most likely has never been used with birds. However, when the use of an essential oil is considered for difficult cases or life threatening situations, it may be an important option to pursue. Certainly, the use of common sense, a very conservative start, and cooperation and testing with an avian veterinarian is advised whenever you may choose to explore the use of an essential oil that does not have much data behind it. However, in severe situations such as self-mutilation or with conditions that may result in the ultimate death of a bird, great discoveries are often made with natural remedies that benefit avian medicine as a whole. I felt it was important to share potential avenues with you, however, please understand that some of these treatments would qualify as "breaking new ground," and should be explored with great detail and care.

DIFFUSION:
Diffusion from water-based diffusers is recommended in households with birds. Air diffusers have been utilized, however require a much farther distance from the bird, or use in a much larger room (such as a barn or large aviary). For the most part, I currently recommend against the use of air-style diffusers with birds. In general, most oil use would start with 3 drops of oil added to the water of the diffuser (approximately 8oz). Monitor the bird(s) closely for the first 5-10 minutes of diffusion. Increase the amounts and frequency of diffusion gradually; most homes find that they can diffuse on an almost continual basis - bringing amazing health and benefits to their birds. Please read the chapter on Diffusion for more detailed instructions.

WATER MISTING:
A favorite technique that is being used currently in thousands of birds is the Feather Spray Recipe. This amazing spray was created by Leigh Foster, and had been used on her rescue and wildlife birds prior to its introduction into mainstream bird care. I use this recipe as a fundamental tool for my avian patients. The components of the spray layer so many different properties into a very well-loved application. Benefits for everything from bacterial, viral, and fungal conditions to even immune system support can be found within this spray.

Feather Spray Recipe:
- Place 20 drops of Lavender, 20 drops of Lemon, and 20 drops of Orange essential oils into a 4 ounce (120 mL) glass spray bottle.
- Add distilled water to fill the bottle. Shake well before each application, then mist the bird with the spray up to twice a day. Birds love this spray, and even those who routinely dislike a shower with a traditional spray bottle are attracted to being sprayed in this manner.
- When desired, an additional essential oil or two, may be added to this recipe, for example a drop or two of Frankincense.
- When adding more than just a couple drops to the recipe, you may wish to omit several drops of the base oils in replacement for the new oils. For example, you may add 15 drops of Lemon instead of 20, replacing those

drops with 5 drops of Frankincense. This is not always necessary, but if you might add an additional 10 drops or more of essential oil(s) to the recipe, it is wise to attempt to keep the concentration, and thus dilution, of the essential oils to water similar in nature.

Copaiba & Frankincense Spray:
This water-misting recipe is wonderful for many things, and can be used whenever these oils are indicated or for general anti-inflammatory or anti-cancer benefits. Frankincense carterii species is recommended for use with birds. This is the basic starting recipe, however variations of it can be made.
- Place 10 drops of Frankincense, and 5 drops of Copaiba essential oils into a 4 ounce (120 mL) glass spray bottle.
- Add distilled water to fill the bottle. Shake well before each application, then mist the bird with the spray up to twice a day.

Copaiba, Frankincense, Helichrysum Spray:
This spray adds the additional healing benefits of Helichrysum.
- Add 5 drops of Helichrysum to the Copaiba & Frankincense Spray recipe, and use as directed.

ADDING ESSENTIAL OILS TO DRINKING WATER:
This is generally done at a rate of 1 drop per liter of water. See the chapter on adding oils to drinking water for more detailed instructions.

ADDING ESSENTIAL OILS TO FOODS:
Please see the chapter Mixing Oils into Food for more detailed instructions.

AVIAN DRIP & RUB TECHNIQUE:
Birds present a unique situation for Drip & Rub. Not only do they have feathers instead of fur, but they are also more sensitive to oils and have less data collected on them to date.

In my practice I have reserved the use of Drip & Rub sort of applications, to birds that have more serious conditions, for which other essential oil protocols have not yielded enough results.

This technique has not been used in thousands of birds like the Feather Spray or diffusion. Likewise it has not been used in hundreds of birds. I encourage everyone who will use this technique to have tried other methods first, and to also follow and monitor the cases carefully to provide further data and advancement of avian aromatherapy.

Drip & Rub Techniques in birds is likely only to occur in birds that are fairly handleable. Chickens are actually quite easy to give an application to, and respond beautifully. Certainly, restraint can be used to allow for the application.

For animals cat sized and smaller, the Drip & Rub Technique is generally going to consist of applying a diluted blend of oils – such as the Small Animal Supportive Blend – in which all of the oils that will be used are mixed into one diluted mixture. Please read the chapter on Body Supportive Blends and Drip & Rub Techniques for more details on this and its use in animals.

Calming & Balancing (optional): Apply a bird-diluted calming blend to the bottom of the feet. This can be directly applied, or be applied by having the bird perch on your hand, which is moistened with oil. Alternately, you may apply to the perch. Perch application should be light and care should be taken to not create too moist of an application.

Avian Drip & Rub Technique Solution: This recipe is a bit stronger than the Small Animal Supportive blend, and can be used in more severe situations or when the Small Animal Supportive Blend has not had enough results. Start with the less concentrated solution and gradually increase the concentration used as needed or indicated.

- Add 1-2 drop each of Oregano, Thyme, Basil, Cypress, Copaiba, Marjoram, and Peppermint oils into 30 mL (1 ounce) of carrier oil (Fractionated Coconut Oil).
- If you feel especially cautious with an individual, please start with 1 drop of each oil in 60 mL (2 ounces) of carrier oil. You can always add more later.
- To modify the Avian Drip & Rub Recipe – add 1-2 drops of an additional essential oil to the above recipes. In general, up to 3 additional essential oils can be added.
- Rock the solution to mix thoroughly. Part the feathers, as best you can, over the back. Drip the Drip & Rub Avian Solution from the tail to neck. Generally 2-3 drops of the solution will be used for most birds. Gently massage the oil into the spine.
- Monitor skin for any irritation or redness. Repeat use of this technique can result in a dry, flakey skin. This is usually non-irritated, and not painful or inflamed. Likely, it is mostly due to the drying effects of the

essential oils. The condition is temporary and resolves when the technique is applied less often or diluted further.
- Alternately, this blend can just be rubbed into and onto feet as needed.

We have used this technique up to daily in parrots and chickens, and most commonly 2-3 times per week. One parrot received a similar recipe for a serious condition 2-3 times per week, for over a year. Her blood work had no abnormal changes or variations due to the essential oil use, however we did note that her skin became flakey at times.

Variations in Species:
In my practice, I have worked on parrots worth in excess of $30,000. These are the situations in which we start with REALLY light and conservative methods, and gradually work our way to more aggressive approaches. It is a sound recommendation to use common sense and caution as you progress.

It is important to mention that passerines and psittacines (finches, canaries, parakeets, budgies, parrots, and the like) are often treated with much more of a delicate touch. This may or may not be founded at this time, and we continually are impressed with how they handle essential oil administration when we need to explore new options. However, since they are relatively new to the use of essential oils medically, we will recommend a more cautious advancement for now.

Chickens, Pea Fowl, Turkeys, and other forms of poultry appear far more hardy in their use of essential oils. With these species, I generally do not hesitate to apply the stronger version of the Avian Drip & Rub Recipe especially to areas of concern such as bumble foot. They also tolerate administration of essential oils by ingestion quite well. These birds are likely to pave the way for more advanced use of essential oils in the avian species.

AVIAN CONDITIONS

ARTHRITIS
(See also BUMBLEFOOT)

Arthritis is a condition of inflammation of the joints. As birds are rarely radiographed or evaluated for arthritis in the traditional sense, one can assume that older birds, or birds with any form of discomfort, may fall into this category of having pain that affects their mobility.

FIRST LINE RECOMMENDATIONS:
WATER MISTING: With a solution of 10 drops of Frankincense and 5 drops of Copaiba in 4 ounces (120 mL) of distilled water. Shake well, and mist directly onto the bird, 1-2 times a day.
INGESTION: Copaiba can be added to foods or drinking water.

Single Oils:
Balsam Fir, Black Spruce, Copaiba, Frankincense, German Chamomile, Ginger, Helichrysum, Lavender, Lemon, Marjoram, Myrrh, Nutmeg, Orange, Peppermint, Vetiver

ASPERGILLOSIS
(See also RESPIRATORY CONDITIONS)

Aspergillosis is a serious fungal infection that usually affects the lungs and air sacs of the avian species – including parrots, raptors (birds of prey), and more. Symptoms may be varied and include labored breathing, respiratory clicking, tail bobbing, general illness, etc... Aspergillosis is a serious condition that is difficult to treat traditionally, essential oils hold true answers to defeating this condition.

AVIAN CONDITIONS

FIRST LINE RECOMMENDATIONS:
WATER DIFFUSION: Three Part Blends created with diffusion appropriate antifungal oils can be diffused in an open room, as well as by tenting or caging up to multiple times per day.
AVIAN SUPPORTIVE BLENDS: Small Animal Supportive Blend or the Avian Drip & Rub Recipe can be applied up to once daily, when indicated and possible.
INGESTION: Copaiba, Oregano, and Thyme may be considered for oral use.

Single Oils:
Black Spruce, Cinnamon, Clove, Copaiba, Eucalyptus globulus, Eucalyptus radiata, Geranium, Lavender, Lemon, Lemongrass, Marjoram, Melaleuca alternifolia, Oregano, Rosemary, Thyme

BEHAVIORAL CONDITIONS
(See also HORMONAL CONDITIONS)

Any behavioral concern can be assisted by the use of essential oils. The capability of the oils to affect the physical as well as the emotional, is holistically complete. Nutritional supplements are often underestimated in behavioral concerns, and should always be added. Standard Process whole food supplements, tuna omegas, and minerals can be explored with your holistic veterinarian.

FIRST LINE RECOMMENDATIONS:
WATER DIFFUSION: Rotational diffusion of emotional Three Part Blends.
TOPICAL: Feather Spray Recipes in a water-mist, daily to twice daily or as needed.

Single Oils:
Black Spruce, Bergamot, Chamomile (German), Chamomile (Roman), Frankincense, Geranium, Grapefruit, Lavender, Lemon, Marjoram, Melissa, Myrrh, Orange, Patchouli, Spikenard, Tangerine, Valerian, Vetiver, Ylang Ylang

BLEEDING

Bleeding of any sort is enough to send a bird owner into a state of panic. It is often described that birds can bleed to death, in a very short amount of time. In practice, this is a little less than accurate. However, it remains important to stop bleeding when it occurs. Veterinary attention is always recommended.

FIRST LINE RECOMMENDATIONS:
TOPICIAL: Cistus or Helichrysum
ORAL: Cistus

Single Oils:
Cistus, Geranium, Helichrysum, Lavender

Caution:
Avoidance of oils such as Cinnamon, Clove, Nutmeg, Wintergreen – and other oils that have anticoagulant effects, is wise.

BLOOD FEATHER, BROKEN
(See also BLEEDING)

As an avian veterinarian, I rarely recommend the pulling of a blood feather, broken or otherwise. When pulled out, the body will just start the creation of a brand new immature feather, which may be prone to being broken again in the future. When possible, allowing the broken feather to continue its "life cycle," stops the continuation of the problem.

BONES - BROKEN
(See also PAIN MANAGEMENT)

FIRST LINE RECOMMENDATIONS:
See PAIN MANAGEMENT for methods of pain control.
TOPICAL: Three Part Blends diluted, Feather Spray with added Copaiba, other indicated oils safe for water-misting
WATER DIFFUSION: Three Part Blends for calming

Single Oils:
Balsam Fir, Black Spruce, Copaiba, Helichrysum, Lavender, Myrrh

BORNA VIRUS
(See PROVENTRICULAR DILATATION DISEASE, VIRAL CONDITIONS)

There is still some debate whether Borna Virus is the true cause of Proventricular Dilatation Disease (PDD), or if it simply is a factor in its development. Regardless of the relationship, essential oils support the entire body in many ways. Giving the body tools for complete healing and immune system health will support the correction of the problem on many levels.

BUMBLEFOOT
(See also ARTHRITIS, WOUNDS)

Bumblefoot is an inflammatory condition of the foot, which is often caused by chronic pressure related to perches. Inadequate perch diameter, bearing weight on one leg more than another, poor perch variety, and many other husbandry issues contribute to this condition. Lesions may appear as open wounds, pressure sores, or general swelling and distortion of the foot. This condition is quite common in raptors. Bumblefoot can also become secondarily infected, increasing the complications of this difficult issue.

FIRST LINE RECOMMENDATIONS:
TOPICAL: 1 Tablespoon of natural ointment with 1 drop each of Helichrysum, Balsam Fir, Copaiba, Melaleuca alternifolia, Palmarosa, Myrrh, Rosemary, and Frankincense mixed into it. Apply sparingly to wound, 1-2 times a day. Do not use if the wound is creating a beneficial dry scab, as these heal better when allowed to remain dry.
WATER MISTING: Place 5 drops Helichrysum, 10 drops Frankincense, 5 drops Copaiba into 4 ounces of distilled water. Shake well, mist directly onto feet 1-2 times a day.

Single Oils:
Balsam Fir, Black Spruce, Copaiba, Frankincense, Geranium, Helichrysum, Lavender, Lemon, Marjoram, Myrrh, Nutmeg, Orange, Oregano, Palmarosa, Patchouli, Spikenard, Vetiver

CANCER

Cancer is a difficult condition, which certainly needs to be addressed on many levels. Please see the descriptions in Feline Conditions for an explanation of the holistic approach to cancer. The recommendations made in any of the conditions listings, no matter what the animal species, can be used as described for birds in their individual single oil description.

FIRST LINE RECOMMENDATIONS:
WATER DIFFUSION: Rotational diffusion of emotional blends. Frankincense diffusion up to 24 hours a day.
TOPICAL: Feather Spray Recipe up to twice a day. Avian Drip & Rub Recipe or Small Animal Supportive Blend weekly to daily, or as able.
WATER MISTING: 10-20 drops of Frankincense, and 5 drops of Copaiba in 4 ounces (120 mL) of distilled water. Mist at least twice a day.
INGESTION: Frankincense and Citrus oils in foods and water.

Single Oils:
Copaiba, Frankincense, Grapefruit, Hyssop, Lavender, Lemon, Orange, Sandalwood, Tangerine

CHLAMYDIOSIS, CHLAMYDOPHILA PSITTACI
(See PSITTACOSIS)

CROP INFECTION
(See also REGURGITATION)

A crop infection is a serious concern, and requires proper examination and diagnosis by an avian veterinarian. Essential oils provide an amazing tool for the treatment, prevention, and whole body support with this condition.

FIRST LINE RECOMMENDATIONS:
INGESTION: diluted Three Part Blends of indicated oils

Single Oils:
Black Spruce, Cinnamon, Clove, Copaiba, Lavender, Lemon, Marjoram, Oregano, Patchouli, Peppermint, Spearmint, Tarragon, Thyme

CROP STASIS
(See also CROP INFECTION)

Crop stasis is the poor movement of the initial part of a bird's gastrointestinal tract. This can have many causes, and is most common in baby birds who are being hand fed. The root of the problem should always be addressed, however these recommendations can help with motility.

FIRST LINE RECOMMENDATIONS:
   WATER DIFFUSION: Three Part Blends
   INGESTION: Peppermint, digestive Three Part Blends
   WATER-MIST: Feather Spray Recipe, especially with Copaiba added

Single Oils:
   Copaiba, Ginger, Lavender, Lemon, Marjoram, Orange, Oregano, Patchouli, Peppermint, Spearmint, Spruce, Tangerine, Tarragon

DIARRHEA
(See also GIARDIA)

A thorough work up with a veterinarian is critical to determining the cause for the diarrhea. More specific therapies can be used once the cause is found.

FIRST LINE RECOMMENDATIONS:
   INGESTION: Three Part Blends for digestive concerns
   WATER DIFFUSION: Three Part Blends
   WATER-MIST: Feather Spray Recipe, with Copaiba added

Single Oils:
   Copaiba, Ginger, Lavender, Lemon, Melissa, Oregano, Peppermint, Tangerine, Tarragon, Thyme

EGG BINDING
(See also EGG LAYING- EXCESSIVE, HORMONAL CONDITIONS)

Egg binding is the failure to pass an egg from the reproductive tract. Dehydrated, weak, or malnourished birds are much more prone to this disorder. It is often a veterinary emergency, and medical attention should be sought. Hydration and warmth are the most important factors to be addressed in this condition.

FIRST LINE RECOMMENDATIONS:
WATER DIFFUSION: Lavender, or Three Part Blends
TOPICAL: Three Part Blends, Feather Spray with added Clary Sage

Single Oils:
Clary Sage, Copaiba, Geranium, Hyssop, Lavender, Lemon, Marjoram, Myrrh, Vetiver, Ylang Ylang

EGG LAYING - EXCESSIVE
(See also HORMONAL CONDITIONS)

Excessive egg laying is described as when a bird lays so many eggs that it becomes detrimental to their health. Attention to light cycles is incredibly important when attempting to have companion birds stop laying.

FIRST LINE RECOMMENDATIONS:
WATER DIFFUSION: Clary Sage, or Three Part Blends
WATER MISTING: Feather Spray Recipe with 1 drop of Clary Sage added.

Single Oils:
Clary Sage, Marjoram, Nutmeg, Orange, Ylang Ylang

EGG LAYING – INADEQUATE PRODUCTION
(See also HORMONAL CONDITIONS)

This is most commonly a concern for those who raise laying hens. Making sure there is adequate nutrition, low stress, and proper light cycles.

FIRST LINE RECOMMENDATIONS:
INDIRECT DIFFUSION: Three Part Blends may be sprinkled in chicken shavings or nest boxes (often diluted)
WATER MISTING: Feather Spray Recipe with 1 drop of Clary Sage added.
INGESTION: Some oils may be added to drinking water or food to support general health and normal laying function.

Single Oils:
Clary Sage

FATTY LIVER DISEASE
(See also LIVER DISEASE)

FIRST LINE RECOMMENDATIONS:
INGESTION: Grapefruit, Copaiba, Three Part Blends
WATER MISTING: Feather Spray Recipe with Helichrysum.
WATER DIFFUSION: German Chamomile, Geranium

Single Oils:
Chamomile (German), Copaiba, Geranium, Grapefruit, Helichrysum, Juniper, Lavender, Ledum, Lemon, Myrrh, Myrtle, Nutmeg, Orange, Rosemary, Spearmint, Tangerine

FEATHER LOSS
(See also FEATHER PICKING)

Feather loss may not always be the same as feather picking. Feather loss may occur when a bird is housed with another bird who plucks the other's feathers. Or, feather loss can also be a result of a medical condition. Loss of feathers from areas that the bird cannot actively reach (the head) is a prime indicator of actual feather loss. A quality medical work up with an avian veterinarian should be sought. Treat specific underlying problems if discovered – such as parasites, bacterial skin infection, or viral infection. Separation from other birds may be helpful in determining the cause. Chickens and poultry are commonly picked and attacked by flock mates.

FIRST LINE RECOMMENDATIONS:
  WATER MISTING: Feather Spray Recipes 1-2 times a day.
  INGESTION: Melissa in drinking water.
  WATER DIFFUSION: Diffuse listed oils in Three Part Blends up to 24 hours a day. Follow directions for rotational diffusion of emotional blends.

Single Oils:
  Chamomile (Roman), Copaiba, Frankincense, Geranium, Helichrysum, Lavender, Ledum, Lemon, Melissa, Orange, Patchouli, Rosemary, Sandalwood, Tangerine, Ylang Ylang

FEATHER PICKING
(See also FEATHER LOSS, HORMONAL CONDITIONS)

Feather picking is an unfortunately common problem amongst companion birds. Causes range from emotional distress to medical conditions such as heart disease. It is important to seek as accurate of a diagnosis as is possible, however even with the most experienced avian veterinarian, often a thorough work up still leaves one clueless. Feather picking is important to differentiate from feather loss. With feather picking, the bird themselves is actually plucking or damaging their feathers. This means that areas that the bird cannot reach are still feathered (for example the head). The most successful treatment of feather picking involves discovery and treatment of the underlying condition responsible. For example – if a bacterial infection of the skin initiated the feather plucking – then exposure to anti-bacterial essential oils would be the most beneficial. If heart disease was suspected, then exposure to essential oils that are beneficial to the heart would be indicated.

In all cases, nutritional support is of the utmost importance. This cannot be ignored, and should be ranked very high on the list of things to do.

FIRST LINE RECOMMENDATIONS:
  TOPICAL: Feather Spray Recipes up to 1-2 times a day. Avian Drip & Rub or Small Animal Supportive Blend may be indicated for some cases.
  WATER DIFFUSION: Diffusion of Three Part Blends up to 24 hours a day. Rotational diffusion of emotional blends is also recommended.
  DRINKING WATER: Melissa

Single Oils:
Basil, Black Spruce, Chamomile (German), Chamomile (Roman), Copaiba, Frankincense, Geranium, Grapefruit, Helichrysum, Laurus nobilis, Lavender, Ledum, Lemon, Melissa, Marjoram, Myrrh, Orange, Patchouli, Rosemary, Tangerine, Valerian, Vetiver, Ylang Ylang

GASTROINTESTINAL CONDITIONS
(See CROP INFECTION, CROP STASIS, DIARRHEA, REGURGITATION)

GIARDIA
(See also DIARRHEA)

Contamination of drinking water is often the culprit in the spread and continuation of Giardia in bird flocks. Adding essential oils to the water can help disinfect, as well as treat the condition. Research has shown the effectiveness of essential oils such as Clove against Giardia.

FIRST LINE RECOMMENDATIONS:
INGESTION: Clove, Oregano
DRINKING WATER: Three Part Blends

Single Oils:
Basil, Clove, Lavender, Lemon, Melaleuca alternifolia, Nutmeg, Oregano, Patchouli, Peppermint, Rosemary, Spearmint, Tangerine, Tarragon, Thyme

GOUT
(See also ARTHRITIS, KIDNEY DISEASE, PAIN MANAGEMENT)

Gout is the accumulation of uric acid deposits within the joints. It is a painful condition, often secondary to kidney disease in birds. The use of oils to encourage drinking of water is strongly recommended, as well as increasing hydration in general.

FIRST LINE RECOMMENDATIONS:
DRINKING WATER: Three Part Blends, especially with citrus
INGESTION: Three Part Blends
WATER MISTING: Feather Spray Recipe with 1 drop of Juniper, 2 drops of Copaiba, and 1 drop Helichrysum added.

Single Oils:
Black Spruce, Copaiba, Grapefruit, Juniper, Lemon

HEAD TRAUMA
(See also NEUROLOGIC CONDITIONS)

The most common scenario for this condition is a bird who flies into a window. Often dazed and stunned, they can benefit from essential oils until they are ready to fly away again. The recommendations have been used on countless wild birds to get them up and flying again soon. Providing a warm quiet place to rest is also important.

FIRST LINE RECOMMENDATIONS:
INDIRECT: Place 1-2 drops of neat Frankincense into the palms of your hand. Rub together, and allow to absorb completely, then cup the bird within your hands. You can allow them to smell it, and they will absorb minute amounts through their feet and by inhalation.
TOPICAL: diluted Three Part Blends or Small Animal Supportive Blend
WATER DIFFUSION: With caging or tenting, diffuse Frankincense, Helichrysum, and Copaiba (3 drops of each) for at least 20 minutes or as needed. Repeat or continue diffusion based on responses. Diffusion with Three Part Blends.

Single Oils:
Copaiba, Frankincense, Helichrysum, Lavender, Rose

HEAVY METAL POISONING

FIRST LINE RECOMMENDATIONS:
INGESTION: Helichrysum in food and/or drinking water.
DRINKING WATER: Grapefruit, Tangerine
TOPICAL: Feather Spray Recipe made with Tangerine instead of Orange oil. Add 3 drops of Helichrysum, and 1 drop of Juniper.
WATER DIFFUSION: Three Part Blends

Single Oils:
Chamomile (Roman), Cilantro, Grapefruit, Helichrysum, Hyssop, Juniper, Lavender, Ledum, Lemon, Nutmeg, Tangerine

HORMONAL CONDITIONS
(See also BEHAVIORAL CONDITIONS)

Hormonal conditions can encompass many things, but in birds this most commonly will mean behavioral concerns or sexual and reproductive behaviors. Males may masturbate, females may lay eggs, and even feather picking and screaming can be related to hormonal surges. Sometimes these actions are completely normal, however when they become disruptive or unhealthy, the exaggerated responses should be softened.

FIRST LINE RECOMMENDATIONS:
Marjoram is particularly helpful in calming over active sexual activity, particularly masturbation.
WATER MISTING: Feather Spray Recipe with 2 drops of Clary Sage added.
WATER DIFFUSION: Any of the suggested oils, Three Part Blends

Single Oils:
Clary Sage, Geranium, Lavender, Marjoram, Melissa, Myrrh, Nutmeg, Orange, Spikenard, Tarragon, Ylang Ylang

KIDNEY DISEASE

With Kidney Disease it is important that hydration stays increased. If essential oil use in the drinking water increases water consumption, this is a wonderful bonus. It is important to not add too many new things into a protocol all at once, as if elimination occurs too quickly for the compromised kidneys to process, an individual could feel more uncomfortable. Go very slowly, adding items gradually in compromised individuals.

FIRST LINE RECOMMENDATIONS:
DRINKING WATER: Three Part Blends, especially of citrus oils
TOPICAL: Feather Spray Recipe made with 10 drops of Orange and 10 drops of Grapefruit instead of the entire 20 drops of Orange oil. Add 2 drops of Juniper.
WATER DIFFUSION: Three Part Blends

Single Oils:
Geranium, Grapefruit, Helichrysum, Juniper, Lavender, Ledum, Lemon

LEAD POISONING
(See HEAVY METAL POISONING)

LIVER DISEASE

FIRST LINE RECOMMENDATIONS:
INGESTION: Helichrysum in food and/or water
WATER DIFFUSION: Any selected oils, Three Part Blends
TOPICAL: Feather Spray Recipe made with Tangerine instead of Orange oil. Alternately, replace some of the drops of oil in the recipe with 5 drops of Helichrysum or 5 drops of Roman Chamomile.

Single Oils:
Chamomile (German), Chamomile (Roman), Geranium, Grapefruit, Helichrysum, Juniper, Lavender, Ledum, Lemon, Myrtle, Nutmeg, Rosemary, Spearmint, Tangerine

MACAW WASTING DISEASE
(See PROVENTRICULAR DILATATION DISEASE)

MALNUTRITION

The word malnutrition often makes bird owners feel uncomfortable, or like they have fallen short of caring properly for their bird. However, the vast majority of birds in captivity today suffer from malnutrition. The simple fact is that we cannot duplicate an adequate diet for them, no matter how hard we try. Eggs are laid and hatched with already-deficient little beings. Malnutrition is labeled when physical or laboratory findings actual confirm that the body is in a state of lack. It is more true that all birds are in this state already, we just don't diagnose it until there are tangible values to detect.

FIRST LINE RECOMMENDATIONS:
WATER DIFFUSION: Any selected oil, Three Part Blends
WATER MISTING: Feather Spray Recipes

Single Oils:
Grapefruit, Helichrysum, Lavender, Ledum, Lemon, Orange, Spearmint, Tangerine, Tarragon

MUTILATION, SELF
(See also FEATHER LOSS, FEATHER PICKING, PAIN MANAGEMENT)

Self-mutilation is a disturbing disorder in which a bird bites and chews their own skin to the point of causing damage, sometimes severe in extent. Most commonly this area of mutilation is on the chest area, but can include other locations. Although often linked with emotional concerns, this condition is most certainly grounded in physical conditions. An accurate diagnosis and extensive diagnostic testing is worthwhile. Any concern such as Arthritis, Heart Disease, or Hormonal Conditions should be addressed as they may be a potential cause for the mutilation behavior.

FIRST LINE RECOMMENDATIONS:
Use the basic recommendations for FEATHER PICKING and also slowly incorporate one or all of the following:

WATER MISTING: With 4 drops of Helichrysum, 4 drops of Copaiba, 10 drops of Frankincense, and 4 drops of Myrrh in 4 ounces (120 mL) of distilled water. Shake well, spray mutilated area up to 4 or more times per day.

WATER DIFFUSION: Rotational diffusion of emotional Three Part Blends. Tented diffusion with Three Part Blends for physical purposes may be helpful to ease infection and discomfort of the lesion.
INGESTION: Use oils indicated for any medical concerns noted. Also see PAIN MANAGEMENT for methods to control discomfort.
TOPICAL: Mix 1 drop each of Helichrysum, Myrrh, and Frankincense into 1 tablespoon of a natural ointment. Apply sparingly to wound. Avian Drip & Rub Recipes or Small Animal Supportive Blend may be indicated for some cases.

Single Oils:
Basil, Chamomile (German), Chamomile (Roman), Copaiba, Frankincense, Geranium, Grapefruit, Helichrysum, Laurus Nobilis, Lavender, Ledum, Lemon, Marjoram, Melissa, Myrrh, Nutmeg, Orange, Palmarosa, Patchouli, Spikenard, Tangerine, Valerian, Vetiver, Ylang Ylang

NEUROLOGIC CONDITIONS

Neurologic conditions can be caused by many different things, heavy metal poisoning, liver disease, viruses, and more. An accurate diagnosis is critical to addressing the foundation of the problem, however these recommendations build and support normal nerve health and regeneration.

FIRST LINE RECOMMENDATIONS:
WATER MISTING: Feather Spray Recipe made with exchanging 6 drops of base oils, with 2 drops Roman Chamomile and 4 drops Helichrysum. Rotationally, also use the Copaiba, Frankincense, and Helichrysum Spray Recipe.
WATER DIFFUSION: Any of the recommended oils, Three Part Blends
DRINKING WATER: Melissa
TOPICAL: Three Part Blends, Small Animal Supportive Blend, or Avian Drip & Rub Recipe can be considered.

Single Oils:
Black Spruce, Chamomile (German), Chamomile (Roman), Copaiba, Frankincense, Helichrysum, Juniper, Laurus Nobilis, Lavender, Lemon, Marjoram, Melissa, Vitex

PAIN MANAGEMENT

Pain management is critical for any bird. Any symptom can be demonstrated as a response to pain, and we should never forget that although an animal cannot communicate that they are painful, pain does exist and is a significant source of stress, immune dysfunction, and delayed healing.

FIRST LINE RECOMMENDATIONS:
INGESTION: Add 1 drop each of Helichrysum, Myrrh, and Copaiba to 1 teaspoon of fractionated coconut oil. Feed one drop of this mixture, gradually increasing amount and frequency of feeding, based on response.
WATER MISTING: Copaiba, Frankincense, and Helichrysum Recipe.

Single Oils:
Black Spruce, Clove, Copaiba, Frankincense, Helichrysum, Lavender, Myrrh, Peppermint

PAPILLOMATOSIS

Papilloma was one of the first conditions I treated aggressively with essential oils for a bird. The incredible and significant responses revolutionized the medical use of essential oils for birds. Often times, these cases have been struggling for many years with the wart-like condition, so responses are not expected over night. Immune systems and basic health must be rebuilt to fully address this disorder.

FIRST LINE RECOMMENDATIONS:
WATER MISTING: Alternate between daily to twice daily use of each spray recipe recommended at the beginning of the chapter.
WATER DIFFUSION: Three Part Blends in rotation, and almost all day long
DRINKING WATER: Melissa essential oil is a must for this condition. Other oils can be used, however it is wise to make sure that ingestion of Melissa oil in particular is achieved.
INGESTION: Rotate ingestion of Melissa, Oregano, and Clove oils mixed into foods.

Single Oils:
Clove, Copaiba, Frankincense, Lavender, Lemon, Melissa, Oregano, Peppermint, Sandalwood, Thyme

PARROT FEVER
(See PSITTACOSIS)

PBFD
(See PSITTACINE BEAK AND FEATHER DISEASE)

PDD
(See PROVENTRICULAR DILATATION DISEASE)

PROVENTRICULAR DILATATION DISEASE
(See also NEUROLOGIC CONDITIONS, VIRAL CONDITIONS)

Proventricular Dilatation Disease is thought to be caused by a virus (see Borna Virus), and causes neurologic damage and inflammation. This damage is mainly noted as a disruption in digestion and gastrointestinal function, however other neurologic signs can be seen. This is a devastating disease, and I feel that true hope lies within essential oils for prevention and treatment. Many affected birds are placed on NSAID therapies, and the use of Copaiba can greatly replace these medications. Slow and careful introduction of oils and supplements must be taken, as these birds are often fragile, are malnourished, and have been on prescription medications long term. Focusing on highly antiviral oils (like Melissa), anti-inflammatory actions, and neurologic repair are important with this condition.

FIRST LINE RECOMMENDATIONS:
WATER MISTING: Rotational spraying with various recipes. Feather Spray Recipe with 2 drops Roman Chamomile added. Copaiba, Frankincense, and Helichrysum Recipe.
DRINKING WATER: Melissa
WATER DIFFUSION: Rotational diffusion of any recommended oils. Up to 24 hours a day, if the bird handles it well. Three Part Blends.
INGESTION: Melissa, Helichrysum, Copaiba. Peppermint may help with peristalsis and movement of the gastrointestinal system.

TOPICAL: Small Animal Supportive Blend or Avian Drip & Rub Recipe may be indicated in some cases.

Single Oils:
Chamomile (Roman), Copaiba, Helichrysum, Hyssop, Laurus Nobilis, Lavender, Lemon, Melissa, Patchouli, Peppermint, Sandalwood, Spearmint, Tarragon, Thyme

PSITTACINE BEAK AND FEATHER DISEASE
(See also FEATHER LOSS, VIRAL CONDITIONS)

Psittacine Beak and Feather Disease is a viral infection that causes abnormal feather growth, feather loss, and can also affect many other body systems. It is a contagious disease, and continued diffusion of essential oils is likely to reduce transmission and boost immune function in flock situations.

FIRST LINE RECOMMENDATIONS:
Follow the recommendations outlined for VIRAL CONDITIONS and FEATHER LOSS for items that support this disorder.

WATER DIFFUSION: Three Part Blends should be diffused on a continual basis as tolerated. Rotating through diffusion of several versions for health and environmental decontamination is suggested.
DRINKING WATER: Melissa
WATER MISTING: Feather Spray Recipes
TOPICAL: Small Animal Supportive Blend or Avian Drip & Rub Recipes may be indicated.

Single Oils:
Eucalyptus globulus, Eucalyptus radiata, Helichrysum, Hyssop, Lavender, Lemon, Melissa, Rosemary, Sandalwood, Thyme

PSITTACOSIS

Psittacosis is caused by a bacteria, and is contagious to humans. Traditional therapies include treatment with Doxycycline antibiotics. Prevention is the ideal course, with the use of natural cleaners containing essential oils and continual diffusion helping to boost immune systems and reduce environmental contamination.

FIRST LINE RECOMMENDATIONS:
WATER DIFFUSION: Three Part Blends in the room, and also via tenting or caging when needed. Rotate through several recipes.
INGESTION: can be considered of indicated appropriate oils.
WATER MISTING: Feather Spray Recipes
TOPICAL: Small Animal Supportive Blend or Avian Drip & Rub Recipes can be considered.

Single Oils:
Black Spruce, Cinnamon, Copaiba, Eucalyptus globulus, Eucalyptus radiata, Helichrysum, Laurus Nobilis, Lavender, Ledum, Lemon, Oregano, Rosemary, Thyme

REGURGITATION
(See also CROP INFECTION, CROP STASIS, HORMONAL CONDITIONS)

Regurgitation can occur for many reasons, so it is important to have a thorough examination by an avian veterinarian to help determine the cause. If the cause seems hormonal in nature, please see HORMONAL CONDITIONS. Laboratory testing is ideal and can show if kidney, liver, or gastrointestinal systems may be implicated. Once the underlying cause is determined, using recommendations specific to these needs, will aid in healing more thoroughly.

FIRST LINE RECOMMENDATIONS:
WATER DIFFUSION: digestive Three Part Blends
WATER MISTING: Feather Spray Recipe, especially with Copaiba

Single Oils:
Black Spruce, Copaiba, Ginger, Juniper, Laurus Nobilis, Lavender, Lemon, Marjoram, Patchouli, Peppermint, Spearmint, Tangerine, Tarragon

RESPIRATORY CONDITIONS
(See also ASPERGILLOSIS, SINUS INFECTIONS)

FIRST LINE RECOMMENDATIONS:
WATER DIFFUSION: Three Part Blend via caging or tenting. Diffuse for up to 20 minutes, 3 or more times per day, depending on response. Diffusion via open room, can occur 24 hours a day when tolerated, with any oil recommendation.
WATER MISTING: Feather Spray Recipes

Single Oils:
Balsam Fir, Black Spruce, Copaiba, Cedarwood, Eucalyptus globulus, Eucalyptus radiata, Hyssop, Laurus nobilis, Lavender, Lemon, Lemongrass, Marjoram, Melaleuca alternifolia, Melissa, Myrtle, Oregano, Rosemary, Thyme

SCALY FACE MITES

Scaly face mites are common in Budgerigars (Budgies, Common Parakeets), and often cause a grainy overgrowth on the nasal area (cere) and beak. Often the beak is distorted in growth. Infections can be undetected for years, until they become severe enough to warrant a veterinary exam. Mite protection products sold on the avian market, are completely toxic, and generally useless as well. Diffusion of anti-parasitic oils from the acquirement of a bird, would likely help this problem from festering.

FIRST LINE RECOMMENDATIONS:
TOPICAL: diluted Three Part Blends can be carefully applied to the cere (nasal tissue area) and affected beak. Care is taken to avoid contact with the eyes. Monitor responses carefully, and with a veterinarian. Repeat the application daily for 7-14 days, depending on how the bird is handling it. Then use direct application every few days to every week, along with other methods of application.
WATER DIFFUSION: Three Part Blends via tenting can be performed at least once a day to help permeate the infected tissues with essential oil.
WATER MISTING: Feather Spray Recipes can be used, and addition and use of indicated oils by water misting (4 drops in 4 ounces of distilled water to start). Birds can be misted once to several times per day. This is a long term problem, and when beak and tissue deformity is present, it can take a long time to repair.

Single Oils:
Black Spruce, Catnip, Citronella, Copaiba, Eucalyptus citriodora, Lavender, Lemon, Orange, Palmarosa

SEIZURES
(See also SEIZURES in CANINE CONDITIONS)

FIRST LINE RECOMMENDATIONS:
WATER MISTING: Feather Spray Recipe daily, add additional oils as indicated.
WATER DIFFUSION: Water diffusion of neurologic Three Part Blends up to 24 hours a day (ideally rotating through many different oils.) Tenting or caging is usually not necessary, but having the diffuser close by the bird is nice.
DRINKING WATER: Melissa or another indicated oils.
TOPICAL: Small Animal Supportive Blend or Avian Drip & Rub Recipes may be indicated.

Single Oils:
Balsam Fir, Black Spruce, Chamomile (German), Chamomile (Roman), Copaiba, Frankincense, Helichrysum, Laurus nobilis, Lavender, Lemon, Melissa

SINUS INFECTIONS
(See also RESPIRATORY CONDITIONS)

FIRST LINE RECOMMENDATIONS:
WATER DIFFUSION: Three Part Blends via caging or tenting. Open room diffusion up to 24 hours a day. Caging or tenting for 20 minutes at a time, 3-4 times a day is common.
SINUS FLUSH: In severe situations, sinus flushes can be prepared with essential oils added to them. Sinus flushes should only be performed by extremely experienced avian handlers or veterinarians. The person performing the flush will generally have solutions and recipes which they use for the sinus flush. In general, the medically appropriate agents are included and chosen by the professional to disperse the essential oil.

A very dilute solution can be used initially, increasing in concentration only if indicated and needed.

Single Oils:
Black Spruce, Copaiba, Hyssop, Laurus nobilis, Lavender, Lemon, Lemongrass, Marjoram, Melaleuca alternifolia, Melissa, Myrtle, Oregano, Thyme

VIRAL CONDITIONS

Any disorder that is affected or caused by a virus, can use these methods to support the body in healing.

FIRST LINE RECOMMENDATIONS:
DRINKING WATER: Melissa drinking water is provided.
WATER MISTING: Feather Spray Recipe is used daily.
WATER DIFFUSION: 3-4 drops of Three Part Blends is diffused up to 24 hours a day.
TOPICAL: Small Animal Supportive Blend or Avian Drip & Rub Recipes may be indicated for some cases, up to once a day in severe situations.

Single Oils:
Black Spruce, Copaiba, Geranium, Helichrysum, Hyssop, Laurus nobilis, Lavender, Lemon, Melissa, Mountain Savory, Oregano, Peppermint, Sandalwood, Spikenard, Thyme

WARTS
(See PAPILLOMATOSIS)

WASTING DISEASE
(See PROVENTRICULAR DILATATION DISEASE)

WOUNDS
(See also BUMBLEFOOT)

FIRST LINE RECOMMENDATIONS:
TOPICAL: 1 drop (or more) of Helichrysum is mixed into 1 tablespoon of natural ointment and applied to the area sparingly. Care needs to be taken to not over use ointments, or to get it onto the feathers.
WATER MISTING: Spraying with the Feather Spray Recipes (even twice a day or more), is also very beneficial. Just the Feather Spray Recipe can be used if it is difficult to handle the bird or to apply ointment. Using sprays containing Helichrysum, or adding several drops to the Feather Spray is also suggested.
INGESTION: If painful wounds are noted, see PAIN MANAGEMENT.
WATER DIFFUSION: Diffusion can also be used to permeate the injured area and decrease stress.

Single Oils:
Chamomile (German), Chamomile (Roman), Copaiba, Frankincense, Geranium, Helichrysum, Lavender, Lemon, Myrrh, Oregano, Palmarosa, Patchouli, Spikenard

ZINC POISONING
(See HEAVY METAL POISONING)

ESSENTIAL OILS: FERRETS

In general, most ferrets are administered essential oils very similarly to cats. In many ways, ferrets are actually easier to give oils orally, topically, and in food. If a similar condition is listed in the Feline Section – using these protocols with a ferret is generally recommended.

As Ferrets are very prone to certain conditions, the use of essential oils and nutrition to aid in the prevention of these disorders is strongly suggested. Waiting until the condition is obvious is not ideal.

FIRST LINE RECOMMENDATIONS:
WATER DIFFUSION: Rotational diffusion of anti-cancer and endocrine supportive oils should be continual. Various Three Part Blends are ideal. Odor Eliminating and Air Freshening Three Part Blends are an excellent choice for odor control.
TOPICAL: Regular applications of either the Small Animal Supportive Blend or Feline Supportive Blend is suggested. Diluted Three Part Blends are also appropriate.
BATHING: Essential oils can be added to natural shampoo to add additional health benefits to routine bathing. Adding additional Frankincense or other preventive oils is a convenient way to add health.
LITTER BOX RECIPES: Just like cats, Ferrets can also benefit from the addition of essential oils to their litter boxes.

Single Oils:
Balsam Fir, Black Spruce, Copaiba, Frankincense, Helichrysum, Lemon, Nutmeg, Orange, Tangerine

FERRET – ADRENAL TUMORS

Adrenal disease and tumors are far too common in Ferrets, and almost expected to occur in aged Ferrets. Resulting in hair loss as the most obvious symptom, Ferrets tend to live with this condition on a chronic basis. Household chemicals, food toxins, and preservatives are high on the list of contributing factors. Preventive measures should be followed from kithood, for the best scenario of health.

FIRST LINE RECOMMENDATIONS:
WATER DIFFUSION: Three Part Blends, Balsam Fir, Black Spruce, Frankincense
PETTING: Three Part Blends, Frankincense daily
TOPICAL: Small Animal Supportive Blend or Feline Supportive Blend, with added adrenal supportive oils.

Single Oils:
Balsam Fir, Black Spruce, Copaiba, Frankincense, Helichrysum, Lemon, Nutmeg, Orange, Rosemary, Sandalwood, Tangerine

FERRET – DIARRHEA, HELICOBACTER PYLORI

Ferrets can exhibit bloody diarrhea and illness with this bacterial condition of the gastrointestinal tract. Antibiotics are generally prescribed, and occasionally veterinary hospitalization is also required. Since there can be significant amounts of blood in the stools, both digested (melena) or fresh, use caution with essential oils which carry anticoagulant actions. Helichrysum is helpful for intestinal pains and bleeding.

FIRST LINE RECOMMENDATIONS:
WATER DIFFUSION: Three Part Blends (digestive)
INGESTION: Oregano
PETTING: Three Part Blends (digestive)
TOPICAL: Small Animal Supportive Blend or Feline Supportive Blend, with additional Helichrysum or gastrointestinal oils added.

Single Oils:
Cistus, Clove, Copaiba, Ginger, Helichrysum, Laurus nobilis, Lemon, Melaleuca alternifolia, Nutmeg, Oregano, Patchouli, Peppermint, Tangerine, Tarragon, Thyme

FERRET - INSULINOMA

An Insulinoma is a pancreas based tumor that is generally active and causes excess insulin to be secreted into the body. This can result in severe hypoglycemia episodes. Surgery is often performed to remove the tumors. Essential oils have been helpful in balancing pancreatic function, however careful monitoring should be taken with blood sugar levels.

FIRST LINE RECOMMENDATIONS:
 INGESTION: Black Cumin
 PETTING: Diluted Three Part Blends up to twice a day or more depending on the severity of the case.
 WATER DIFFUSION: Any of the selected oils, Three Part Blends.
 LITTEROMA: Can also be utilized to layer exposure to beneficial oils.

Single Oils:
 Black Cumin, Copaiba, Frankincense, Geranium, Grapefruit, Lemon, Lemongrass, Myrrh, Myrtle, Nutmeg, Orange, Sandalwood, Spearmint, Tangerine, Ylang Ylang

FERRET – LYMPHOMA, LYMPHOSARCOMA

Ferrets are also particularly prone to developing malignant enlargement of the lymph nodes. Juvenile onset of this disorder carries a poor prognosis. Prevention measures are critical. Supporting health, eliminating household toxins, and providing indicated essential oils and nutritional supplements PRIOR to the disease eruption, is a strong recommendation.

FIRST LINE RECOMMENDATIONS:
 WATER DIFFUSION: Diffuse the recommended oils within Three Part Blends on a regular basis to aid in prevention as well as disease.
 INGESTION: Grapefruit, Lemon, Orange, in water or foods has been used, as well as Frankincense.
 TOPICAL: Small Animal Supportive Blend or Feline Supportive Blend applied monthly for prevention, adding various anti-cancer oils. During times of disease, daily or more frequent administration with additional indicated oils has been used.

Single Oils:
 Black Spruce, Copaiba, Frankincense, Grapefruit, Lemon, Orange, Sandalwood, Tangerine

FERRET – PROSTATIC DISEASE

Male Ferrets can be affected by an enlarged prostate, which can also be infected. This condition often results in discomfort and straining to urinate.

FIRST LINE RECOMMENDATIONS:
TOPICAL: Diluted Three Part Blends, Small Animal Supportive Blend, or Feline Supportive Blends can be used. Additional Copaiba and Sage may be added.
WATER DIFFUSION: Three Part Blends

Single Oils:
Black Spruce, Copaiba, Frankincense, Sage, Tarragon, Thyme

FERRET – DRIP & RUB RECIPE
(See also FELINE DRIP & RUB RECIPE)

Ferrets receive the Feline Supportive Blend application in the same way as Cats. All of the descriptions, techniques, and modifications all apply to use in Ferrets.

FIRST LINE RECOMMENDATIONS:
Mix 4 drops each of Oregano, Thyme, Basil, Cypress, Marjoram, Lavender, Copaiba, Helichrysum, and Peppermint oils into 30 mL of Fractionated Coconut Oil. Apply 5-8 drops up the spine, and stroke in as described for cats. Balancing prior to the application can be performed, but is optional. Modifications and additions to the Feline Supportive Blend can be made in the same ways as described for cats. Generally adding 4 drops of the desired oil to the recipe. See descriptions for individual oils, Body Supportive Blends, and Drip & Rub Techniques for more instructions.

ESSENTIAL OILS: RABBITS

Most remedies for rabbits will be used with a very gentle approach initially. Starting with water-based diffusion for every recommended oil is wise. Since rabbits are hind gut fermenters, the use of antibacterial essential oils must be used with caution to avoid killing their natural gut flora. Essential oils that are the most mild are recommended for use first, but it is refreshing to know that in severe cases that are non-responsive to other methods – the use of essential oils is becoming more and more wide spread, and "aggressive" in end stage cases, with good results.

I would recommend starting with rabbits in a few, well documented ways, then advancing to more aggressive administration if these protocols fail you. Reading through all of the conditions, and becoming familiar with Rabbit friendly recommendations, is a wonderful way to incorporate more natural health into your rabbit's life.

RABBITS - BREEDING

Basic disease prevention, stress reduction, healthy immune systems, easy delivery, and a healthy milk supply can all be supported with the use of essential oils.

FIRST LINE RECOMMENDATIONS:
WATER DIFFUSION: Three Part Blends for immune support and disease prevention. Three Part Blends for delivery. Fennel can be used to increase milk production.
DRINKING WATER: Tangerine and Orange have been used to boost immune systems.
PETTING: Even newborn baby bunnies have been handled with essential oils absorbed into the human hands. An extremely small amount is absorbed through the wet newborns, but significant enough for health benefits.
CLEANING: All cleaning should be done with natural cleaning recipes with essential oils added.
TOPICAL: Small Animal Supportive Blend

Single Oils:
Copaiba, Fennel, Frankincense, Geranium, Lavender, Lemon, Orange, Rose, Rosemary, Tangerine, Ylang Ylang

RABBITS - DIARRHEA

Diarrhea can have many causes, and of course dysbiosis, or the disruption of normal intestinal flora must be considered. Probiotics are generally not of the same bacterial culture that is present in the Rabbit digestive tract, however they still may appear helpful. Transfaunation (the feeding of morning stools from normal rabbits) remains the best route to repopulate a rabbit's gut. Care must be taken to never use stools from a sick or potentially contagious rabbit. Baby rabbits and rabbits who are housed together, may occasionally eat each other's morning stools, which is a common occurrence in rabbits. Depending on the cause of the diarrhea, recommendations may vary.

FIRST LINE RECOMMENDATIONS:
TOPICAL: Small Animal Supportive Blend, diluted Three Part Blends (digestive)
WATER DIFFUSION: Three Part Blends (digestive)

Single Oils:
Copaiba, Ginger, Laurus nobilis, Lemon, Orange, Peppermint, Tangerine, Tarragon

RABBITS – EXTERNAL PARASITES, MITES

There are many forms of external parasites in Rabbits. The most common include Cheyletiella Mites (walking dandruff), Psoroptes cuniculi (ear mites), and Cuterebra larvae. Cuterebra is contracted through flies, and a grub worm actually develops within the skin. Care must be taken with Cuterebra to not rupture or harm the worm inside the body, as anaphylaxis may result. Prevention with the recommendations is the best suggestion for Cuterebra, with veterinary attention and extraction required for the presence of the actual worm. Topical and area use of essential oils and products are helpful.

FIRST LINE RECOMMENDATIONS:
BATHING: Add 5 drops of Three Part Blends for parasites, to 1 tablespoon of natural shampoo and bathe as needed, approximately weekly is suggested.
WATER MISTING: 20 drops of Three Part Blends for parasites in 4 ounces (120 mL) of distilled water. Shake well and thoroughly mist the rabbit, taking caution near the face and eyes.
PETTING: With diluted Three Part Blends on your hands, up to twice a day. Occasionally to avoid greasiness to fur, neat oils completely absorbed into your hands may be used for petting applications.
TOPICAL: diluted Three Part Blends for parasites, Small Animal Supportive Blends can be applied directly, Pet onto locations, or swabbed into the ears. With ear mites, diluted Three Part Blends have been swabbed into the ears. It is still important to treat the entire body for mites, not only the ears.
WATER DIFFUSION: Regular diffusion of Three Part Blends for parasites can keep insects to a minimum.
AIR DIFFUSION: For large barns or areas containing rabbits, air diffusion may be called for.
CLEANING: The use of natural cleaning products with added essential oils for cleaning as well as area control of insects is highly recommended.

Single Oils:
Catnip, Eucalyptus citriodora, Citronella, Lavender, Palmarosa

RABBITS – PASTEURELLOSIS

Infection with Pasteurella multocida bacteria in Rabbits can present in several ways. There can be respiratory infections called "Snuffles," infection that affects the nervous system called "Wry Neck" or torticollis, and there can also be abscesses that form in a variety of locations. Some strains are mild and rabbits will naturally recover, and some strains are more severe and can result in permanent symptoms or even death. Long term antibiotic use is common traditionally. In more severe cases, more aggressive regimens with essential oils can be considered, however it is important to always be mindful of the intestinal flora of the rabbit. For neurologic involvement, oils such as Helichrysum and Frankincense are especially indicated.

Starting with diffusion alone initially is recommended. Then gradually adding and layering application methods is suggested. If tented water diffusion does not yield enough results, then moving onto Petting applications is encouraged, and so forth. The main object with Rabbits is to move slowly, and start mildly. However, in life threatening situations, many Rabbits have received quite aggressive treatments with essential oils and have benefited.

FIRST LINE RECOMMENDATIONS:
WATER DIFFUSION: Three Part Blends with indicated oils. Rotate with several blend versions. Caging or Tenting can be performed as needed.
TOPICAL: Small Animal Supportive Blend, Lemon, Lavender, Laurus nobilis. To abscesses directly diluted Lavender, Lemon, or diluted Three Part Blends. Administration up to daily or twice a day may be indicated for some cases.
INGESTION: Starting with ingestion of oils such as Lemon is suggested. If use of stronger oral antibiotic oils is deemed necessary, proceed slowly and monitor stools carefully. Placing 1 drop of Lemon in 1 tablespoon of vegetable baby food, and gradually increasing to feeding 1 mL of this mixture two to three times a day is a suggested.
CLEANING: Disinfect things well with natural cleaners with essential oils within them. Abscesses can be flushed and cleaned with solutions containing essential oils as well.

Single Oils:
Frankincense, Helichrysum, Laurus nobilis, Lavender, Lemon, Melaleuca alternifolia, Oregano, Thyme

RABBIT – DRIP & RUB TECHNIQUE

Being hindgut fermenters, Rabbits represent a distinct challenge and require a bit of care when strong antibacterial agents are administered, whether they are natural or chemical in nature. Many Rabbits have tragically been killed when an unknowing veterinarian prescribed a harmful antibiotic for them. With all Rabbits, Guinea Pigs, and Chinchillas starting with the very mildest of oils (ones that you would use on a human baby or on your face) is recommended. Then progressing to stronger or more aggressive oils if needed is suggested. The Small Animal Supportive Blend is a perfect start for these animals.

FIRST LINE RECOMMENDATIONS:
SMALL ANIMAL SUPPORTIVE BLEND: Add 1 drop each of Copaiba, Frankincense, Lavender, Lemongrass, Helichrysum, Tangerine, Ginger, Basil, and Marjoram to 30 mL (1 ounce) of Fractionated Coconut Oil. Apply 3-6 drops of this solution up the back and stroke in. Balancing with calming blends beforehand is optional. This blend may be applied to other locations of need as well, or applied in a general Petting application.

STRONGER RABBIT DRIP & RUB RECIPE: Add 1 drop each of Oregano, Thyme, Copaiba, Frankincense, Basil, Cypress, Lavender, Marjoram, and Peppermint to 30-60 mL (1-2 ounces) of Fractionated Coconut Oil. Balancing with a calming blend beforehand is optional as described previously. Apply 3-6 drops of this solution up the back, from tail to head. Stroke the oils in. Starting with the more diluted solution, and then making it stronger if needed, is recommended. Application via Petting can also be used.

Single Oils:
Chamomile (German), Chamomile (Roman), Copaiba, Dill, Frankincense, Helichrysum, Lavender, Lemon, Myrrh, Orange, Tangerine

RABBITS - SNUFFLES
(See PASTEURELLOSIS)

RABBITS - SYPHILIS

Syphilis, also known as Vent, is a sexually transmitted disease caused by Treponema cuniculi. This is a spirochete bacteria similar to that which causes Syphilis in humans. It lives in the bloodstream and can cause lesions, scabs, and weeping sores on the face, mouth, and genitals. Many Rabbits are killed when this diagnosis is made, especially in breeding situations. The disease is difficult to eliminate, even with traditional antibiotics. Hygiene and cleanliness of the environment is very important, and constant diffusion as well as cleaning with natural cleaners containing disinfecting essential oils is a must. The same recommendations and increases in aggressiveness of treatment that are made for Pasteurellosis, is suggested for Syphilis.

FIRST LINE RECOMMENDATIONS:
Follow the suggestions and recommendations listed for Pasteurellosis. It is likely that Syphilis may require the Stronger Rabbit Drip & Rub Recipe and possibly oral oils to completely eliminate the disorder.
DIFFUSION: In a Rabbitry, air diffusion may be indicated. Strong Antimicrobial Three Part Blends are suggested in rotation.
WATER MISTING: Add 5 drops Helichrysum, 5 drops Copaiba, 5 drops Frankincense, 5 drops Lemon, and 10 drops Lavender to 4 ounces (120 mL) of distilled water. Shake well and mist onto sores, mainly on the genital area. Use caution and common sense if other locations need application.
TOPICAL: Mixing various oils into natural ointments for application to wounds is recommended. Start with 1 drop per tablespoon. Multiple oils can be used, and stronger concentrations when indicated.

Single Oils:
Copaiba, Frankincense, Helichrysum, Lavender, Lemon, Oregano, Thyme

RABBITS – TUMORS, WARTS, PAPILLOMA

Shope's Papilloma is a viral wart condition that can cause the growth of tumors in Rabbits. The virus is contagious and thought to be spread by insects. Insect control through the use of essential oils (see External Parasites) is helpful. The immune system is important to support to prevent and care for this disorder. Below are recommendations specific to the tumors.

FIRST LINE RECOMMENDATIONS:
DIFFUSION: Reduction of insects by air or water diffusion of insect repelling Three Part Blends. Air diffusion is only recommended for large areas such as Rabbitries.
WATER MISTING: 20 drops of Three Part Blends (against insects) in 4 ounces (120 mL) of distilled water. Shake well and thoroughly mist the rabbit, taking caution near the face and eyes.
PETTING: With insect repelling Three Part Blends up to twice a day. For reduction of insects.

TOPICAL: Various essential oils can be applied to warts directly, especially Frankincense. Caution needs to be followed based on the location and ability to apply the oils. Often, neat oils are applied to warts and tumors. One can start with mild and diluted oils (1 drop per 5 drops of carrier oil), and gradually build up in concentration based on responses. Small Animal Supportive Blends or the Stronger Rabbit Drip & Rub Recipes can be applied to the rabbit, and to tumors and warts directly as well.
DRINKING WATER: Melissa

Single Oils:
Blue Cypress, Copaiba, Frankincense, Grapefruit, Helichrysum, Lavender, Melissa, Orange, Oregano, Peppermint, Sandalwood, Tangerine

RABBITS - VENT
(See RABBITS - SYPHILIS)

RABBITS – WRY NECK
(See RABBITS – PASTEURELLOSIS)

ESSENTIAL OILS: EXOTIC ANIMALS

AMPHIBIANS

Amphibians require very light and special techniques when using oils. A fundamental trait of frogs, toads, salamanders, and newts is that they readily absorb things through their skin. Often known as strong indicators of environmental health, the exposure of amphibians to the residues of hand lotions, hand purifiers, cleaners, tap water, and pollutants can be harmful to their health. Aquatic amphibians can be exposed to essential oils much as fish are, starting with a toothpick dip of essential oil added to their water source. Water-based diffusion of essential oils is often enough to provide systemic absorption of the oil through the skin. Topical administration of oils should involve the complete absorption of the essential oil (neat) into our hands, and then the amphibian can be gently cupped within our hands. Neat oils are recommended for this purpose, as a carrier oil is not compatible with amphibian skin, and is best left off of it. Aquariums and environments can be cleaned with natural cleaners containing essential oils, although these should be thoroughly rinsed afterwards for most amphibians. Topical applications of Three Part Blends or Small Animal Supportive Blends is not recommended for these animals.

FIRST LINE RECOMMENDATIONS:
TOPICAL: Only if strictly indicated, and when water-based diffusion has not been enough, we can consider the placement of 1 drop of neat oil (often starting with Frankincense) into the palm of your hand. Rub your hands together until the oil is completely absorbed into your skin. Cup the animal in the palms of your hand. They will absorb the essential oil!
WATER SOAKING: Add 1 toothpick dip of a Three Part Blend or single essential oil into 1 Liter of water, use as their soaking or swimming water source. Increase concentration only if needed, and based on responses.

WATER MISTING: 1 toothpick dip to 1 drop of essential oil can be placed in 1 Liter of water and the amphibian or the environment can be misted.

WATER DIFFUSION: Place 1-4 drops of essential oil or Three Part Blend into a water diffuser. Generally, do not diffuse "hot" oils within a room containing an amphibian. Diffusion in an open room setting is generally adequate for these animals.

Single Oils:
Copaiba, Frankincense, Grapefruit, Helichrysum, Lavender, Lemon, Orange, Tangerine

CATS LARGE (LIONS, TIGERS, COUGARS...)

Large cats can use essential oils in all of the same methods described for domestic cats. Feline Supportive Blend is still utilized for these larger felines, however many more drops can be dispensed. Diffusion may be the most easily administered method, depending on how much the cat can be handled. Air diffusion may be used in large areas such as zoo confinements. For cats who may have a swimming pool or water area, essential oils can be added to the water for absorption. Some large cats may ingest essential oils in food or water. Petting can be used when the technique is possible.

FIRST LINE RECOMMENDATIONS:
DIFFUSION: Water or Air Diffusion is recommended on a consistent basis for health. Rotation through various essential oils and blends are recommended, and especially being considerate of emotional health.

Single Oils:
Bergamot, Copaiba, Frankincense, Geranium, Grapefruit, Helichrysum, Lavender, Melissa, Orange, Valerian, Vetiver, Ylang Ylang

CHINCHILLAS

See more information about hindgut fermentation and the special care with essential oils within the Rabbit descriptions. Chinchillas contain the most hair follicles per square inch of skin, of any land animal. This means that even diffusion of an essential oil into the air, is likely to achieve systemic levels within their body. Chinchillas should have an especially light touch with the use of oils, and water diffusion is likely all they may need. Some Chinchillas have even enjoyed licking essential oils off of their owner's hands, and this is fine if they choose to do so. Oils can also be added to their drinking water. Petting can be utilized in more critical situations, however the oils should be applied to your hands neat, and completely absorbed into your skin prior to handling the Chinchilla. Carrier oils should not be used on Chinchilla fur. In dire situations, Small Animal Supportive Blend has been applied to the hairless areas near the groin and scrotal areas of Chinchillas.

FIRST LINE RECOMMENDATIONS:
WATER DIFFUSION: Start with 1 drop of essential oil added to the diffuser. Open room diffusion is suggested, and only very rarely would tenting or caging be used.
DRINKING WATER: Starting with a toothpick dip into 1 Liter of water, gradually increase to 1 drop per Liter. Citrus oils are suggested.

Single Oils:
Copaiba, Frankincense, Grapefruit, Helichrysum, Lavender, Lemon, Orange, Tangerine

ELEPHANTS

Elephants can mainly use essential oils in the ways described for large animals. Air Diffusion can be used, especially due to the large and open environment that is likely to be occupied. While it would seem logical that elephants require huge amounts of essential oils, quite the opposite is true. And very small amounts and dilutions, even worn on their handlers, can be of great benefit and effect for these large, wonderful creatures. Rotational diffusion of oils for health and emotional well-being is often suggested. Care should be taken with elephants who may have severe emotional concerns, and safe handling practices should always be observed. Zoopharmacognosy is likely to be most fascinating with Elephants. They seem to be most knowledgeable in their own needs, and I feel we should respect them immensely, especially in regards to emotions.

Essential oils most certainly help and calm the emotional turmoil that may reside within a particular individual. Since we may not always be able to judge the response to a particular essential oil use, allowing for some "alone time" when performing emotional work and support, is advisable. All of the Body Supportive Blends can be utilized with Elephants – from the Small Animal Supportive Blend to the Large Animal Supportive Blend. It is a wonderful gradient that each Elephant may be exposed to, depending on their needs. Pre-diluted oils are most commonly recommended for topical skin use, regardless of the large size or tough skin.

Common conditions of Elephants include foot infections and degeneration, arthritis, tooth and oral issues, emotional traumas, gastrointestinal upset and concerns, and various skin issues. In my work with Global Sanctuary for Elephants in Brazil, we have noted some interesting responses to essential oil use. One elephant greatly increases her desire to eat, after administration of Copaiba. While this might be an excellent trait for some elephants, for her it seems a bit excessive and unnecessary.

Certainly, each elephant seems to have particular favorites in terms of essential oils for emotional concerns.

FIRST LINE RECOMMENDATIONS:
DIFFUSION: Rotational diffusion of any essential oils, often within Three Part Blends. Water-misting can be utilized when diffusion is not possible. Both air-style and water-based diffusion can be considered.
INDIRECT DIFFUSION: Placement of essential oils and blends can be made on bedding and around enclosures. Also handlers can also wear oils to benefit elephants.
SOAKING WATER: Elephants who have a swimming pool or water area to play in, will greatly benefit from the addition of essential oils to the water.
INGESTION: Just as with horses and other large animals, elephants enjoy oils such as Peppermint or Tangerine added to their water. Oils such as Copaiba can also be added to foods or water for inflammation support.
TOPICAL: Most commonly we use essential oil blends for a variety of mists for insect control, foot treatments, and skin conditions. Sprays are often easier to administer, and elephants are commonly trained to accept applications to their feet, and both water mists and oil based mists can be considered. Rather strong concentrations of oils can be used for applications to the feet, and experimentation may be necessary to find the correct ratios for a particular individual.

Single Oils:
Balsam Fir, Bergamot, Black Spruce, Cassia, Catnip, Cinnamon, Copaiba, Frankincense, Geranium, German Chamomile, Ginger, Grapefruit, Helichrysum, Lavender, Lemon, Lemongrass, Marjoram, Myrrh, Orange, Oregano, Peppermint, Roman Chamomile, Rose, Tangerine, Thyme, Valerian, Vetiver, Ylang Ylang

FISH

Adding essential oils to the aquarium or ponds of fish is a wonderful way to expose them to essential oils but to also rid them of fungus, bacteria, viruses, and other health concerns. Glass aquariums should be used, and avoiding plastic components of aquariums, as much as possible, is advised. Many oils have been used with fish, however the oils listed below have been used most commonly. I recommend starting with these well used oils, and only moving onto others when needed. Starting with a toothpick dip into the water, and gradually building concentrations is suggested. It is not uncommon for 2-5 drops of oil to be used in a 10 gallon aquarium. With very large areas of water such as ponds, results are often seen with even a few drops added (10-20 per large pond.) Fish have been seen ingesting droplets of oil from the water's surface, and I have changed my stance to not prefer this to happen. There is risk of the gills becoming topically irritated, and fish are likely only responding to something on the surface of the water. Ideally, essential oils can be added to a separate water supply first, such as 1 drop to 1 Liter of water in a glass jar or bottle. This water can then be used to fill a fish bowl, or to add to the existing water environment. Essential oils can serve as a broad spectrum approach against parasites, bacteria, fungi, tumors, and viruses. Carrier oils are not suggested for use within aquariums.

FIRST LINE RECOMMENDATIONS:
Add a toothpick dip of a Three Part Blend to a glass aquarium. Refresh as needed. Some fish receive oils on a weekly and sometimes even daily basis, depending on their need. Gradually increase amounts added to water.

Single Oils:
Copaiba, Frankincense, Grapefruit, Helichrysum, Lavender, Lemon, Melaleuca alternifolia, Orange, Peppermint, Tangerine

GUINEA PIGS

Please see the description regarding hindgut fermenters in the Rabbit section. Guinea Pigs have a particular need for Vitamin C to be provided through their diet, however citrus essential oils do not carry Vitamin C within them. Water diffusion is always suggested, and most of the ailments that Guinea Pigs confront can be treated in a similar manner to what is recommended for Rabbits. Guinea Pigs are quite commonly affected with Pneumonia, and following the guidelines for Pasteurellosis within Rabbits, is suggested. If topical oils are considered for a Guinea Pig, it should be provided with the same recommendations as made for Rabbits.

FIRST LINE RECOMMENDATIONS:
WATER DIFFUSION: Generally in an open room, but tenting and caging can be used for respiratory conditions. Three Part Blends can be utilized when their oils are appropriate for use with Exotic Species.
TOPICAL: Applications of the Small Animal Supportive Blend can be utilized as needed. Additional oils can be added, when indicated.
DRINKING WATER: Guinea Pigs have consumed small amounts of essential oils in their drinking water. Start with 1 drop per Liter or less, see the chapter on Adding Oils to Drinking Water for more information.

Single Oils:
Copaiba, Frankincense, Grapefruit, Helichrysum, Lavender, Lemon, Orange, Tangerine

HEDGEHOGS

Hedgehogs require a "hands off" sort of application technique most often. Water diffusion and water misting are methods that work very well for these critters. Mites and fungal skin infections are common in hedgehogs, and misting with 4 drops of anti-parasitic Three Part Blends within 4 ounces (120 mL) of water up to twice a day is suggested. Tumors and cancers are also quite common in hedgehogs, so routine water-based diffusion or occasional misting of Three Part Blends with Frankincense is also suggested. The Small Animal Supportive Blend can also be used with Hedgehogs, as can the stronger Avian or Ferret Drip & Rub Recipes if needed.

FIRST LINE RECOMMENDATIONS:
WATER DIFFUSION: With appropriate Three Part Blends.
WATER MISTING: As needed with 4 drops of a Three Part Blend (often for external parasites) in 4 ounces of water for mites or fungal infections. Mist with Frankincense for tumor related issues.
DRINKING WATER: Orange, Grapefruit or other tasty anti-cancer oils
CLEANING: Clean caging well with essential oil blends and recipes for natural cleaners.

Single Oils:
Copaiba, Frankincense, Grapefruit, Helichrysum, Lavender, Lemon, Orange, Tangerine

HIPPOPOTAMUS

Hippos are not always the friendliest of creatures. When treating these animals, we are most often limited to diffusion, misting applications, or by adding essential oils to their swimming water. Due to the large amount of time spent in the water, adding oils to their environment is often the best route of exposure for a hippo. Start with a small amount of the chosen oil, and add it to the water up to once or more per day. The hippopotamus that I treated had a chronic skin condition, for which they would routinely apply a mineral oil based baby oil. This was unfortunately likely adding to the problem. Adding several drops of Lavender essential oil to the water supply, as well as cleaning the environment thoroughly with essential oil based natural cleaning recipes, was suggested. Other non-toxic massage oils could also be used in place of the baby oil, and would have had wonderful therapeutic benefits from the essential oils contained within them. Selecting any appropriate oil for the condition at hand is suggested, and then the basic advice is to find an easy method of application for your particular individual. Once you start to look, it is often easy to find multiple routes of exposure that is appropriate for the species you are trying to treat. Depending on the situation and the individual, if topical applications were desired it is likely that the Feline Supportive Blend or even the Feather Spray recipes could have been used easily.

FIRST LINE RECOMMENDATIONS:
SOAKING WATER: Add your chosen essential oil to the water. Start with small amounts and gradually increase. Lavender is a first suggestion.

Single Oils:
Bergamot, Copaiba, Frankincense, Grapefruit, Helichrysum, Lavender, Lemon, Orange, Tangerine, Valerian, Vetiver

INSECTS, ARACHNIDS, INVERTEBRATES

Care should be taken with insects to not use heavily insecticidal or insect repelling essential oils. Species that are most commonly exposed to essential oils by a human would be Honey Bees, Butterflies, Tarantulas, Ant Farms, Hermit Crabs and other household "pet" critters. Most people may focus on repelling problem insects, however in households where insects may be a part of the family, it is important to respect their needs and health as well. If the species you are considering is from a certain continent or may be exposed to certain foods (such as citrus), then selecting essential oils from the region or from the food category is suggested. So as Hermit Crabs who would naturally eat an orange, would generally tolerate exposure to Orange essential oil very well. Our Hermit Crabs greatly enjoy a misting with the Avian Feather Spray! Honey Bees in Arabian countries, just so happen to frequent the flowers of Frankincense blossoms, so a drop of Frankincense oil on a piece of natural cardboard or organic paper stock, can be placed inside a hive for immune system benefits. With Honey Bees, it is common that Thymol is being used within hives. These solutions are applied to cardboard, and the bees are exposed during their efforts to remove the foreign item. Of course, my preference is for exposure to natural and whole essential oils, and not a fraction such as Thymol. For most of these critters, water or indirect diffusion should be used.

FIRST LINE RECOMMENDATIONS:
WATER DIFFUSION: Should be in an open room environment, and starting with only 1 drop of oil added to the diffuser. Monitor the animal closely for signs of dislike or discomfort. Frankincense and Orange are starting suggestions.
INDIRECT DIFFUSION: Frankincense, Orange

Single Oils:
Copaiba, Frankincense, Helichrysum, Lavender, Lemon, Orange, Tangerine

PRIMATES

Primates can be treated in the same manner as human babies, children, or adults based on their size. The creative portion to administration lies within the ability to handle or work with the individual primate. Use any method which suits your particular needs and ability, even if it is described for a completely different type of animal. Feline or Canine Supportive Blends can be utilized and applications performed similarly to a human or dog.

FIRST LINE RECOMMENDATIONS:
WATER DIFFUSION: Rotate through various oils for physical and emotional health, just as we would for humans.
BATHING: Use natural shampoos with essential oils added.
TOPICAL: Feline or Canine Supportive Blends, or diluted Three Part Blends can be used.

Single Oils:
Copaiba, Frankincense, Helichrysum, Lavender, Orange

REPTILES

Reptiles such as snakes, lizards, alligators, and crocodiles can greatly benefit from the use of essential oils. Burns from inappropriate heating sources are unfortunately common, and can greatly benefit from Lavender application combined with natural ointments, within water-mists, in soaking water, or even neat in some situations. Skin mites and ticks can be common, and Three Part Blends for parasites can be used via misting applications or in soaking water. Water-based diffusion is helpful for respiratory infections. Oral flushes, washes, and topical applications for various mouth rot situations are extremely beneficial, and the addition of essential oils into various veterinary flush solutions has been effective for even resistant infections.

Metabolic Bone Disease (MBD) is an unfortunately common disorder which is generally caused by poor husbandry practices. Working with a reptile veterinarian is important to determine how to correct your situation. Essential oils may be helpful for MBD, but will not correct the underlying cause of poor nutrition, calcium and phosphorus imbalance, and lack of sunlight and Vitamin D.

Reptiles often require deworming, and fecal tests should be performed at least annually with a veterinarian. Essential oils have been attempted for deworming, however follow up testing must be performed to ensure elimination. Great care must be taken so that a reptile does not aspirate (or inhale) the deworming solutions into their lungs. Inexperienced handlers have done great harm in forcing liquids into the mouths of these animals. Deworming has not been widely successful with essential oils, and it is our recommendation at this time, that direct oral administration as an attempt at deworming be avoided.

Water misting greens and vegetables for herbivorous reptiles is a great way to allow for ingestion of essential oils.

Reptiles have had applications of the Small Animal or Feline Supportive Blends when necessary. The Avian Drip & Rub recipe can also be considered. 3-6 drops of the solution is generally applied along the spine, or to an area of concern. Occasionally, scale discoloration has been noted. The application can be repeated up to once a day.

FIRST LINE RECOMMENDATIONS:
WATER DIFFUSION: Rotate through a variety of essential oils, or choose those indicated for a specific health concern.
WATER MISTING: Add approximately 4 drops per 4 ounces (120 mL) of distilled water and mist the reptile, caging, or food items as needed.
SOAKING WATER: Reptiles often soak in their own drinking water or are provided with an opportunity to soak in a larger area of water. Adding essential oils to these water sources is an excellent method of application.

Single Oils:
Copaiba, Frankincense, Grapefruit, Helichrysum, Lavender, Lemon, Orange, Tangerine

RODENTS

Rodents can use essential oils in many ways, and are a bit more tolerant of oils than Rabbits or Guinea Pigs. The Small Animal Supportive Blend is most recommended for use as a topical application. Approximately 3 drops of this solution is generally applied and stroked into the spine area as needed, based on response.

Due to the common occurrence of tumors and cancers in rodents, exposure to oils containing antitumoral benefits is highly recommended as a preventive measure. There have been reports in the past of some rodents having difficulty in tolerating diffusion, however doing quite well with licking neat essential oils off of their owner's hands. I do believe sometimes synthetics or over-use of oils may factor into this. With animal appropriate blends and recipes, we do not tend to see aversion issues. Please see the chapter on Diffusion, monitor with any new exposure, and adjust for individual needs and responses.

FIRST LINE RECOMMENDATIONS:
DRINKING WATER: Copaiba, Orange, Tangerine
WATER DIFFUSION: Frankincense, Orange, Tangerine
TOPICAL: Small Animal Supportive Blend

Single Oils:
Copaiba, Frankincense, Grapefruit, Helichrysum, Lavender, Lemon, Orange, Tangerine

SUGAR GLIDERS

Sugar Gliders are quite unique little animals, and can greatly benefit from the use of essential oils. They commonly mark areas with their scent glands, but also from their cloaca, which can promote the occurrence of fecal contamination of food, water, and the general environment. Common issues that respond well to essential oil use include Giardia, bacterial diarrhea, skin infections, and parasites. Salmonella and Leptospirosis are two conditions that can actually be shed from healthy Sugar Gliders and given to humans. Good hygiene is the main tool to prevent zoonosis (the spread of disease from animal to human), so cleaning with natural cleaners with essential oils added, as well as routine water-based diffusion can help to disinfect the environment and reduce risks. Washing your hands with essential oil containing soaps or disinfecting with natural hand purifier after handling your "Suggie" is a wonderful and non-toxic way to reduce contamination and risk of infection. Bites from Sugar Gliders can become quite infected, and so immediate application of an essential oil to any bite wound is recommended. Sugar Gliders eat a variety of foods, and their live prey such as mealworms and crickets can be "gut-loaded" by feeding foods misted with essential oils prior to ingestion. The Small Animal Supportive Blend has been used topically for some Sugar Gliders.

FIRST LINE RECOMMENDATIONS:
WATER DIFFUSION: Three Part Blends
TOPICAL: Small Animal Supportive Blend
INDIRECT DIFFUSION: Wear essential oils yourself while handling and spending time with your Sugar Glider.
CLEANING: Use natural recipes containing essential oils as a cage cleaner as well as to wash bedding, toys, and dishes.

Single Oils:
Copaiba, Frankincense, Grapefruit, Helichrysum, Lavender, Lemon, Orange, Tangerine

TAUNTAUNS

Native to the icy planet of Hoth, these snow lizards are quite hardy. However, a common complaint of their human companions is their odor. Essential oils are perfect for this problem, and indeed impart their health benefits along with their deodorizing potential. Being reptilian, it is quite important that quality standards are strict in regards to essential oil selection. While these oils are being used for odor control, fragrance grade or lesser quality oils would most certainly kill the Tauntaun. Care should be taken to never use oils that are "cooling" in nature. This can result in a drop in body temperature, which can be a significant risk to both Tauntaun and rider. The following recipe is suggested to be made with only pre-screened animalEO Essential Oils, as these specific oils have been additionally screened for use with Tauntauns. The other wonderful "side effect" of this essential oil application, is that it confuses Wampa, making the Tauntaun less trackable as a prey species.

TOPICAL: Due to the oily nature of the Tauntaun, dilution of the essential oils is rarely necessary, as they come equipped with their own natural carrier oil. There is no concern for the Tauntauns delicate and intricate respiratory system, and this recipe has proven safe and effective for hundreds of the species. While attracting mates, this recipe has not interfered with the Tauntauns ability to sense pheromones or other Tauntauns. Combine equal parts Cilantro, Catnip, and Eucalyptus citriodora. It is ideal if this mixture can meld for 3 days prior to application. Larger batches can be prepared in advance, and is recommended. Bottling into 5mL bottles is recommended, as this is generally the amount needed for one average sized Tauntaun. Freely drip the recipe over the entire creature, making sure in this instance, to especially concentrate on the neck area where the rider will be most exposed to odors. The natural fatty oils on the Tauntaun will allow the essential oil to spread all over the body, however they do enjoy it massaged in when possible.

TORTOISES

Tortoises can use essential oils in all of the manners described for Reptiles. Please see their description for more information. Topical Drip & Rub applications are not readily used for this species due to the presence of the shell, however some of the topical recipes can be applied to legs, shell, or skin lesions when needed. Small Animal Supportive Blend, Avian Drip & Rub Recipes, and even the Feline Supportive Blend and other Three Part Blends can be used when indicated.

FIRST LINE RECOMMENDATIONS:
WATER DIFFUSION: Rotate through a variety of essential oils, or choose those indicated for a specific health concern.
WATER MISTING: Add approximately 4 drops per 4 ounces (120 mL) of distilled water and mist the tortoise, caging, or food items as needed.
CLEANING: Natural cleaning recipes with essential oils added is recommended

Single Oils:
Copaiba, Frankincense, Grapefruit, Helichrysum, Lavender, Lemon, Orange, Tangerine

TURTLES

Turtles should use oils in the same manners as those described for Reptiles and Fish. Please see those descriptions for more information. Topical applications of diluted oils are not readily used in this species due to the presence of the shell as well as their tendency to be in water, however the same solutions as described for tortoises, can be applied to legs, shell, or skin lesions if indicated.

FIRST LINE RECOMMENDATIONS:
SOAKING WATER: Add 1 toothpick dip to several drops of essential oil to aquarium water.
WATER DIFFUSION: Three Part Blends
CLEANING: Natural Cleaner Recipes with essential oils added

Single Oils:
Copaiba, Frankincense, Grapefruit, Helichrysum, Lavender, Lemon, Orange, Tangerine

UNICORNS

It is incredibly important to recognize certain conditions exclusive to these creatures. Unicorns have recently been faced with a devastating condition known as doubt mites. A relative of the sarcoptic mite found in humans and domestic animals, the sarcastic mite (Sarcraptes unifiei) infests the horns of unicorns, and indeed can cause their horns to appear invisible, thus compounding the issue. Called doubt mites by common folk, unicorns experience great stress when they experience disbelief in their species. Thus, when stress is present, cortisol levels rise, and the natural immune system suffers. It is well documented in the veterinary community that stress plays a vital role in health, healing, and the immune system. One of the most important factors in healing an infected unicorn, is to first believe. After the belief process has completed, the horn will become more visible to you, and then you must apply the following oils. Please note – do not attempt normal scrapings for this mite. Unicorn horns (even if invisible) are impervious to scalpels or instruments.

PRECISE RECOMMENDATIONS:
Not referred to as First Line Recommendations in this instance, as this is the only recipe that can be used or considered for Unicorn Doubt Mites at this time. The recipe must be followed exactly, with no alterations. Quality is of the utmost importance, therefore only pre-screened animalEO Essential Oils are recommended for use.

TOPICAL: 11 drops of Melissa, 11 drops of Frankincense, and 11 drops of Catnip are combined in a crystal dish. The older this dish is the better. One Herkimer Diamond should be added to the oils. Allow the mixture to sit for exactly 11 minutes. Whenever possible, if treatment can occur on the 11th day of the month, this is ideal. Apply the essential oil blend neat to the horn, using the Herkimer Diamond. This can seem difficult, but in the presence of the unicorn horn, the diamond will transform and become the perfect applicator. Apply the entire amount to the full length of the horn. The horn should become more visible as the application proceeds. One application is usually all that is needed.

ZOO ANIMALS

Depending on the species of Zoo Animal, there are many ways in which to use essential oils. Hopefully, at this point, you have discovered many creative and beneficial ways to incorporate essential oils into the lives of various animals. Zoo animals will greatly benefit from the physical, as well as the emotional, properties of essential oils. Rotational diffusion is likely to be the easiest route of administration. Non-toxic and healthful cleaning with natural cleaning recipes containing essential oils is very important. For animals who may participate in petting zoo situations, be sure to provide natural hand purifier instead of the typical toxic products on the market. Adding essential oils to foods, drinking water, as well as soaking and swimming water is likely to be very easy for these animals. Water misting applications to the animal and to foods is also well accepted. The possibilities are endless, and the most important factor is that these animals obtain exposure to essential oils. If Topical applications are desired, most often starting with the Feline Supportive Blend is suggested.

FIRST LINE RECOMMENDATIONS:
CLEANING: Natural Cleaning Recipes with Essential Oils added
WATER DIFFUSION: Rotate diffusion with any essential oil of choice. Recommendations include Frankincense, Orange, and Three Part Blends
SOAKING WATER: Frankincense, Lavender

Single Oils:
Copaiba, Frankincense, Grapefruit, Helichrysum, Lavender, Lemon, Orange, Tangerine, Valerian, Vetiver, Ylang Ylang

ESSENTIAL OILS: FELINE

Cats present their own unique controversies and requirements to essential oil use. Most cat owners would agree that cats have distinct opinions of the world, and this certainly holds true for aromatherapy. Cats are likely a little proud of the fact that they are indeed, the most contested topic in the world of essential oil use. Human viewpoints of this subject range from the adamant stance that essential oils cannot be used safely for cats, to those who use contraindicated essential oils on a daily basis for their felines.

After hearing all of the cautions and warnings from the veterinary community, I had concerns for my own multi-cat household. Routine blood and urine evaluations calmed the concerns, and no detrimental effects have been shown with over 10 years of almost constant diffusion in my home. What I eventually found to be true, was that the veterinarians who were so carefully warning other veterinarians and owners not to use essential oils, had in fact, never used them themselves. The oils that were linked to killing cats and harming animals were also never graded or evaluated by the veterinarians who condemned them.

My recommendations when I started considering essential oil use for cats was to choose oils that were already being used often, have been used with many cats, and to use them with techniques that cats enjoy. Tea Tree Oil, or Melaleuca alternifolia, is another feline controversy which fascinates me. I have directly communicated with people who have sadly exposed their cat to a poor grade Melaleuca oil topically, resulting in subsequent seizures and death. Conversely, I have also witnessed firsthand a cat receiving 4 drops of Melaleuca oil orally twice a day, followed it clinically with blood work, and it showed no ill events. I do not use this example as a recommendation for everyone to use Melaleuca for their cats, as there are many essential oils that can be used in place of this particular oil. It is the best choice to first select an oil which is known to be very safe and well tolerated in cats. However, it remains a fascinating conundrum as to what makes the essential oil safe to use, and what doses and routes are important as we consider toxicity.

Traditional chemical flea and tick preparations are very similar to essential oils in regards to quality, effectiveness, and risk. In the veterinary community, we have seen horrific side effects to the use of over-the-counter, lower cost flea and tick products. The use of better quality products, typically results in a reduction of significantly harmful reactions. Although not completely benign, this is a very different scenario from the reactions of seizuring and drooling cats, neurologic symptoms, dying kittens, or pets who are frantically trying to rub the product off of themselves. Even the most traditional vets can usually relate to this parallel concerning quality variations. Essential oils can vary in quality, much like other veterinary products, and poor quality can equal toxicity.

One factor that is true for cats, is that they are notoriously deficient in the Cytochrome p450 liver metabolism pathway. This particular pathway is utilized for the metabolism and excretion of all sorts of chemicals from their body, including traditional medications. A cat's liver just does not metabolize items in the same manner or efficiency as a large dog or a human. This fact has made cats unique in veterinary medicine, no matter what the substance may be that we are exposing them to. For example, certain traditional Non-Steroidal Anti-Inflammatory (NSAID) drugs can be used in dogs, but if given to a cat, has a high likelihood of causing significant damage to organs and even death.

Medically, I have found that we can actually use many of the contraindicated essential oils in cats. If there are other oil choices for treatment that carry similar benefits and activities, which are more appropriate for cats, then those should be a first choice. However, when needed and indicated, the use of more aggressive essential oils is completely possible for cats. Please see the chapters on Metabolism Theory and Just the Science for more information on cats.

Presented in this chapter, are the application methods most commonly used with many thousands of cats worldwide. There are many ways to administer oils to cats, but these remain the most cat friendly. It is important to remember that animals are still individuals, and there could be a specific cat that will not respond well to one application method, or may prove more sensitive to use than another feline. Common sense and a tailored approach to each individual is important. Consulting with a veterinarian, and having blood and urine evaluations prior to starting the use of essential oils is a good policy.

Litter Box Recipes:

I developed this technique after observing my outdoor cats using pine needles as their "litter box." I began to realize all of the wonderful ways that animals would naturally expose themselves to essential oils in the "wild," and use of essential oils in the litter box was born. Litter box recipes are perhaps one of the easiest methods in which to expose cats to the health benefits of essential oils. It not only replaces the toxic fragrances found in commercial kitty litter, but offers a way to provide preventive and continued health benefits from essential oils on a regular basis.

Start with unscented kitty litter - staying within the same brand that you currently use is often advisable. Add 1-3 drops of your chosen essential oil or essential oil blend to 1 cup of baking soda - store this mixture within a glass jar, and allow it to "marinade" and blend overnight, shaking the mixture several times. Later, you may find you can add more essential oil drops to this recipe. Starting with a small portion (1-2 Tablespoons depending on your box size and amount of litter) - sprinkle the baking soda mixture onto your kitty litter. You can mix it up a bit, but not so much that all of the baking soda sifts to the bottom of the box. Provide a separate litter box that does not contain essential oils, to make sure that your cat does not have an aversion to the essential oil that was selected. Once you are sure your cat is using the litter box with your oil selection and concentration, you can then omit the use of the "plain" litter box.

An interesting fact relating to the world of Zoopharmacognosy, is that when we allow cats to select to use different litter boxes, with different essential oils added to them, we will often see them select the box in which they are most in need of support. So if we create a box designed for relief of upset stomach – we might see an IBD cat use that box preferentially. However, if we create a litter box recipe for support of the thyroid, a cat with thyroid imbalance may select that box. It has been an interesting journey to witness, and with the ease in which this method exposes cats to regular benefits, this method should be offered to every cat. Still, if you find a cat who always selects use of the "plain" unscented box – then honor that decision. We do not wish to ever create an aversion to use of the litter box.

Selecting and rotating various oils can bring big benefits to your cat. For the most part, Three Part Blends can be created and used to bring even more synergy to the table. But single oils and even more extensive blends can also be considered. Copaiba can aid with arthritis pains and gastrointestinal issues, Ginger and Peppermint are commonly used for nausea, poor eating, and GI concerns, and Frankincense may bring anticancer benefits. The addition of Catnip essential oil to any litter box recipe can bring additional attraction to the litter box for cats as well, and may be incredibly helpful in training kittens or encouraging use of the litter box in situations of inappropriate elimination. Be careful not to use too much Catnip within a blend, it is a strong oil, and just a little is more than enough. If too much is used, we have seen cats who prefer to lay in their litter box, or roll around to enjoy the scent. The choices are endless, and can provide powerful preventive measures to your feline friends.

Examples of Litter Box Recipes: Most recipes can be used in equal parts, however with some oils that are stronger in nature, you may wish to reduce the total contribution to the blend. For example Peppermint or Melissa oil, or those with very strong scents, could be added at 10% of the total blend, instead of 33%. The addition of a small fraction of Catnip can be considered for addition to any of the recipes as well. Once you have made your base blend, you can add it to your baking soda as described previously.

For Gastrointestinal Support:
Copaiba, Ginger, Peppermint (often smaller amounts needed)

For Thyroid Support:
Copaiba, Myrrh, Ledum

For Cardiac Support:
May Chang, Copaiba, Helichrysum

For Sugar Handling Support:
Black Cumin Oil, Myrtle, Anise

For Liver Support:
Ledum, Copaiba, Helichrysum

For Virus Support:
Melissa (often smaller amounts needed), Copaiba, Geranium

For Renal/Kidney/Urologic Support:
Juniper, Copaiba, German Chamomile

Water-Based Diffusion:

Diffusion is usually a method that is well tolerated by all cats, especially from water-based "ultrasonic" diffuser models. Many misconceptions have been placed on what cats "like" or "don't like" - and it appears that these generalizations may have been made based on individual reports, and not from cats as a whole. The dislike of citrus oils or certain blends may hold true for one cat, but then another cat is found to be attracted the diffusion. Allowing a cat to show you their individual preference is a good idea. If a cat can leave the room when you diffuse a certain essential oil, you will quickly find out if they tend to leave the room every time that particular oil is diffused, or if they tend to enter a room to be closer to the diffuser. Some cats even lay right next to the diffuser or sniff the vapors directly. Tenting and caging is commonly used for cats with respiratory concerns when a more intense therapy is desired. See the chapter on Diffusion for more information, as well as the chapters on Metabolism and the science of cats for additional information.

Petting the Cat:

This method is generally well tolerated by cats, and for some may be preferred over dripping diluted oils directly onto the cat. Due to the fact that hair follicles may enhance absorption, spreading the essential oils over a larger area of the cat, proves quite effective. This method involves placing the oil to be applied into your hand. Circling your hands together, the essential oils are allowed to absorb to varying degrees into your skin. Once you have the amount of oil on your hands that you desire - which can vary from completely absorbed, to a thin coating - you simply "pet your cat". Even with oils completely absorbed into your hand - if you smell your cat after "petting" - you will find that they smell like essential oils. Adding the fact that cats groom themselves, oral absorption ingestion of the essential oil is likely to occur. Grooming actions after Petting applications are a wonderful way to obtain buccal and oral exposure to essential oils for antibacterial actions, anti-inflammatory actions, anticancer actions and more. See the chapter on Topical Applications for more information.

Oral Administration:

Although not as commonly used for cats, occasionally oils are given directly in the mouth or via capsule. When capsule administration is given, small gelatin capsules can be found for purchase on the internet through various suppliers. There are various sizes of capsules that can be purchased, and size "3" or "4" are often appropriate for use in cats (the higher the number, the smaller the capsule). When oils are dripped directly into the mouth of a cat, or they are unfortunate enough to bite into a capsule, the cat will often salivate profusely. Some cats shake their heads and paw at their mouths as well. This is usually a short-lived event, but some cats salivate for 15 minutes or more. In general, the oral route is used only after other methods have not yielded enough results, or in critical situations (such as severe pain, hemorrhage, or while under anesthesia.) Most commonly when ingestion of oils is desired, cats should be exposed to oils through topical applications and the resulting grooming process. For many cats, this amount of ingestion is adequate to create a therapeutic response.

FELINE SUPPORTIVE BLEND

This blend has evolved over the last 10 years to become the mainstay of cat essential oil therapies worldwide. Originally, a similar recipe was created by Leigh Foster, and had been used on many of her own rescue cats prior to finding its way into my veterinary practice. Although this recipe includes oils that are typically contraindicated for use with cats by various, often uneducated sources, veterinarians and cat owners alike have witnessed amazing health benefits with use of this recipe. Because of its consideration specifically for cats, it has been remarkable to watch cats actually enjoy and ask for the application. While there are still cats who distinctly express their disgust with any oil application, I often find the vast majority to enjoy the application and massage process. I have personally documented the safe and even long term use of the Feline Supportive Blend and its modified recipes, in thousands of cats including blood work and veterinary monitoring. Even twice daily use, for over 3 years, yielded no negative response. Used properly, this blend can be a huge help to many cats.

Feline Supportive Blend Solution:
To create a base blend – combine equal parts of Oregano, Thyme, Basil Cypress, Marjoram, Lavender, Copaiba, Helichrysum, and Peppermint to a bottle. This blend can then be used to create a variety of concentrations for individual use. In general, I recommend a final concentration of 3-5% for most cats. If additional oils are chosen to be used within the blend, add them to the base blend first, then dilute to the desired concentration. See the chapter on Dilution Rates for more instructions on how to create a proper concentration of essential oil blends.

Alternately, you may add 4 drops each of Oregano, Thyme, Basil, Cypress, Marjoram, Lavender, Copaiba, Helichrysum, and Peppermint - to a 30mL (1 ounce) glass essential oil bottle. Add Fractionated Coconut Oil to fill the remainder of the bottle. Mix by rocking the bottle, and ideally, allow the blend to meld for 1-3 days or more. You will find with experience, blends that are allowed to "marry" for a while, often have a wonderful quality to them. However, when necessary, freshly made blends can be used.

Apply approximately 5-8 drops of the prepared solution up the spine of the cat, from tail to head. Next, gently stroke, pet, or massage the essential oil solution up the back of the cat. Amazingly enough, cats often enjoy the recommended backwards stroke, and there is some evidence to suggest that it plays a part in reprogramming the body to detect different nerve information. For example, a cat with hyperesthesia, may have additional pain reduction or "confusion" to the nerves through encountering a different sensation that the body is not used to receiving. However, if you encounter a cat that does not enjoy a backwards stroke, just pet them normally. Some cats may not be able to be touched at all, as in the case with feral cats. In these situations, I allow the solution to just drip onto their back while they are distracted, and allow the drops to "fall where they may". I basically ignore the cat completely, and it will soak in on its own or be groomed off. The solution can also be applied or "pet" onto bedding, cat trees, or even other cats to gain exposure to especially difficult cats.

When indicated, repeat applications can be made as needed. We have had many sickly and fading kittens who would only eat after a Feline Supportive application was given. For some of these tiny kittens, we would even apply oils four times a day. There has been only help in using the oils to the proper interval that the cat shows is necessary. While I am a firm believer in using the "lowest effective dose" – I also find that most people do not use oils often enough. You should strive to apply one application, then monitor the animal closely to see if you notice beneficial signs, and for how long they last. Timing your next application to when the effects wear off is ideal. During an acute episode, I may find that I have to apply more often initially, but then with time may be able to decrease the frequency of applications.

Balancing, grounding, or calming the cat with a calming blend is optional, and not as widely used anymore. For energy work, this may still be desired. See the chapter on Drip & Rub Techniques for more information. Energy work, massage, or reflexology is always welcome to be incorporated into any essential oil application.

Modification of the Feline Supportive Blend:

Additional oils may be desired for use based on their individual properties, and may be suggested for addition into the Feline Supportive Blend. In general, you should add additional essential oils into the base blend, prior to diluting it to its final concentration. This eliminates any errors in calculation, which may occur through the addition of drops to an already diluted application solution. You may need to consider the individual properties, qualities, and strength of the essential oil you wish to add, as some may be so intense, it would make sense to add it in less than equal parts to the blend. Oils such as Melissa, are quite strong, and within the single oil descriptions for them, it will indicate if less oil is generally used for addition to the Feline Supportive Blend. If an oil makes a recommendation to add directly to the fully created Feline Supportive Blend, then you are fine to follow those directions. However, if in your reading you feel you would really love to add a specific oil for an individual, add it to your base blend first.

In general, I would suggest not adding more than 3 additional oils to your base blend until you have extensive experience in blending or aromatic therapies.

Frequency of Application:

The chapter How Much, How Often should be referred to for more information. With almost every situation in which the Feline Supportive Blend is suggested, no matter what species of animal, I will always recommend the same procedure for the initial use of this technique. First, give the animal one application as typically directed of the Feline Supportive Blend. So for a cat, 5-8 drops may be applied. You can apply less if you feel your cat may be excessively sensitive, or if you are just cautious by nature. Then, you will monitor the cat or animal for signs of improvement or response. If there is no response, then we can administer the application again either more frequently, or with more drops applied. If there was a noticeable response, the length of that response is evaluated, then the application frequency can be repeated at the length of that time interval.

For example, a cat with arthritis is given an application of the Feline Supportive Blend. The cat enjoyed it, and the owner reported that she felt more comfortable for about 4 days after the application. Even though this cat "could" get an application daily, giving the application every 3-4 days is a great next step; spacing the timing of the repeat application to the ideal needs of the individual cat.

FELINE CONDITIONS

ABSCESS
(See also PAIN MANAGEMENT)

An abscess is a pus filled pocket of infection, most commonly created from a bite wound from another cat. Cat bites are the most serious in their transmission of bacteria, and cause of serious infections. Cat bites to humans have resulted in infections severe enough to require surgical debridement of the wound. Symptoms of swelling, heat at location, drainage of pus, fever, lethargy, as well as others can develop within hours of the injury and resultant infection. When animals feel poorly, this can be an emergency situation, and often traditional antibiotics are encouraged.

FIRST LINE RECOMMENDATIONS:
Seek Veterinary care when an animal feels poorly or when infection is severe. See also PAIN MANAGEMENT for suggestions regarding discomfort.

TOPICAL: Apply Feline Supportive Blend to the abscess head, up to twice a day. Hot pack the abscess with a very warm, damp wash cloth to help bring the abscess to a "head" or to drain. Once the "head" has opened and drainage is occurring, the wound can be flushed with solutions containing essential oils as well.

FELINE SUPPORTIVE BLEND: Apply as usual to cat, generally up to once per day. This solution can also be applied to the abscess directly.

Single Oils:
Copaiba, Laurus nobilis, Lavender, Lemon, Lemongrass, Melaleuca alternifolia, Oregano, Spikenard, Thyme

ACNE - FELINE
(See also CANINE CONDITIONS - SKIN INFECTIONS)

Feline Acne is often seen as small blackheads on the chin. Commonly, this condition is due to food residues, plastic dishes, food allergies, and exposure to household toxins. Changing the diet, using glass, stainless steel, or ceramic food and water dishes, washing dishes daily, and washing the chin area is helpful.

FIRST LINE RECOMMENDATIONS:
TOPICAL: Wipe chin gently with a very dilute water solution of selected essential oils. A water-mist can be created to spray onto cotton pads for wiping.
FELINE SUPPORTIVE BLEND: Apply as usual to cat. After rubbing into the back, residue on the hands can be used to pet the cats face (most cats enjoy this) and coat the chin slightly. Be careful to not use too much carrier oil on the chin with this condition.

Single Oils:
Copaiba, Frankincense, Helichrysum, Lavender, Myrrh

ALLERGIES

Allergies have many different causes, and secondary skin infections can continue the occurrence of symptoms, even after the allergen has been removed. Careful veterinary exams, and accurate diagnosis must be made to effectively treat the allergy complex of symptoms. Diet is often the culprit in cats, and a grain, egg, soy, wheat, corn, and dairy free diet is recommended. Many holistic grain free diets still contain egg products, and we find this to be a common offender in our veterinary practice.

FIRST LINE RECOMMENDATIONS:
FELINE SUPPORTIVE BLEND: Apply as usual to cat, up to once a day or as needed for the individual. Addition of Melissa oil is especially recommended.
WATER DIFFUSION: Three Part Blends, especially containing Clove
LITTER BOX RECIPES: Black Spruce, Copaiba, Melissa

Single Oils:
Basil, Black Spruce, Cinnamon, Clove, Copaiba, Frankincense, Geranium, Helichrysum, Lavender, Ledum, Melissa, Oregano, Thyme

AORTIC THROMBOEMBOLISM
(See SADDLE THROMBUS)

ANEMIA

Anemia is usually defined as the low count of red blood cells. There are many causes of anemia including iron and nutritional deficiency, renal failure, Feline Leukemia Virus, autoimmune destruction of red blood cells, decreased production of red blood cells by the bone marrow, as well as blood loss due to hemorrhage and bleeding, parasitic infections, intestinal parasites, flea infestation, and more. Anemic cats generally have pale gums or foot pads, are lethargic, and may show signs of dyspnea – or respiratory stress. As an interesting note in the veterinary community, it is recognized that cats with certain types of Pica (eating abnormal things) are often found to have anemia. The ingestion of kitty litter seems to be commonly related to anemia.

FIRST LINE RECOMMENDATIONS:
Ensure accurate diagnosis and work up with your veterinarian. If a diagnosis can be reached, include regimens for those issues (for example: renal disease, intestinal parasites, autoimmune disorders…)

FELINE SUPPORTIVE BLEND: Apply as usual to cat, often up to once a day. Consider addition of Cistus, Frankincense.
WATER DIFFUSION: Three Part Blends
LITTER BOX RECIPES: Cistus, Black Spruce, Frankincense

Single Oils:
Black Spruce, Frankincense, Cistus, Copaiba, Helichrysum, Juniper, Ledum, Orange, Oregano, Thyme

ANOREXIA

Anorexia is a term used to describe poor or no eating by an animal. Many times it is accompanied by feelings of nausea or discomfort. There are many reasons for an animal to be anorexic, and an accurate veterinary diagnosis is important. These recommendations generally stimulate appetite and ease digestive concerns and nausea.

FIRST LINE RECOMMENDATIONS:
WATER DIFFUSION: Three Part Blends of digestive oils
FELINE SUPPORTIVE BLEND: Apply as needed, consider adding Ginger.

Single Oils:
Copaiba, Ginger, Laurus nobilis, Lavender, Ledum, Lemon, Patchouli, Peppermint, Tarragon

ARTHRITIS
(See also CANINE CONDITIONS - ARTHRITIS)

FIRST LINE RECOMMENDATIONS:
FELINE SUPPORTIVE BLEND: Apply as needed. Consider addition of Frankincense.
TOPICAL: Diluted applications of Three Part Blends.
LITTER BOX RECIPES: Copaiba, Frankincense, Myrrh

ASTHMA

FIRST LINE RECOMMENDATIONS:
WATER DIFFUSION: Three Part Blends up to 24 hours a day in the home. Tenting or caging can be used when needed.
LITTER BOX RECIPES: Copaiba, Melissa, Frankincense
FELINE SUPPORTIVE BLEND: Apply as needed, often up to once a day. Consider addition of Frankincense and Melissa.

Single Oils:
Basil, Black Spruce, Cinnamon, Clove, Copaiba, Cypress, Eucalyptus globulus, Eucalyptus radiata, Frankincense, Laurus nobilis, Lavender, Lemon, Marjoram, Melissa, Myrtle, Oregano, Thyme, Peppermint

AUTOIMMUNE DISORDERS

FIRST LINE RECOMMENDATIONS:
FELINE SUPPORTIVE BLEND: Apply as needed, often up to once a day. Consider addition of Frankincense, Melissa.
LITTER BOX RECIPES: Copaiba, Black Spruce, Frankincense
WATER DIFFUSION: Three Part Blends up to 24 hours a day. Rotation through several blends suggested.

Single Oils:
Balsam Fir, Black Spruce, Copaiba, Frankincense, Helichrysum, Laurus nobilis, Melissa, Oregano, Thyme

BEHAVIORAL CONDITIONS

FIRST LINE RECOMMENDATIONS:
WATER DIFFUSION: Rotational diffusion of emotionally based Three Part Blends.
FELINE SUPPORTIVE BLEND: Apply as needed, consider additions of Frankincense, Melissa, German Chamomile.
LITTER BOX RECIPES: Valerian, Lavender, Clary Sage

Single Oils:
Bergamot, Black Spruce, Catnip, Chamomile (German), Chamomile (Roman), Clary Sage, Frankincense, Geranium, Grapefruit, Lavender, Lemon, Marjoram, Melissa, Orange, Rose, Spikenard, Tangerine, Valerian, Vetiver, Ylang Ylang

BLADDER INFECTIONS
(See URINARY CONDITIONS)

BLOCKED - URINARY
(See also PAIN MANAGEMENT, URINARY CONDITIONS)

Male cats can commonly suffer from a blocked urethra, which is an emergency situation. The inability to urinate creates a very toxic and dangerous situation, and death can occur. Immediate veterinary attention is required if you suspect your cat has a urinary blockage. These recommendations are to be used to complement veterinary care.

FIRST LINE RECOMMENDATIONS:
FELINE SUPPORTIVE BLEND: Apply as needed, consider additions of Vetiver, Juniper.
DIFFUSION: By any method, sometimes even just letting the cat sniff the bottle. Rose and Frankincense has been used in critical situations to raise the life force, and have been incredibly effective.
LITTER BOX RECIPES: Copaiba, Lavender, German Chamomile.

Single Oils:
Black Spruce, Copaiba, Chamomile (German), Juniper, Laurus nobilis, Lavender, Lemon, Lemongrass, Marjoram, Myrrh, Tangerine, Tarragon, Vetiver, Ylang Ylang

BLOOD CLOT
(See SADDLE THROMBUS)

CANCER

There are many different kinds of cancer, and each type may have a different specific focus for essential oil recommendations. However there is a basic foundation of items that must be met in order for an immune system to function to the fullest, and to give an animal the utmost possibility of clearing cancer. These recommendations apply to all animals, not just cats. However, listed below are cat friendly methods for using essential oils and supplements with cancer.

It is very important in conditions such as cancer, to incorporate as many layers of care as possible. This is one situation, where starting with small amounts of items, but building up to using many and in relatively high amounts (sometimes quickly) is fully warranted.

FIRST LINE RECOMMENDATIONS:
DIET: Every cat with cancer should have their diet fully evaluated and likely changed. Unprocessed and raw whole foods are recommended, but products and recipes available are not always properly balanced or desired by many cats. Work with a holistic veterinarian or nutritionist to determine the best diet option for your cat.

KETOGENIC DIET: While more and more is being discovered about the ketogenic diet and dog cancer, less is known for cats at this time. However, please do your research fully, as more and more information is learned daily. See the resource section for more information.

DRINKING WATER: Tap and city water should be avoided at all costs. Spring water is the best recommendation, and even high quality bottled water should be used if needed.

ELIMINATE HOUSEHOLD TOXINS: The use of natural cleaners and household products should be a standard recommendation. Scented kitty litter, air fresheners, fabric softeners, household cleaners, human perfumes, lotions, hairsprays, etc… <u>must</u> be eliminated from the home. Microwave ovens should also be completely removed from the household. Electromagnetic fields (cell phones, computers, Wi-Fi) should be evaluated and be lessened or eliminated. This is especially important for the cat that enjoys lying on top of a warm computer!

OMEGA FISH OILS: A good quality fish oil is strongly recommended. Standard Process Tuna Omega-3 Oil, Standard Process Calamari Oil, Nordic Naturals, Mercola Healthy Pets, and several other reputable veterinary brands can be selected from. Capsules can be "popped" and 1-2 drops placed into foods.

DIGESTIVE ENZYMES: Digestive enzymes are incredibly important for health, but especially in cases of cancer. Work with your holistic veterinarian on sources and suggestions. Mercola Healthy Pets has an excellent digestive enzyme. Start with a small amount, mixed into moist food, generally with each meal. I typically use caution towards products that combine probiotics with digestive enzymes. This has become a popular trend, however to me it seems logical that the enzyme could digest and destroy the items combined with it, rendering it less beneficial. I would prefer to supply these items separately.

WHOLE FOOD SUPPLEMENTS: One important recommendation that must be made in cases of cancer, is to also include raw whole food supplements that contain non-vegetarian products and glandulars. Since cats are obligate carnivores, I recommend the use of Standard Process Supplements for all cases. Recommended Standard Process formulas for cats with cancer include: Feline Whole Body Support and Feline Immune System Support. Adding in other specific formulas is advised if other body systems are showing stress or need support (liver, renal, enteric, etc...).

WATER DIFFUSION: Rotational diffusion of emotional oils is recommended. See also the chapter on Emotional Work with Oils for more information. Diffuse any anti-cancer oils up to 24 hours a day. Rotation through a variety of oils is recommended.

FELINE SUPPORTIVE BLEND: Apply up to twice a day, consider additions of Frankincense, Tangerine, and Melissa. Small amounts of the Feline Supportive Blend may be applied directly to some types of tumors.

LITTER BOX RECIPES: Frankincense, Copaiba, Melissa

INGESTION: For most cats, ingestion of essential oils will occur through normal grooming. For some cats who may feel too ill to groom, or have oral tumors limiting grooming ability, topical applications and water-based diffusion of oils will often start to deliver desirable results. Cats will rarely tolerate oral administration of oils for long periods of time, if capsule administrations are attempted. As the resolution of cancer can be a longer term adventure, direct oral administration is often not used. Many cats reject the flavor of essential oils in food or water, however if you are lucky enough to have a cat that will ingest oils in these ways – these routes can be considered in cases of dire need.

DRINKING WATER: Essential oils can be considered for addition to drinking water, and may especially be helpful to coat the mouth. Dilute the essential oil or blend in Fractionated Coconut Oil to at least 50% before addition to water. Many cats enjoy coconut oil, and so they will often lick a film off the top surface of water readily. Frankincense is often considered, and 1-2 drops of the diluted oil can be added to 1 liter of spring water.

FOODS: In soft moist favorite foods, dip a toothpick into the essential oil (Frankincense) and mix into the food. Gradually increase the amounts mixed in as tolerated. Raw Coconut Oil is often a favorite for cats to eat, as is Sardines. Essential oils can be diluted within these fatty items, to help gain contact with oral tumors especially.

Single Oils:
Balsam Fir, Black Spruce, Copaiba, Frankincense, Grapefruit, Helichrysum, Lemon, Melissa, Myrrh, Oregano, Orange, Sandalwood, Tangerine, Thyme

CARDIOMYOPATHY, HYPERTROPHIC
(See HEART DISEASE)

CAVITY
(See FELINE ODONTOCLASTIC RESORPTIVE LESION)

CERVICAL LINE LESIONS, CERVICAL NECK LESIONS
(See FELINE ODONTOCLASTIC RESORPTIVE LESIONS)

CONJUNCTIVITIS
(See also UPPER RESPIRATORY INFECTIONS)

FIRST LINE RECOMMENDATIONS:
WATER DIFFUSION: Three Part Blends up to 24 hours a day, including tenting or caging.
WATER MISTING: If tolerated (most cats do not appreciate this) – mist the eye area with 4 drops of Lavender, in 4 ounces (120 mL) of distilled water.
LITTER BOX RECIPES: Copaiba, Melissa, Lavender
FELINE SUPPORTIVE BLEND: up to once a day.

Single Oils:
Basil, Black Spruce, Copaiba, Frankincense, Lavender, Melissa, Oregano, Thyme

CRYSTALS - URINARY
(See URINARY CONDITIONS)

CYSTITIS
(See also FLUTD, URINARY CONDITIONS)

DECLAW SURGERY
(See also PAIN MANAGEMENT)

It is unfortunate that many animal caretakers are not informed of the fact that this procedure is unnecessary and traumatic. There is much information to be found on how to keep cats comfortably in homes without declawing, and I encourage you to seek reputable advice from holistic veterinarians or cat organizations.

Cats who have been declawed, not only have healing to deal with, but emotional and physical traumas as well. Both aspects are important to address. See the chapter on Emotional Work with Oils for more information.

FIRST LINE RECOMMENDATIONS:
WATER DIFFUSION: Rotational diffusion of Three Part Blends for emotional clearing and calming.
LITTER BOX RECIPES: Copaiba, Helichrysum, Myrrh
FELINE SUPPORTIVE BLEND: Apply as needed, consider addition of Frankincense and Myrrh. Ledum can be added especially to support anesthesia clearance and recovery. After application, residue on the hands can be massaged down the leg area for added comfort. Ingestion of this blend from normal grooming practices, is often adequate for pain support.

SECOND LINE RECOMMENDATIONS:
PETTING: For discomfort and healing: Place 1 drop each of Helichrysum, Myrrh, and Copaiba into 1 teaspoon of fractionated coconut oil. Mix together, then place 10 drops of this solution into your hand, rub together, and pet onto the leg and foot area. Ideally this is done as close as possible to the completion of surgery.
WATER MISTING: Alternately, Helichrysum, Myrrh, and Copaiba can be added to a water-mist for spritzing onto the foot area if tolerated.

Helichrysum is an important oil for the prevention and treatment of phantom pain syndrome. Oral Helichrysum has been used to help manage pain and can be used with or without other traditional medications.

Single Oils:
Black Spruce, Copaiba, Frankincense, Helichrysum, Lavender, Marjoram, Myrrh

DENTAL DISEASE
(See also FELINE ODONTOCLASTIC RESORPTIVE LESIONS)

FIRST LINE RECOMMENDATIONS:
FELINE SUPPORTIVE BLEND: Apply as needed, with the distinct goal of grooming to inoculate the oral cavity with beneficial oils. Consider addition of Catnip, Frankincense, Myrrh.
LITTER BOX RECIPES: Copaiba, Myrrh, Catnip.
DRINKING WATER: Copaiba or Three Part Blends of selected oils can be diluted in Fractionated Coconut Oil to at least 50:50, and added to drinking water. Some cats will lap up the water, coating the oral cavity with beneficial oils. Read the chapter on adding essential oils to drinking water for further directions.
ORAL: Addition of Copaiba or the Feline Supportive Blend to natural or DIY toothpaste recipes is wonderful for cats who allow brushing or oral applications.
TOPICAL: Raw Organic Coconut Oil can be rubbed and massaged onto the gum areas. After the cat tolerates this well, tiny amounts of essential oil can be added to the Coconut Oil and gradually increased in concentration. Copaiba is a wonderful selection. The grooming of Feline Supportive Blend remains the best way to gain oral exposure to many essential oil benefits.
PETTING: Through grooming cats will ingest various oils off of their fur. This is a great way to get oils into the mouth, however some cats with dental disease do not groom due to pain. Myrrh is suggested.

Single Oils:
Catnip, Copaiba, Frankincense, Laurus nobilis, Lavender, Melaleuca alternifolia, Myrrh, Oregano, Thyme

DEWORMING

While I would love to tell you that we have made great advances in natural methods for deworming, the true answer is that we have not. Natural remedies remain inconsistent at best, and while we can often support the symptoms of parasitic infections, true deworming actions are hard to come by.

FIRST LINE RECOMMENDATIONS:
FELINE SUPPORTIVE BLEND: Apply as needed, consider addition of Ginger, Copaiba, Tarragon
LITTER BOX RECIPES: Copaiba, Ginger, Tarragon

Single Oils:
Eucalyptus globulus, Hyssop, Lemon, Lemongrass, Melaleuca alternifolia, Oregano, Peppermint, Tarragon

DIABETES

Diabetes can be difficult to gain control over, and working with a qualified holistic veterinarian is very important to fully address the entire foundation of the cat's health. Dietary changes alone have eliminated Diabetes for some cats, and is incredibly important. See the recommendations within the chapter on Drug Interactions for more information regarding the introduction of essential oils for diabetics. Veterinary cooperation is imperative for animals who are on Insulin.

FIRST LINE RECOMMENDATIONS:
LITTER BOX RECIPES: Copaiba, Geranium, Black Cumin
FELINE SUPPORTIVE BLEND: Apply as needed, consider addition of Black Cumin, Lemongrass.

Single Oils:
Black Cumin, Chamomile (German), Geranium, Lemongrass, Myrrh, Myrtle, Spearmint, Ylang Ylang

DIARRHEA
(See also TRITRICHOMONAS FOETUS)

FIRST LINE RECOMMENDATIONS:
FELINE SUPPORTIVE BLEND: Apply as needed, consider addition of Ginger.
LITTER BOX RECIPES: Copaiba, Ginger, Peppermint
WATER DIFFUSION: Three Part Blends, especially with Ginger, Anise, Peppermint

Single Oils:
Anise, Black Spruce, Copaiba, Ginger, Fennel, Lemon, Marjoram, Melaleuca alternifolia, Melissa, Peppermint, Tarragon, Ylang Ylang

DISTEMPER - FELINE
(See VIRAL CONDITIONS)

EAR MITES

It is important to recognize that ear mites do not live in the ear alone. They are indeed, all over a cat's body, so treatment of the entire cat is often necessary for clearance. We have performed clinical studies with blends containing Catnip essential oils, and found it quite effective.

FIRST LINE RECOMMENDATIONS:
FELINE SUPPORTIVE BLEND: Add Catnip essential oil to the Feline Supportive Blend. Apply to cat as a whole, at least every three days. This blend can also be swabbed or coated into the ear up to twice a day or as indicated.
TOPICAL: Create a Three Part Blend diluted to 5-10% concentration rates. Swab or coat inside the ear up to twice a day.
LITTER BOX RECIPES: Catnip, Copaiba, Melissa

Single Oils:
Catnip, Citronella, Eucalyptus citriodora, Eucalyptus polybractea, Lavender, Melaleuca alternifolia, Palmarosa, Peppermint

FADING KITTEN SYNDROME

Fading kittens are often cold and/or hypoglycemic. Warming of the kitten is the primary activity that must occur. No oral supplement should be given to a kitten who is too cold to properly digest and absorb the nutrient. Hydration, warmth, nutrition, and proper veterinary care are key factors in saving kittens from this condition. The use of life force oils is incredibly beneficial.

FIRST LINE RECOMMENDATIONS:
WATER DIFFUSION: Have the kitten inhale Rose and Frankincense to raise life force energy. Water-based diffusion of Three Part Blends.
FELINE SUPPORTIVE BLEND: Apply as needed to stimulate eating. Even the youngest of cats have received this blend 4 or 5 times a day when it showed that they ate right after application. Consider addition of Frankincense, Ginger, and Melissa.
LITTER BOX RECIPES: Once awake and using the box, add a layer of oil exposure through litter box recipes. Frankincense, Melissa, Ginger.

Single Oils:
Black Spruce, Copaiba, Frankincense, Ginger, Helichrysum, Melissa, Orange, Oregano, Peppermint, Rose, Thyme

FATTY LIVER DISEASE
(See also LIVER DISEASE)

Fatty Liver Disease is specific to the mobilization of fat into the Liver of sick cats. This is most common in cats who are overweight (even slightly), and who stop eating for one reason or another. Veterinary care and diagnostics are very important. Addressing any other underlying cause (such as Kidney Disease) is important.

FIRST LINE RECOMMENDATIONS:
FELINE SUPPORTIVE BLEND: Apply as needed, consider additions of Ledum, German Chamomile, Ginger.
WATER DIFFUSION: German Chamomile, Geranium, Helichrysum
LITTER BOX RECIPES: Ledum, Copaiba, Helichrysum
ORAL: Helichrysum when indicated, and for severe Liver Failure.

Single Oils:
Anise, Chamomile (German), Copaiba, Fennel, Geranium, Ginger, Grapefruit, Helichrysum, Juniper, Ledum, Lemon, Melissa, Myrrh, Myrtle, Nutmeg, Rosemary, Spearmint, Tangerine

FELINE LEUKEMIA
(See VIRAL CONDITIONS)

FELV
(See VIRAL CONDITIONS)

FELINE IMMUNODEFICIENCY VIRUS
(See VIRAL CONDITIONS)

FELINE INFECTIOUS PERITONITIS
(See also VIRAL CONDITIONS)

Feline Infectious Peritonitis (FIP) is a very severe condition which is caused by the mutation of the Corona Virus in cats. Prevention and good health is the best stance for this disease, as once symptoms have fully developed, reversal is very difficult. This is one disease in which extremely aggressive protocols are often attempted, and the prognosis is generally poor. Regular use of the Feline Supportive Blend, nutritional supplements, water-based diffusion, and litter box recipes to support general health and immune function is recommended for every feline.

FIRST LINE RECOMMENDATIONS:
FELINE SUPPORTIVE BLEND: Apply as needed, consider adding Melissa, Hyssop, Sandalwood, and Frankincense. Even up to twice a day or more, in symptomatic cats.
LITTER BOX RECIPES: Copaiba, Melissa, Frankincense
WATER DIFFUSION: Rotate with Three Part Blends

Single Oils:
Copaiba, Eucalyptus globulus, Eucalyptus radiata, Frankincense, Helichrysum, Hyssop, Laurus nobilis, Melissa, Sandalwood, Thyme

FELINE LOWER URINARY TRACT DISEASE
(See FLUTD – FELINE LOWER URINARY TRACT DISEASE)

FELINE ODONTOCLASTIC RESORPTIVE LESION
(See also DENTAL DISEASE, PAIN MANAGEMENT)

Feline Odontoclastic Resorptive Lesions, also known as FORL's, are often described as a cavity in the tooth of a cat. They are different from human cavities, and are not caused by decay and bacteria as with human teeth. There is much controversy regarding this disorder, and no agreement has been made regarding causes or consistent treatments. Holistically, one can be sure that eliminating toxins, detoxifying the body, and providing foundational tools of health (essential oils and supplements) are key for prevention and treatment. Currently, affected teeth are often best extracted from the mouth, as they are painful and continue to worsen despite our best attempts. Prevention of additional teeth succumbing to the disorder is a primary focus, as well as decreasing pain and inflammation associated with the condition.

FIRST LINE RECOMMENDATIONS:
FELINE SUPPORTIVE BLEND: Apply as needed, often up to once a day. Consider adding Myrrh, Catnip, and Frankincense.
LITTER BOX RECIPES: Myrrh, Copaiba, Catnip
TOPICAL: Coconut Oil – see Dental Disease for further information.
DRINKING WATER: Copaiba, see further instructions

Single Oils:
Catnip, Copaiba, Frankincense, Helichrysum, Laurus nobilis, Myrrh

FEVER OF UNKNOWN ORIGIN
(See also PAIN MANAGEMENT)

As the name suggests, this condition is a fever in a cat, for which the cause cannot be determined. In this situation, an approach of providing tools against every cause of a fever is recommended. The Feline Supportive Blend is ideal for this need. It is important to address pain if that may also be a contributing factor.

FIRST LINE RECOMMENDATIONS:
>FELINE SUPPORTIVE BLEND: Applied up to twice a day, or as needed. Consider addition of Frankincense, Melissa, Ginger.
>WATER DIFFUSION: Rotation of Three Part Blends, determining which may be more beneficial for your individual.
>LITTER BOX RECIPES: Copaiba, Melissa, Ginger

Single Oils:
>Black Spruce, Copaiba, Frankincense, Ginger, Helichrysum, Lavender, Lemon, Marjoram, Melissa, Myrrh, Oregano, Peppermint, Thyme

FIP
>(See FELINE INFECTIOUS PERITONITIS, VIRAL CONDITIONS)

FIV
>(See VIRAL CONDITIONS)

FLEAS

Fleas are one of the most difficult parasites to eliminate. Often many multiple layers of prevention are needed. All animals in the household must be treated for fleas, not just one or two.

FIRST LINE RECOMMENDATIONS:
>DIFFUSION: See the description for Pepper (Black), for directions for a household Flea Bomb Recipe.
>FELINE SUPPORTIVE BLEND: Add oil such as Catnip, Geranium, Eucalyptus citriodora. Apply up to once a day. Fleas particularly dislike the Feline Supportive Blend solution, and it is helpful to apply this solution to locations where the fleas are the worst (rear end.)
>TOPICAL: Bathe with natural shampoos containing Catnip, Geranium, Eucalyptus citriodora or others intended for topical use.

CLEANING: Cleaning, laundering, and spraying with essential oils added to recipes indoors and out is suggested.

Single Oils:
Black Spruce, Catnip, Citronella, Eucalyptus citriodora, Eucalyptus polybractea, Geranium, Lavender, Melissa, Orange, Oregano, Thyme

FLUTD – FELINE LOWER URINARY TRACT DISEASE
(See also PAIN MANAGEMENT, URINARY CONDITIONS)

FLUTD is a poorly understood condition that could have underlying viral and stress related causes. Cats experience periods of bladder inflammation (idiopathic cystitis), and often strain and pass bloody urine during an episode. Good hydration and the feeding of foods with additional moisture (canned, raw, or otherwise) is helpful for the condition. Often courses of antibiotics are prescribed, but are not truly indicated as there is usually no bacterial infection present. Given time, the cat will generally get over the episode on their own, but may flare up again at a later date. A holistic approach to this disorder is mandatory for correction. Stress appears to be a certain factor in the occurrence and flare of this condition for cats, so the use of essential oils in their home, is especially helpful. Some vets do feel that there may be a viral connection with the bladder inflammation, the ability of essential oils to not only contribute to physical health and comfort, but emotional wellbeing is of great importance for this condition.

FIRST LINE RECOMMENDATIONS:
FELINE SUPPORTIVE BLEND: Apply as needed, consider adding Melissa, Frankincense, and Juniper
INGESTION: Copaiba in drinking water or foods can be considered in severe situations. However topical absorption and grooming is likely to be adequate.
LITTER BOX RECIPES: Copaiba, Frankincense, Juniper
WATER DIFFUSION: Rotational diffusion of Three Part Blends especially focusing on stress relief as well as antiviral actions may be indicated.

Single Oils:
Black Spruce, Copaiba, German Chamomile, Helichrysum, Juniper, Laurus nobilis, Lavender, Lemon, Melissa, Marjoram, Myrrh, Oregano, Thyme, Valerian, Vetiver, Ylang Ylang

FORL
(See FELINE ODONTOCLASTIC RESORPTIVE LESION)

FUO
(See FEVER OF UNKNOWN ORIGIN)

GASTROINTESTINAL CONDITIONS
(See INFLAMMATORY BOWEL DISEASE)

GINGIVITIS
(See also DENTAL DISEASE, FELINE ODONTOCLASTIC RESORPTIVE LESIONS, STOMATITIS)

HAIRBALLS

Hairballs are not a normal occurrence in cats. As much as we have been lead to believe that this is an expected event, I have found that dietary changes, support of greater health, and removal of household chemicals and toxins often eliminate the expulsion of hairballs. There may still be an occasional episode, but these should be few and far between, and mainly limited to very long haired cats.

FIRST LINE RECOMMENDATIONS:
DIET: Grain free or raw. Eliminate egg, corn, soy, wheat, and dairy. Some protein sources may need to be eliminated.
FELINE SUPPORTIVE BLEND: Apply as needed, consider addition of Ginger.

WATER DIFFUSION: Three Part Blends for digestive concerns, or for calming
LITTER BOX RECIPES: Copaiba, Ginger, Marjoram

Single Oils:
Anise, Copaiba, Fennel, Ginger, Juniper, Lavender, Marjoram, Patchouli, Peppermint, Tarragon

HCM – HYPERTROPHIC CARDIOMYOPATHY
(See HEART CONDITIONS)

HEART CONDITIONS

FIRST LINE RECOMMENDATIONS:
FELINE SUPPORTIVE BLEND: Apply as needed, consider addition of Cistus and Melissa.
WATER DIFFUSION: Three Part Blends. Consider Helichrysum, Copaiba, May Chang.
LITTER BOX RECIPES: Helichrysum, Cistus, May Chang

Single Oils:
Cistus, Copaiba, Helichrysum, Lavender, Ledum, Marjoram, May Chang, Melissa, Nutmeg, Orange, Patchouli, Spikenard, Ylang Ylang

HEART MURMUR
(See HEART CONDITIONS)

HERPES VIRUS
(See also VIRAL CONDITIONS)

FIRST LINE RECOMMENDATIONS:
FELINE SUPPORTIVE BLEND: Apply as needed. Always include the addition of Melissa essential oil, other oils may be considered.
LITTER BOX RECIPES: Melissa, Geranium, Copaiba
WATER DIFFUSION: Three Part Blends for respiratory help, or antiviral properties can be diffused on a rotational basis.

Single Oils:
Copaiba, Eucalyptus polybractea, Frankincense, Geranium, Helichrysum, Marjoram, Melaleuca ericifolia, Melissa, Mountain Savory, Oregano, Peppermint, Rose, Sandalwood, Thyme

HIT BY CAR
(See also PAIN MANAGEMENT)

FIRST LINE RECOMMENDATIONS:
WATER DIFFUSION: For lung trauma Tent or Cage Diffuse with the following recipe: 3 drops Helichrysum, 2 drops Frankincense, 1 drop Lavender, 1 drop Copaiba.
ORAL: Helichrysum – see PAIN MANAGEMENT
FELINE SUPPORTIVE BLEND: Apply as needed, consider addition of Myrrh, Frankincense
LITTER BOX RECIPES: Copaiba, Helichrysum, Myrrh

Single Oils:
Cistus, Copaiba, Frankincense, Helichrysum, Lavender, Marjoram, Myrrh, Rose

HORNER'S SYNDROME
(See also NEUROLOGIC CONDITIONS)

FIRST LINE RECOMMENDATIONS:
FELINE SUPPORTIVE BLEND : Apply as needed, consider addition of Frankincense, Roman Chamomile, and German Chamomile.
LITTER BOX RECIPES: Helichrysum, Copaiba, Frankincense
WATER DIFFUSION: Three Part Blends in rotation.

Single Oils:
Balsam Fir, Black Spruce, Chamomile (German), Chamomile (Roman), Frankincense, Geranium, Helichrysum, Juniper, Laurus nobilis, Marjoram, Melissa, Spikenard

HYPERESTHESIA
(See also ARTHRITIS, NEUROLOGIC CONDITIONS, PAIN MANAGEMENT)

Hyperesthesia is the over-sensitivity of a cat to touch. This is generally associated with pain, however it can be hard to determine the exact cause. Supporting multiple levels of nutrition, detoxification of the household, and pain control is suggested. See the other condition listings for further recommendations.

FIRST LINE RECOMMENDATIONS:
FELINE SUPPORTIVE BLEND: Apply as needed, consider addition of Frankincense, Myrrh, and Melissa.
LITTER BOX RECIPES: Copaiba, Helichrysum, Myrrh
WATER DIFFUSION: Three Part Blends

Single Oils:
Black Spruce, Copaiba, Frankincense, Helichrysum, Marjoram, Melissa, Myrrh, Oregano, Peppermint, Thyme, Ylang Ylang

HYPERTENSION
(See also KIDNEY DISEASE)

FIRST LINE RECOMMENDATIONS:
FELINE SUPPORTIVE BLEND: Apply as needed, consider additions of Melissa, Frankincense
LITTER BOX RECIPES: Ylang Ylang, Copaiba, Lavender
WATER DIFFUSION: Three Part Blends

Single Oils:
Cistus, Helichrysum, Lavender, Lemon, Marjoram, Melaleuca alternifolia, Melissa, Nutmeg, Orange, Patchouli, Rose, Ylang Ylang

HYPERTHYROIDISM

FIRST LINE RECOMMENDATIONS:
LITTER BOX RECIPES: Myrrh, Copaiba, Frankincense
FELINE SUPPORTIVE BLEND: Apply as needed, with addition of Myrrh
WATER DIFFUSION: Three Part Blends

Single Oils:
Myrrh

HYPERTROPHIC CARDIOMYOPATHY
(See HEART CONDITIONS)

IBD
(See INFLAMMATORY BOWEL DISEASE)

INNAPROPRIATE ELIMINATION
(See also BEHAVIORAL CONDITIONS, FLUTD, KIDNEY DISEASE, URINARY CONDITIONS)

Cats may urinate or defecate outside of their litter box for a number of reasons. It is important to have a thorough evaluation with a holistic veterinarian to rule out medical causes. Common things that are helpful include getting a brand new litter box, changing styles of litter boxes, adding additional litter boxes, changing locations of litter boxes, and making sure that other animals are not ambushing the elimination event. Most commonly there is some sort of underlying issue that can be found. Even though we may desire to have the litter box "out of sight" within our basement, our cat with arthritis may have a hard time getting to that location. Or, a cat just may decide they do not like our chosen bathroom location, so they will create their own. Daily cleaning of the litter box (or more) is mandatory, as well as providing one litter box for each cat in the household, plus one additional litter box for good measure.

FIRST LINE RECOMMENDATIONS:
WATER DIFFUSION: Three Part Blends for emotional support, odor control, or health support in rotation.
FELINE SUPPORTIVE BLEND: Apply as needed, consider addition of Juniper, Melissa, Myrrh
LITTER BOX RECIPES: Catnip, Copaiba, Melissa
WATER MISTING: Odor eliminating Three Part Blends or other recipes can be made to spray on household areas (not on the cat). For odor elimination, often the mixture can be made quite strong – 50-60 drops into 4 ounces (120 mL) of distilled water. Shake well and mist areas of concern. Test an area of carpet or fabric prior to treatment with the solution.

Single Oils:
Black Spruce, Catnip, Frankincense, German Chamomile, Melissa, Orange, Roman Chamomile, Spikenard, Tangerine, Valerian, Vetiver, Ylang Ylang

INFLAMMATORY BOWEL DISEASE
(See also DIARRHEA)

FIRST LINE RECOMMENDATIONS:
FELINE SUPPORTIVE BLEND : Apply as needed, the addition of Ginger is recommended.
INGESTION: Copaiba in foods can be considered, but is rarely necessary. Grooming of the Feline Supportive Blend is often adequate for antibacterial, anti-inflammatory, and GI soothing needs.
LITTER BOX RECIPES: Copaiba, Ginger, Black Spruce
WATER DIFFUSION: Rotate with any Three Part Blend, especially those for GI concerns and inflammation.

Single Oils:
Anise, Black Spruce, Copaiba, Fennel, Ginger, Helichrysum, Lemon, Myrrh, Nutmeg, Tarragon, Ylang Ylang

KIDNEY DISEASE

FIRST LINE RECOMMENDATIONS:
WATER DIFFUSION: Three Part Blends
FELINE SUPPORTIVE BLEND: Apply as needed, addition of Juniper is always recommended. Other oils may be added.
LITTER BOX RECIPES: Helichrysum, Juniper, Grapefruit

Single Oils:
Copaiba, Grapefruit, Helichrysum, Juniper, Marjoram

FELINE CONDITIONS

LIMPING KITTEN SYNDROME
(See also PAIN MANAGEMENT, VACCINATION DETOXIFICATION)

FIRST LINE RECOMMENDATIONS:
ORAL: Follow suggestions in Pain Management if needed.
FELINE SUPPORTIVE BLEND: Apply as needed, addition of Frankincense and Myrrh is suggested.
WATER DIFFUSION: Three Part Blends, especially calming and anti-inflammatory (Copaiba, German Chamomile, Black Spruce)
LITTER BOX RECIPES: Copaiba, Myrrh, Helichrysum

Single Oils:
Balsam Fir, Black Spruce, Copaiba, Frankincense, German Chamomile, Helichrysum, Lavender, Marjoram, Melissa, Myrrh, Oregano, Peppermint, Spikenard, Thyme

LIVER DISEASE

FIRST LINE RECOMMENDATIONS:
FELINE SUPPORTIVE BLEND: Apply as needed, additions of Ledum and Grapefruit can be considered.
ORAL: Helichrysum when indicated, and for severe Liver Failure.
LITTER BOX RECIPES: Helichrysum, Ledum, Copaiba
WATER DIFFUSION:

Single Oils:
Copaiba, Geranium, Grapefruit, Helichrysum, Juniper, Ledum, Myrrh, Myrtle, Nutmeg, Rosemary, Sage, Spearmint, Tangerine

LYMPHOCYTIC PLASMACYTIC STOMATITIS/GINGIVITIS
(See STOMATITIS)

NEUROLOGIC CONDITIONS

FIRST LINE RECOMMENDATIONS:
FELINE SUPPORTIVE BLEND: Apply as needed, consider addition of Frankincense, German Chamomile.
WATER DIFFUSION: Three Part Blends (Roman Chamomile, Melissa, Copaiba)
LITTER BOX RECIPES: Roman Chamomile, Helichrysum, Copaiba

Single Oils:
Black Spruce, Chamomile (German), Chamomile (Roman), Copaiba, Frankincense, Helichrysum, Juniper, Laurus nobilis, Marjoram, Melissa

PAIN MANAGEMENT

Pain is an important item to address. The presence of pain is not only uncomfortable for an animal, but it will actually suppress the immune system and inhibit healing. All of the recommendations can be used alongside of traditional medications when they are being used. Careful monitoring and care with a veterinarian is recommended to make sure that adequate control of pain is always met.

FIRST LINE RECOMMENDATIONS:
FELINE SUPPORTIVE BLEND: Apply as needed, adding Myrrh.
WATER DIFFUSION: Copaiba, Myrrh, Helichrysum
LITTER BOX RECIPES: Copaiba, Lavender, Myrrh

SECOND LINE RECOMMENDATIONS:
ORAL: In the past, the cat Pain Recipe started with 5 drops each of Myrrh, Helichrysum, and Copaiba per 2 mL of fractionated coconut oil. This solution was given orally directly, by capsule, or within foods if the cat is willing. 5 drops or more of this dilution could be given, 3 or more times per day. Cats often salivate when given any essential oil orally, and this was an expected event. However, cats rejoiced everywhere (as well as their owners), when we recognized that simple topical applications, topical absorption, inhalation absorption, and grooming actions resulted in comfort without all the hassle. While we can still consider use of the oral Pain Recipe for cats in severe need, it should be used mainly as a last resort.

Single Oils:
   Copaiba, Helichrysum, Lavender, Marjoram, Myrrh

PANCREATITIS

FIRST LINE RECOMMENDATIONS:
   FELINE SUPPORTIVE BLEND : Apply as needed, addition of Ginger is recommended.
   WATER DIFFUSION: Rotation of Three Part Blends, especially for GI concerns, inflammation, and stress
   LITTER BOX RECIPES: Copaiba, Ginger, Black Spruce

Single Oils:
   Anise, Balsam Fir, Black Spruce, Copaiba, Fennel, Frankincense, Geranium, Ginger, Helichrysum, Lemon, Oregano, Patchouli, Peppermint, Spearmint, Tarragon, Thyme

PARASITES - INTERNAL
   (See DEWORMING)

PARVO VIRUS - FELINE
   (See VIRAL CONDITIONS)

PILLOW PAW
   (See AUTOIMMUNE CONDITIONS)

PLASMA CELL PODODERMATITIS
   (See AUTOIMMUNE CONDITIONS)

PREGNANCY & DELIVERY

We have had many litters of kittens delivered in our home, and most of them directly next to a water-based diffuser. Although I was very cautious at first, and attempted to not have my Queen near essential oils, she in fact, decided to set up her "nest" right where a diffuser consistently ran. We trusted her instincts, and have never regretted her decision to create what we term "oil babies." The continual diffusion of essential oil selections, created wonderfully healthy kittens and reduced any goopy eyes we may have seen with previous litters who were not exposed to oil use.

Prior to birthing, Three Part Blends can be diffused daily. Rotation through blends is a wonderful idea, and be sure to take note of particular combinations your Queen shows interest in. Although we often stress rotation, when a certain diffusion blend is desired or obtains more results for an individual (no matter what the situation) we should honor that body's need for that particular blend. During birthing, Frankincense, Rose, and Myrrh are top favorites to be included within blends. Read individual oil descriptions, to select oils best suited for diffusion versus topical use.

When oils are desired for topical applications, the Feline Supportive Blend should be selected. This can be dripped or pet onto the Queen, and we have never noted any ill effects or less desire for kittens to snuggle or nurse with oils being present. With cases of mastitis or engorgement, this blend has been massaged directly onto mammary tissue, although we typically try to avoid the nipples directly.

After delivery, kittens have definitely been handled with Frankincense absorbed directly into hands, or even the Feline Supportive Blend with additional Frankincense added. Most often, whichever oil or blend is selected, just handling kittens with the oils absorbed into your hands is sufficient. When there has been concern for umbilical cords, Three Part Blends have been applied directly to the area, both in neat form and diluted. Water-mists can also be considered. Oils such as Helichrysum, Cistus, and Lavender are often selected, as well as Frankincense. Myrrh can also be applied diluted to the umbilical cord after delivery. A huge portion of what I have learned about essential oils and cats, has come from my work with hundreds of rescue cats. We have applied oils to kittens who were still wet from delivery, and we saw significant improvements in health and vitality. As a veterinarian, seeing this connection as well as following their blood work for many years thereafter, and including many additional uses of essential oils, is a very eye-opening experience.

If there are signs of extreme stress or dystocia (difficulty delivering), water-based diffusion or diluted topical applications (Petting) of calming Three Part Blends can have a soothing effect. We have found in practice, that blends were more effective and balanced than diffusion of a single oil alone. Never neglect medical attention for dystocia, however, I am usually quite confident in allowing a client to use some oils while seeking help.

FIRST LINE RECOMMENDATIONS:
WATER DIFFUSION: Three Part Blends (Frankincense, Roman Chamomile, Geranium)
LITTER BOX RECIPES: Myrrh, Frankincense, Geranium
FELINE SUPPORTIVE BLEND: Apply as needed, addition of Frankincense, Myrrh, Roman Chamomile

Single Oils:
Chamomile (German), Chamomile (Roman), Clary Sage, Copaiba, Frankincense, Geranium, Lavender, Myrrh, Orange, Palmarosa, Rose

QUEENING
(See PREGNANCY & DELIVERY)

RESORPTIVE LESIONS
(See FELINE ODONTOCLASTIC RESORPTIVE LESIONS)

RESPIRATORY CONDITIONS
(See ASTHMA, UPPER RESPIRATORY INFECTION)

RINGWORM

Ringworm is a fungal condition of the skin that is contagious to humans. Some Ringworm infections can be quite resistant to treatment, and rotation of different essential oils is suggested, especially if very little results are noted after a week of application. Making "super-charged" Feline Supportive Blend solutions, each with a different combination of antifungal additions, is a great way to treat not only the cat but the lesions themselves. Good health is critical in clearing the infection, and supplements should always be provided.

FIRST LINE RECOMMENDATIONS:
FELINE SUPPORTIVE BLEND: Additions of oils such as Melaleuca alternifolia, Lemongrass, and Myrrh can be considered. Apply at least weekly, and often daily. Application to the site of Ringworm is suggested up to multiple times a day, when located in a position that can be treated topically. Petting may be a more effective way to create widespread coverage.
WATER DIFFUSION: Aid in disinfecting the environment by continually diffusing antifungal essential oils. Cats can be tented with Lavender or appropriate Three Part Blends to permeate the fur as well, this is especially helpful for extensive lesions on the face which are hard to access.
DIRECT TOPICAL: Lavender neat to the lesion, can be considered, at least once a day. Three Part Blends can also be created from appropriate oils, and used for diluted topical applications.
BATHING: Addition of antifungal essential oils to natural shampoo is suggested whenever bathing might occur.
CLEANING: Clean all areas frequently and thoroughly with natural cleaners containing antifungal oils.

Single Oils:
Eucalyptus radiata, Geranium, Lavender, Lemongrass, Marjoram, Melaleuca alternifolia, Melaleuca ericifolia, Myrrh, Oregano, Thyme

ROUNDWORM
(See DEWORMING)

SADDLE THROMBUS

See also PAIN MANAGEMENT for suggestions on how to deal with this painful condition. A Saddle Thrombus is a blood clot, which is generally located in the pelvic area of a cat, and can result in paralysis and pain of one or both back legs. Other areas of the body can also be affected. This disorder generally carries a very poor prognosis traditionally, and aggressive holistic treatments are necessary. This is one condition where "cat friendly" methods are disregarded, and many application techniques are layered together.

FIRST LINE RECOMMENDATIONS:
TOPICAL: Three Part Blends of Cistus, Helichrysum, and Copaiba applied diluted to the site of the clot
FELINE SUPPORTIVE BLEND: Apply up to twice a day, with the additional oils of Cypress, Cistus, and Black Pepper.
WATER DIFFUSION: Three Part Blends in rotation can serve many purposes. From stress relief, to safe exposure to oils with blood thinning properties.

SECOND LINE RECOMMENDATIONS:
ORAL: Cistus, Helichrysum – for the blood clot. Starting with 1 drop of each oil, dilute within 2mL of carrier oil. This dilution can be given multiple times a day, increasing amounts when needed. It is important to closely work with a veterinarian who can help determine if beneficial effects are being noted (return of pulses.)
ORAL: If anticoagulant actions are desired, certain essential oils may facilitate these actions. This is reserved for only the most critical of cases, and only under direct veterinary care and supervision. Dilution of the essential oils is suggested to at least 50%, and historically, up to 5 drops twice a day (or to effect) of the diluted essential oil may be given.

Single Oils:
Black Pepper, Cinnamon, Cistus, Clove, Copaiba, Cypress, Geranium, Helichrysum, Hyssop, Laurus nobilis, Lavender, Marjoram, Nutmeg, Orange

SARCOMA – VACCINE INDUCED, INJECTION SITE
(See also CANCER)

As this form of cancer is often caused from vaccination, both following the recommendations for Cancer as well as for Vaccination Detoxification is important. While we once recognized Sarcomas as related to vaccination sites, we now know that all sorts of injections, especially those designed to last long term (depo or depot injections) – are causing harm to the body, and may give rise to these monstrous tumors. These tumors tend to be very aggressive, and unfortunately surgical removal often results in a more aggressive and faster regrowth. Some specific recommendations are made specifically for this tumor, due to its particularly aggressive nature.

FIRST LINE RECOMMENDATIONS:
FELINE SUPPORTIVE BLEND: Modify by adding Sandalwood, Frankincense, and Hyssop. Apply up to twice a day, and onto the tumor site as well.
LITTER BOX RECIPES: Frankincense, Copaiba, Melissa
TOPICAL: Three Part Blends with antitumoral oils can be applied topically (diluted) multiple times a day.
WATER DIFFUSION: Three Part Blends

Single Oils:
Balsam Fir, Black Spruce, Copaiba, Frankincense, Grapefruit, Helichrysum, Hyssop, Lemon, Melissa, Orange, Sandalwood, Tangerine

SEIZURES
(See also NEUROLOGIC CONDITIONS, and SEIZURES in CANINE CONDITIONS)

For Cats, also follow the recommendations made for Seizures in Canine Conditions, using them in the cat suggested ways. For some cats, performing a Vaccination Detoxification or addressing other forms of illness may be necessary. All recommendations can be used with other medications. Cats are not as commonly affected with Epilepsy, so other causes of seizures such as trauma, toxins, viral infections, or other medical concerns should be fully investigated with a veterinarian.

FIRST LINE RECOMMENDATIONS:
FELINE SUPPORTIVE BLEND: Modified with Frankincense, Melissa, Valerian.
WATER DIFFUSION: Frankincense, Balsam Fir, Copaiba
LITTER BOX RECIPES: Valerian, Roman Chamomile, Lavender
DIRECT INHALATION: During a prolonged seizure, allowing a cat to inhale essential oils can be helpful. Any Three Part Blend can be utilized, this may even be presented neat (undiluted). Lavender, Roman Chamomile, Valerian, Frankincense are excellent suggestions.

Single Oils:
Balsam Fir, Chamomile (German), Chamomile (Roman), Frankincense, Helichrysum, Juniper, Laurus nobilis, Lavender, Melissa, Valerian

SQUAMOUS CELL CARCINOMA
(See also CANCER)

Squamous Cell Carcinoma is unfortunately common, aggressive, and very difficult to treat. It is common within the mouth of cats, and is often not found until it is in the later stages. Very aggressive and layered approaches must be taken with this form of cancer. Incorporating many holistic methods and modalities (such as Acupuncture or Herbals) is encouraged.

FIRST LINE RECOMMENDATIONS:
Follow all of the suggestions within CANCER. Utilizing every supplement and lifestyle change, as well as multiple application methods of essential oils, is strongly recommended.
INGESTION: For this cancer, oral use of essential oils within capsules may be attempted. Start with small amounts of the desired oil, which is indicated for oral use, and gradually increase the amounts given based on responses.
ORAL: Dripping diluted oils directly into the mouth may be helpful to coat oral tumors. Helichrysum, Frankincense, and Copaiba are suggested.

Single Oils:
Copaiba, Frankincense, Grapefruit, Helichrysum, Lemon, Melissa, Orange, Oregano, Sandalwood, Tangerine, Thyme

STOMATITIS
(See also FELINE ODONTOCLASTIC RESORPTIVE LESIONS)

Stomatitis is a particularly horrible inflammation of the mouth, which is usually also complicated by bacterial infection. Treatment with traditional antibiotics is often helpful, however never addresses the underlying cause or healing needed by the cat. Change in diet and the addition of nutritional supplements are very important. Some cats will not groom properly due to this painful condition, however if they do, residual essential oils applied topically are very beneficial to the mouth. Also see the Pain Management recommendations for suggestions.

FIRST LINE RECOMMENDATIONS:
FELINE SUPPORTIVE BLEND: Modified with Myrrh and Catnip; apply up to once a day or as needed. Grooming of this blend is desired to inoculate the mouth, however effects will still be present when grooming is absent.
ORAL: Raw Organic Coconut oil can be fed or rubbed into the mouth. Small amounts of essential oils can be slowly added if the cat will accept them. Coconut Oil or Toothpastes can also have the Feline Supportive Blend added to it.
LITTER BOX RECIPES: Three Part Blends, Copaiba, Frankincense, Myrrh
DRINKING WATER: Diluted Three Part Blends can be added to water if desired. Copaiba especially.

Single Oils:
Black Spruce, Catnip, Copaiba, Helichrysum, Lavender, Lemon, Melissa, Myrrh, Oregano, Thyme

TAPEWORM
(See DEWORMING)

THROMBOCYTOPENIA
(See AUTOIMMUNE CONDITIONS)

TOOTH LESIONS
(See FELINE ODONTOCLASTIC RESORPTIVE LESIONS)

TOXOPLASMOSIS

FIRST LINE RECOMMENDATIONS:
WATER DIFFUSION: Three Part Blends, especially GI related.
FELINE SUPPORTIVE BLEND: Modified by adding Hyssop, Ginger, and Melissa.
ORAL: Ingestion of Feline Supportive Blend via grooming.
LITTER BOX RECIPES: Juniper, Hyssop, Copaiba

Single Oils:
Anise, Copaiba, Fennel, Ginger, Hyssop, Juniper, Lemon, Oregano, Patchouli, Tarragon, Thyme

TRITRICHOMONAS FOETUS
(See also DIARRHEA)

Tritrichomonas is a flagellated protozoan parasite which can create severe and long term diarrhea in cats. The disease is hard to diagnose, and often is overlooked.

FIRST LINE RECOMMENDATIONS:
FELINE SUPPORTIVE BLEND: Modified with Ginger.
LITTER BOX RECIPES: Copaiba, Ginger

Single Oils:
Copaiba, Clove, Lemon, Oregano, Tarragon, Thyme, Vetiver, Ylang Ylang

UPPER RESPIRATORY INFECTION

Upper Respiratory Infections are often chronic in nature, and can seem to never go away. This is always due to nutritional deficiency, as once a cat receives the nourishment they are lacking, the infections go away and stay away. The nutritional deficiency is not always about what diet is being fed currently. It is my opinion that many felines are born in a deficient state, not only in nutrition but in digestive enzymes. No matter which diet you select, you will need to supplement your cat with additional items to make up for lost time. Since generations of cats have been born and raised on deficient, processed diets – their shorter generation cycle reveals their chronic deficiency in the form of disease.

FIRST LINE RECOMMENDATIONS:
WATER DIFFUSION: Via caging or tenting, with 3-4 drops of Three Part Blends for respiratory needs. Diffuse for 20 minutes, 3-4 times a day.
LITTER BOX RECIPES: Copaiba
FELINE SUPPORTIVE BLEND: Modified with Melissa, Frankincense.

Single Oils:
Black Spruce, Cinnamon, Clove, Copaiba, Eucalyptus globulus, Eucalyptus radiata, Hyssop, Laurus nobilis, Lavender, Lemon, Lemongrass, Marjoram, Melaleuca alternifolia, Melissa, Myrtle, Oregano, Rosemary, Thyme

URI – UPPER RESPIRATORY INFECTION
(See UPPER RESPIRATORY INFECTION)

URINARY CONDITIONS

FIRST LINE RECOMMENDATIONS:
LITTER BOX RECIPES: Copaiba, Juniper, Frankincense.
FELINE SUPPORTIVE BLEND: Modified by adding Juniper. This solution may also be applied over the bladder area in a Petting fashion.

Single Oils:
Copaiba, Geranium, Grapefruit, Juniper, Laurus nobilis, Ledum, Lemon, Lemongrass, Spruce, Tarragon, Vetiver

URINATING IN THE HOUSE
(See also FLUTD, INAPPROPRIATE ELIMINATION, URINARY CONDITIONS)

UTI – URINARY TRACT INFECTION
(See URINARY CONDITIONS)

VACCINATION DETOXIFICATION

Vaccinations can cause many health concerns and have even been linked with the formation of cancerous tumors (Sarcomas.) It is likely that any animal can benefit from the described cleansing cycle, whether they have been vaccinated or not. Even asymptomatic animals will benefit from detoxification from past vaccinations. In animals experiencing symptoms such as thyroid imbalance, allergies, asthma, autoimmune disorders, or other chronic illnesses; detoxification from previous vaccines becomes much more critical for healing to occur.

FIRST LINE RECOMMENDATIONS:
FELINE SUPPORTIVE BLEND: Modified by adding Ledum. Apply once a week for 3 months. Apply more frequently if symptoms require it.
LITTER BOX RECIPES: German Chamomile, Roman Chamomile, Helichrysum.

Single Oils:
Chamomile (German), Chamomile (Roman), Copaiba, Geranium, Grapefruit, Helichrysum, Hyssop, Juniper, Ledum, Lemon, Melissa, Oregano, Thyme

VACCINOSIS
(See VACCINATION DETOXIFICATION)

VIRAL CONDITIONS

There are many viral conditions in cats, and thankfully, all of the antiviral essential oils will benefit each condition. There are specific oils that may target Herpes Virus more so than another virus, but thankfully, when providing the body with multiple tools for healing, many benefits are seen. Even when only diffusion of essential oils is provided, we have seen a great reduction in viral infections and transmission of disease where multiple cats are exposed to each other.

FIRST LINE RECOMMENDATIONS:
FELINE SUPPORTIVE BLEND: Modified with addition of Melissa. Apply up to once a day.
LITTER BOX RECIPES: Melissa, Frankincense, Copaiba.
WATER DIFFUSION: in an open room basis, up to 24 hours a day. Tenting and Caging can also be performed, as described in Upper Respiratory Infections.

Single Oils:
Copaiba, Frankincense, Geranium, Helichrysum, Hyssop, Laurus nobilis, Lemon, Melissa, Oregano, Sandalwood, Thyme

VOMITING
(See also HAIRBALLS, PANCREATITIS)

Vomiting can have many causes, and it is important that they be thoroughly explored by a veterinarian. Once you have determined the cause of the vomiting, more exact remedies can be provided.

FIRST LINE RECOMMENDATIONS:
PETTING: Diluted Three Part Blends for GI
LITTER BOX RECIPES: Copaiba, Ginger, Three Part GI Blends
FELINE SUPPORTIVE BLEND: Modify by adding Ginger

Single Oils:
Copaiba, Ginger, Juniper, Lavender, Ledum, Lemon, Patchouli, Peppermint, Spearmint, Tarragon

CANINE SUPPORTIVE BLEND

Please see the chapters on the Drip & Rub Techniques as well as the Body Supportive Blends. The Canine Supportive Blend will be the mainstay for support for most Canines. This blend can also be used for a variety of larger animals such as goats, pigs, and other livestock.

Modifications of this blend, are generally achieved by adding additional oils of interest to the base blend, then diluting the base to the desired end concentration.

Just as described previously – this blend is more appropriate for dogs and larger animals. While cats will be safe if exposed to this blend by laying with a dog, or even grooming it, the concentration and oils contained within are not suitable for use directly on a feline. In general this blend is used between a 10-30% concentration.

To create a neat base blend; combine equal parts Oregano, Thyme, Basil, Cypress, Marjoram, Lavender, Copaiba, Helichrysum, and Peppermint. Add to carrier oil to create the desired concentration. Additional oils often considered to add to the base blend include Frankincense, Myrtle, Catnip, Ginger, Juniper, Ledum, and Melissa.

Alternately, add 10 drops each of Oregano, Thyme, Basil, Cypress, Marjoram, Lavender, Copaiba, Helichrysum, and Peppermint to 30mL of Fractionated Coconut Oil. Apply 8-10 drops of this solution up the back, and stroke in. This blend may also be applied using the Petting Technique.

See the Chapter on Drip & Rub Techniques for more information on balancing and energy work prior to applications.

CANINE CONDITIONS

ABSCESS

An abscess is a pus filled pocket generally located under the skin, however can be located anywhere within the body. Most abscesses contain bacteria of various sorts, although there are conditions in which sterile abscesses form. Abscesses can erupt very quickly and result in severe systemic illness including fever, lethargy, inappetence, and more.

FIRST RECOMMENDATIONS:
TOPICAL: Apply Canine Supportive Blend to the abscess head, up to twice a day or more. If the abscess is open and draining, essential oils can be added to solutions used to clean and flush the abscess.
CANINE SUPPORTIVE BLEND: Can be administered for general immune support and anti-bacterial actions, up to daily.
ORAL: In general, oral use of essential oils is often not necessary. When oral use is considered, see the descriptions under Oregano or Thyme for more information on oral dosing. 1 drop per 25 pounds of dog can be considered once or twice a day (generally of Three Part Blends) for antibacterial action. See also Pain Management for suggestions if indicated.

Single Oils:
Copaiba, Laurus nobilis, Lavender, Lemongrass, Melaleuca alternifolia, Oregano, Spikenard, Thyme

ACNE
(See also ALLERGIES, HOT SPOTS, SKIN INFECTIONS, and FELINE CONDITIONS - ACNE)

ADDISON'S DISEASE
(aka HYPOADRENOCORTICISM, ADRENAL INSUFFICIENCY)

Addison's Disease is the under-activity of the adrenal gland, resulting in low levels of critical hormones. Symptoms include weakness and generalized, "crashing" due to electrolyte disorders. In critical situations, veterinary care is almost certainly needed – with IV electrolyte replacement via fluids. Steroid medications are also given in attempts to normalize the critical patient.

FIRST RECOMMENDATIONS:
CANINE SUPPORTIVE BLEND: Modified with Nutmeg, Frankincense, and Black Spruce. Apply as needed, even up to daily for some cases.

Single Oils:
Black Spruce, Chamomile (German), Clove, Copaiba, Frankincense, Nutmeg, Spikenard

ALLERGIES
(See also SKIN INFECTIONS)

Allergies are a complex problem, however many fundamental basics of holistic health will benefit the condition. There are definite, multi-factorial issues involved with allergies – and often a multi-layer approach is needed. Secondary skin infections must be detected and treated, or symptoms will continue to be seen, even if the allergies are improved. Diet is important to address, as well as liver health and cleansing.

FIRST LINE RECOMMENDATIONS:
CANINE SUPPORTIVE BLEND: Up to once a day, as needed for comfort. Consider additions of Melissa, Ledum, Catnip.
CLEANING & BATHING: Three Part Blends can be added to natural shampoos, and to cleaning recipes
DIFFUSION: Three Part Blends, especially containing Clove

Single Oils:
Basil, Black Spruce, Clove, Copaiba, Lavender, Ledum, Melissa, Oregano, Thyme

ALOPECIA X

Alopecia X is a condition mainly of hair loss, that is currently poorly understood. A direct cause or treatment has not been discovered. Melatonin has been recommended from many references as being a treatment option, but with variable results. The best answer for this condition is a complete holistic approach, to give the body the tools it needs to correct the "undiscovered" problems at hand.

FIRST LINE RECOMMENDATIONS:
CANINE SUPPORTIVE BLEND: Monthly for general health, adjust as indicated. Daily to weekly applications may be indicated for some.
DIFFUSION: With any suggested oil, or Three Part Blend.

Single Oils:
Balsam Fir, Black Spruce, Clary Sage, Copaiba, Frankincense, Oregano, Rosemary, Sandalwood, Thyme, Ylang Ylang

AMYLOIDOSIS
(See also COGNITIVE DYSFUNCTION, KIDNEY DISEASE)

Amyloidosis occurs when abnormal proteins are deposited within various body tissues. This can happen in other animals, such as cats and horses, and some breeds are more prone to this disease than others, and display hereditary and genetic tendencies. It is commonly found in the spleen and kidneys however the liver, brain, and other body tissues can be affected. Amyloid in the brain is a major factor in Cognitive Dysfunction of senior dogs, as well as Alzheimer's in humans. Inflammation appears to play a primary role in stimulating the deposition of this material, and providing holistic tools that are anti-inflammatory, should be an integral part to prevention and treatment. Enzymes are incredibly important to be supplemented, as the only way to break down these deposits, is with the enzymes within the body. High doses of enzymes, especially containing Protease, should be provided.

FIRST LINE RECOMMENDATIONS:
ORAL: Copaiba, Helichrysum, Frankincense
CANINE SUPPORTIVE BLEND: At least monthly, or as indicated.
Consider addition of Melissa, Black Pepper, or other indicated oils.

CANINE CONDITIONS

Single Oils:
Black Pepper, Copaiba, Frankincense, Grapefruit, Juniper, Ledum

ANAL GLANDS
(See also ABSCESS)

The need for routine Anal Gland expression is not normal. Often the act of expression actually causes inflammation and can drive bacteria into the gland, resulting in bacterial infection and possibly the formation of an abscess. Abnormal stools, either too soft or too hard, can cause the glands to not express adequately upon defecation. Addressing the diet, providing tools for health, and addressing other conditions such as allergies or skin infections is important.

FIRST LINE RECOMMENDATIONS:
CANINE SUPPORTIVE BLEND: At least monthly, or as indicated.
WATER MISTING: Place 20 drops of Lavender, 10 drops of Copaiba, and 10 drops of Melaleuca alternifolia in 4 ounces (120 mL) of distilled water and mist the anal area twice a day or as needed.
TOPICAL: Three Part Blends added to natural ointments
ORAL: Copaiba, or recipes for pain

Single Oils:
Copaiba, Helichrysum, Laurus nobilis, Lavender, Lemon, Melaleuca alternifolia, Oregano, Thyme

ANAPLASMA
(See TICK BORNE DISEASE)

ANESTHESIA DETOXIFICATION
(See EQUINE CONDITIONS)

ANOREXIA

Anorexia is often used to describe poor or no eating by an animal. Many times it is accompanied by feelings of nausea or discomfort. There are many reasons for an animal to be anorexic, and an accurate veterinary diagnosis is important. These recommendations generally stimulate appetite and ease digestive concerns and nausea.

FIRST LINE RECOMMENDATIONS:
PETTING: Three Part Blends, diluted, for GI concerns
ORAL: Ginger for extreme nausea
CANINE SUPPORTIVE BLEND: Add Ginger, apply as needed.
WATER DIFFUSION: Three Part Blends for GI concerns

Single Oils:
Anise, Copaiba, Fennel, Ginger, Juniper, Laurus nobilis, Lavender, Marjoram, Patchouli, Peppermint, Tarragon

ANTIHISTAMINE-LIKE ACTIONS
(See also STEROIDS - REPLACMENT)

Some essential oils can be used for their antihistamine type of actions. These suggestions can be used when an antihistamine would be called for.

FIRST LINE RECOMMENDATIONS:
CANINE SUPPORTIVE BLEND: As indicated for comfort. Consider addition of Melissa.
PETTING: Basil or Black Spruce
ORAL: Melissa, Basil, or Vetiver

Single Oils:
Balsam Fir, Basil, Black Spruce, Copaiba, Lavender, Melissa, Vetiver

ANXIETY
(See also BEHAVIORAL CONDITIONS)

Anxiety can be helped specifically through the supplementation of minerals and enzymes. Pack leadership and good training is the foundation of correction of all anxiety issues, but addressing physical needs are important as well.

FIRST LINE RECOMMENDATIONS:
WATER DIFFUSION: Of any selected oil, Three Part Blend. See also the chapters Emotional Work with Oils.
CANINE SUPPORTIVE BLEND: Even a full body supportive blend can help emotions. Consider additions of other emotionally beneficial oils.
TOPICAL: diluted Three Part Blends can be applied in a variety of ways

Single Oils:
Anise, Bergamot, Black Spruce, Frankincense, Grapefruit, Lavender, Lemon, Melissa, Orange, Rose, Tangerine, Valerian, Vetiver, Ylang Ylang

ARTHRITIS
(See also PAIN MANAGEMENT)

This regimen has been used successfully in our veterinary practice to eliminate and replace the use of traditional NSAIDs.

FIRST LINE RECOMMENDATIONS:
ORAL: Copaiba
CANINE SUPPORTIVE BLEND: Regular applications of a full body supporting blend, can support relief of arthritis
PETTING: Copaiba or other selected oils, diluted within Three Part Blends for musculoskeletal concerns can be helpful on location.

Single Oils:
Balsam Fir, Black Spruce, Copaiba, Frankincense, Helichrysum, Lavender, Lemongrass, Marjoram, Myrrh, Nutmeg, Peppermint, Vetiver

ASCITES
(See also LIVER DISEASE)

Ascites is an accumulation of fluid within the abdomen, most commonly related to advanced liver or heart disease. Providing additional support to any body system that is involved is recommended.

FIRST LINE RECOMMENDATIONS:
CANINE SUPPORTIVE BLEND: Consider addition of Ledum, Melissa, and Frankincense.
ORAL: Grapefruit, Ledum, Helichrysum
PETTING: Any selected oil, diluted Three Part Blend.

Single Oils:
Copaiba, Grapefruit, Helichrysum, Juniper, Ledum, Lemon, Lemongrass, Marjoram, Melaleuca alternifolia, Tangerine

ASPIRATION PNEUMONIA
(See COUGH, MEGAESOPHAGUS, RESPIRATORY INFECTIONS)

ATOPY
(See ALLERGIES)

AURAL HEMATOMA

An Aural Hematoma is a blood filled pocket on the ear flap of a dog. This can occur in cats and other animals as well, but is most commonly seen in canines. Often, there is an ear infection (see Ear Infections) that causes repeated shaking of the head and trauma to the ear. The cartilage of the ear separates, and is filled with blood. Other direct trauma to the ear can cause this condition as well. It is very important that any ear infections or other conditions are corrected for this problem to heal. Many veterinarian recommend surgical drainage of the ear, and some are even injecting them with steroids. Ears can become scarred and misshapen if the disorder is allowed to become chronic. If response is not noted to the following suggestions in approximately 2 weeks, veterinary treatment may be necessary.

FIRST LINE RECOMMENDATIONS:
TOPICAL: Helichrysum, Cistus, Cypress onto hematoma 2-3 times a day. Generally diluted. Effects can be amplified by applying diluted Copaiba and Peppermint, after application of other oils.
CANINE SUPPORTIVE BLEND: Can be used as full body support, and may be also massaged onto the ear flap. Consider the addition of Cistus.
EAR SPRAY: Please see the recipe for ears, as many of these conditions may have an ear infection present.

Single Oils:
Cistus, Copaiba, Cypress, Geranium, Helichrysum, Lavender

AUTOIMMUNE CONDITIONS

FIRST LINE RECOMMENDATIONS:
CANINE SUPPORTIVE BLEND: Modified by including Melissa, Frankincense, and Black Spruce.
PETTING: diluted Three Part Blends

Single Oils:
Balsam Fir, Black Spruce, Copaiba, Frankincense, Helichrysum

BEHAVIORAL CONDITIONS
(See also ANXIETY)

FIRST LINE RECOMMENDATIONS:
PETTING: diluted Three Part Blends
DIFFUSION: Three Part Blends
CANINE SUPPORTIVE BLEND: Consider addition of Frankincense, Melissa or other emotional oils.

Single Oils:
Bergamot, Black Spruce, Cedarwood, Chamomile (German), Chamomile (Roman), Geranium, Grapefruit, Lavender, Lemon, Marjoram, Melissa, Patchouli, Rose, Rosemary, Spikenard, Tangerine, Valerian, Vetiver, Ylang Ylang

BELL'S PALSY
(See also NEUROLOGIC CONDITIONS)

FIRST LINE RECOMMENDATIONS:
PETTING: diluted Helichrysum within appropriate Three Part Blends, especially near face.
CANINE SUPPORTIVE BLEND: Add additional oils for neurologic support such as Geranium, Melissa.

Single Oils:
Black Spruce, Copaiba, Frankincense, Geranium, Helichrysum, Juniper, Laurus nobilis

BENIGN PROSTATIC HYPERTROPHY (BPH)
(See PROSTATE CONDITIONS)

BENIGN TUMOR

FIRST LINE RECOMMENDATIONS:
TOPICAL: Apply Frankincense, Copaiba, and Peppermint to the tumor, up to twice a day based on response and tolerance. Dilution is generally recommended. For some situations, neat oil use may be considered.

Single Oils:
Copaiba, Frankincense, Grapefruit, Lavender, Lemon, Orange, Sandalwood, Tangerine

BILIOUS VOMITING

Bilious Vomiting is when a dog vomits due to having an empty stomach. There can be medical reasons behind this event; however it seems to be closely associated with an empty stomach or a delayed meal. Sometimes this issue has been eliminated by simply providing the dog with a late night snack. Providing holistic tools for normal digestive function is likely a better answer.

FIRST LINE RECOMMENDATIONS:
PETTING: with diluted Three Part Blends (digestive)
DRINKING WATER: Peppermint, digestive Three Part Blends
CANINE SUPPORTIVE BLEND: Regular applications of full body support, may address issues more completely. Consider addition of Ginger

Single Oils:
Anise, Copaiba, Fennel, Ginger, Helichrysum, Juniper, Laurus nobilis, Lemon, Marjoram, Melissa, Patchouli, Peppermint, Spearmint, Tangerine, Tarragon, Valerian

BLADDER INFECTION

FIRST LINE RECOMMENDATIONS:
CANINE SUPPORTIVE BLEND: consider addition of Juniper

Single Oils:
Copaiba, Grapefruit, Juniper, Laurus nobilis, Ledum, Lemon, Lemongrass, Oregano, Tarragon, Thyme

BLADDER STONES
(See also BLADDER INFECTION, PAIN MANAGEMENT)

Bladder Stones should be evaluated by a veterinarian for type and cause. Some stones may require surgical removal. Dietary adjustments are important, and increased moisture intake through the diet as well as through drinking is recommended.

FIRST LINE RECOMMENDATIONS:
DRINKING WATER: Lemon may be considered
CANINE SUPPORTIVE BLEND: consider addition of Juniper
ORAL: Oregano may be considered, also Copaiba and recipes for pain and inflammation can be helpful

Single Oils:
Black Spruce, Copaiba, Grapefruit, Juniper, Laurus nobilis, Lavender, Ledum, Lemon, Myrrh, Vetiver

BLASTOMYCOSIS
(See also RESPIRATORY INFECTION)

Blastomycosis is a severe fungal infection primarily of the lungs, but which can affect skin, eyes, and other tissues.

FIRST LINE RECOMMENDATIONS:
WATER DIFFUSION: Three Part Blends via tenting and caging, 3 or more times a day. Diffusion of any oil within an open room is suggested 24 hours a day.
CANINE SUPPORTIVE BLEND: Add additional oils as indicated. Apply up to once or twice a day or as indicated.

Single Oils:
Black Spruce, Cinnamon, Clove, Copaiba, Laurus nobilis, Lavender, Lemongrass, Marjoram, Melaleuca alternifolia, Melaleuca ericifolia, Oregano, Peppermint, Rosemary, Thyme

BLOAT
(See GASTRODILITATION VOLVULUS)

BONE - BROKEN
(See also PAIN MANAGEMENT)

These oils will aid in healing time, inflammation, and can encourage remodeling of the bone.

FIRST LINE RECOMMENDATIONS:
PETTING: diluted Three Part Blends for bone health, inflammation and healing. Consider oils such as Balsam Fir, Spruce, Helichrysum, Copaiba near the fracture area as often as tolerated, generally 2-3 times a day for the first week, then less often later.
CANINE SUPPORTIVE BLEND: Apply as needed for comfort and support, application on the affected limb can be considered.

Single Oils:
Balsam Fir, Black Spruce, Copaiba, Helichrysum, Lemongrass, Marjoram, Myrrh, Thyme

BONE - CANCER
(See CANCER - BONE)

BONE CONDITIONS

These suggestions support bone health in general. Any condition affecting a bone will benefit with these oils.

FIRST LINE RECOMMENDATIONS:
PETTING: Any of the suggested oils, within Three Part Blends, generally diluted.
CANINE SUPPORTIVE BLEND: consider additions of Balsam Fir, Black Spruce, and Frankincense. Apply along spine and to bone of interest.

Single Oils:
Balsam Fir, Black Spruce, Copaiba, Rosemary, Thyme

BRUCELLA CANIS

Brucella Canis, also called Brucellosis, causes abortions and reproductive concerns in breeding dogs. It is transmitted through ingestion of contaminated materials and sexual contact. Many dogs who contract this disease are subsequently sterilized or euthanized. Careful monitoring with a veterinarian is important if you attempt to clear the infection in an intact dog, as it is very difficult. Sterilization is recommended for many cases, where the spread of the disease is hard to prevent.

FIRST LINE RECOMMENDATIONS:
CANINE SUPPORTIVE BLEND: Modify by including Melissa, Frankincense. Up to daily administration may be necessary in some cases.

Single Oils:
Lemon, Melaleuca alternifolia, Melissa, Oregano, Thyme

CALLUS

Elbows and pads of dogs sometimes produce excess skin, become bald or damaged, or over grow with keratin or "corns." Some conditions are quite a normal occurrence for some dogs, however pressure sores and wounds may need veterinary attention. General skin care as well as liver and colon cleansing and support, will aid in the health and resilience of the skin.

FIRST LINE RECOMMENDATIONS:
TOPICAL: Three Part Blends for skin within natural ointments or salves can be used.

Single Oils:
Copaiba, Geranium, Helichrysum, Lavender, Myrrh, Palmarosa, Patchouli, Rose

CANCER
(See also MAST CELL TUMOR, CANCER in FELINE CONDITIONS)

There are many different kinds of cancer, and each type may have a different specific focus for essential oil recommendations. If certain oils are more indicated for specific types of Cancer, they are listed. However there is a basic foundation of items that must be met in order for an immune system to function to the fullest, and to give an animal the utmost possibility of clearing cancer. These recommendations apply to all animals. Please see the Feline Cancer section for further descriptions.

It is very important in conditions such as cancer, to incorporate as many layers of care as possible. This is one situation, where starting with small amounts of items, and building up to using many items, in relatively high amounts (sometimes quickly) is fully warranted.

FIRST LINE RECOMMENDATIONS:
KETOGENIC DIET: See Feline comments. Raw, ketogenic diets can have profound impacts on cancer. Please research this more through the KetoPet Sanctuary (see Resources).

DRINKING WATER: See Feline comments.

ELIMINATE HOUSEHOLD TOXINS: See Feline comments.

OMEGA FISH OILS: A good quality fish oil is strongly recommended. Standard Process Tuna Omega-3 Oil, Standard Process Calamari Oil, Nordic Naturals, Mercola Healthy Pets, and several other reputable veterinary brands can be selected from. Many dogs will approach human dosing suggestions or more.

DIGESTIVE ENZYMES: Digestive enzymes are incredibly important for health, but especially in cases of cancer. See Feline comments.

WHOLE FOOD SUPPLEMENTS: See Feline comments. Recommended Standard Process formulas for dogs with cancer include: Canine Whole Body Support, Canine Immune Support, Boswellia Complex, Burdock Complex, and a variety of other animal and human formulas. I strongly urge working with a holistic veterinarian who is familiar with these products.

WATER DIFFUSION: Rotational diffusion of emotional oils is recommended. See also the chapter on Emotional Work with Oils for more information. Diffuse any anti-cancer oils up to 24 hours a day. Rotation through a variety of oils is recommended.

CANINE SUPPORTIVE BLEND: Modify by addition of Frankincense, Melissa, and Tangerine to the mixture. Apply up to once or twice a day, and at least weekly. Drip & Rub Techniques can also be used in a rotational schedule of different oils (diluted within Three Part Blends).

EMOTIONAL USE OF OILS: It is very important to address emotional cleansing with Cancer. See Emotional Work with Oil. I strongly recommend emotional work and cleansing for the owner as well.

TOPICAL: Topical applications of diluted Three Part Blends can be used in supplemental methods for emotional support, calming, or physical effects. Applications can be as needed, and may include applications to lumps or masses themselves.

ORAL: Frankincense has been given orally in quite high doses for cancer. Dogs have consumed extremely high amounts of Frankincense (60 or more drops per day) with little to no ill effects. GI burn out is a valid issue to contend with, and more often than not, excessive amounts show no more benefits than with the layered applications of Frankincense along with other anti-cancer oils.

DRINKING WATER: Frankincense, Orange, Tangerine, or other desired oils may be given via drinking water when appropriate.

FOODS: Many dogs will ingest essential oils mixed into their foods.

Single Oils:
Balsam Fir, Black Spruce, Copaiba, Frankincense, Grapefruit, Lemon, Melissa, Orange, Oregano, Sandalwood, Tangerine, Thyme

CANCER - BONE

Bone Cancer can benefit from additional support to the bones themselves. Orange oil has also been commonly incorporated into many bone cancer regimens, being added to the Canine Supportive Blend, added to drinking water, or diluted and given by capsule.

FIRST LINE RECOMMENDATIONS:
Also incorporate oil suggestions from BONE CONDITIONS.

CANCER - LIVER

(See also LIVER DISEASE)

Liver Cancer can benefit from additional support to the liver. Please read recommendations for Liver Disease, and incorporate items such as Geranium, Ledum, Helichrysum, and other liver supporting products.

Additional Single Oils:
Chamomile (German), Copaiba, Frankincense, Geranium, Helichrysum, Juniper, Ledum

CANCER - LUNG

Diffusion is especially indicated in cases of Lung Cancer. Adding additional support for lung conditions such as coughs and infections is suggested. Tenting with direct diffusion of Three Part Blends with anti-cancer oils (Tangerine, Frankincense) into the airways is recommended with lung cancer. Do as often, and intensely as the animal will tolerate. This may include air diffusion in some select circumstances.

CANCER – LYMPHOSARCOMA, LYMPHOMA

Follow the basic recommendations for Cancer. Incorporating items that are beneficial for the Lymphatic System is helpful such as Cypress.

Additional Single Oils:
Cypress

CANCER - MAMMARY

Follow the basic recommendations for cancer. Mammary Cancer can specifically benefit from using oils such as Frankincense, Sandalwood, and Myrtle.

CANCER - SPLEEN
(See also HEMORRHAGE – INTERNAL)

Follow the basic recommendations for cancer. If bleeding and hemorrhage are present, the use of Helichrysum and Cistus are recommended for. See Hemorrhage, Internal for more information.

Additional Single Oils:
Cistus, Helichrysum

CANINE INFLUENZA
(See VIRAL CONDITIONS)

CARDIOMYOPATHY
(See also HEART DISEASE)

FIRST LINE RECOMMENDATIONS:
Use the recommendations within Heart Disease, but also add selected oils and supplements which are helpful for muscular conditions – such as Marjoram and Lavender.

Single Oils:
Copaiba, Helichrysum, Lavender, Marjoram, May Chang, Nutmeg, Spikenard, Ylang Ylang

CATARACTS
(See also LENTICULAR SCLEROSIS, EYE CONDITIONS, DIABETES)

The word "cataract" is often misused by owners and occasionally by veterinarians to describe a general cloudy appearance in the eye. It is important not to confuse Lenticular Sclerosis (the clouding of the lens of the eye) with a true cataract, as they are separate conditions. With a true cataract, many dogs will not be visual from the affected eye. Diabetes is a common cause of true cataracts, and once they are formed, it is a difficult condition to reverse. It is very important to obtain an accurate diagnosis, possibly from a veterinary ophthalmologist, and to address the underlying cause of the cataract formation. Prevention of the cataract is the ideal situation.

FIRST LINE RECOMMENDATIONS:
Use recommendations within Lenticular Sclerosis and Eye Conditions.

Single Oils:
Frankincense, Helichrysum

COGNITIVE DYSFUNCTION

Cognitive dysfunction in dogs is becoming more and more common. Possibly due to the older ages that dogs are reaching these days, but more likely to be a result of chronic deficiencies, poor diets, over-vaccination, and toxin exposures. A dog with cognitive dysfunction may forget to go outside to go to the bathroom, may forget that they were just outside and ask to go out again, bark at nothing, whine for no reason, stare off into space, exhibit behavioral changes, and more. Nutritional support is mandatory in this condition, along with essential oils to support the brain. A buildup of plaques within the brain may be the cause of this disorder, and digestive enzyme supplementation is greatly important to support the body's ability to "digest away" these deposits. See also Amyloidosis.

FIRST LINE RECOMMENDATIONS:
WATER DIFFUSION: Diffuse up to 24 hours a day or as comfortable for the animal and their humans. Diffusion especially of Three Part Blends containing oils known for brain function, especially Frankincense.
TOPICAL: diluted applications of Three Part Blends
CANINE SUPPORTIVE BLEND: Modify with inclusion of Melissa, Frankincense, and Black Pepper. Apply as indicated by the response of the animal – approximately every 1-7 days.
ORAL: occasionally, decreasing overall inflammation in the body can be helpful. Copaiba is suggested.

Single Oils:
Cedarwood, Chamomile (German), Chamomile (Roman), Copaiba, Frankincense (Carterii), Grapefruit, Helichrysum, Juniper, Laurus nobilis, Lavender, Lemon, Melissa, Orange, Peppermint, Rose, Rosemary, Spikenard, Valerian, Vetiver, Ylang Ylang

COLLAPSING TRACHEA
(See also COUGH)

A collapsing trachea is a frustrating condition in veterinary medicine. The wind pipe literally collapses upon itself during expiration, inspiration, or both – and causes irritation and reduction in air flow during respiration. There is little that can be done for the condition traditionally, and many attempts have been made to improve the situation with various forms of surgery – which are largely difficult, expensive, and not that helpful. Supporting the correction of inflammation, helping the animal to oxygenate, and nutritionally supporting the structural integrity of the trachea and surrounding tissues is important for improvement of the condition. Although we see improvement in this condition with holistic remedies – lifelong support is often needed and recommended.

FIRST LINE RECOMMENDATIONS:
ORAL: Copaiba
WATER DIFFUSION: Diffuse up to 24 hours a day – Three Part Blends containing oils such as Copaiba, Clove, Frankincense, and Marjoram can be helpful as well as any respiratory supportive oil. Open rooms, small closed rooms, caging, and tenting may be utilized for additional comfort and support.
CANINE SUPPORTIVE BLEND: Modify by including oils such as Black Spruce, Balsam Fir, or other respiratory aids. Apply up to once per day, or as indicated based on response.

Single Oils:
Balsam Fir, Black Spruce, Cedarwood, Clove, Copaiba, Eucalyptus globulus, Eucalyptus radiata, Frankincense, Helichrysum, Laurus nobilis, Lavender, Lemongrass, Marjoram, Rosemary, Vetiver

CONSTIPATION

Constipation is most commonly related to dehydration and improper food choices. Having a quality veterinary exam to look for issues that may contribute to this condition is important. Prostatic disease can often be confused for constipation.

FIRST LINE RECOMMENDATIONS:
Evaluate the dog's diet. Consult with a holistic veterinarian or nutritionist. Add water to every meal, to increase hydration.
PETTING: diluted topical applications of digestive Three Part Blends as needed
ORAL: consideration can be made for administration of appropriate digestive Three Part Blends when necessary. An appropriate blend for ingestion will mean that all oils within that blend are indicated on the singles description as ingestible.

Single Oils:
Anise, Basil, Copaiba, Fennel, Ginger, Juniper, Lavender, Lemon, Marjoram, Peppermint, Spearmint, Tarragon, Vetiver

COPROPHAGIA

Coprophagia is the eating of stool, mainly by dogs but other animals are occasionally witnessed in this activity. For the most part, deficiency in vitamins, minerals, and digestive enzymes are a large component of this occurrence. Make sure to consult with a holistic veterinarian or nutritionist regarding dietary improvements or whole food supplements.

FIRST LINE RECOMMENDATIONS:
CANINE SUPPORTIVE BLEND: Support of the entire body, can be helpful when we do not know if there is an issue at hand. Some animals may eat stools when their physical body is experiencing discomfort.

Single Oils:
Anise, Copaiba, Ginger, Juniper, Spearmint, Tarragon, Vetiver

CORNEA – ABRASION, LACERATION, ULCER, EDEMA
(See also EYE CONDITIONS)

Damage to the Cornea is painful and can be a very dangerous situation. Veterinary attention is always recommended. Diffusion of essential oils via water-based diffusion can provide support for infected corneal conditions.

FIRST LINE RECOMMENDATIONS:
WATER MISTING: See Essential Oils & Eyes for misting recipes for the eyes. Lavender or Therapeutic Eye Spritzers are recommended, 2-3 times a day or as needed for comfort and healing.
WATER DIFFUSION: Frankincense, Helichrysum, and Copaiba via tenting or caging. 20 minutes, 3 times a day or as needed and tolerated for healing and comfort. The mist will contact the surface of the cornea from this application.

Single Oils:
Copaiba, Frankincense, Helichrysum, Lavender, Myrrh

CORNS
(See CALLUS)

COUGH
(See BLASTOMYCOSIS, COLLAPSING TRACHEA, KENNEL COUGH, RESPIRATORY INFECTIONS)

Accurate diagnosis is important to determine the cause of a cough.

FIRST LINE RECOMMENDATIONS:
WATER DIFFUSION: of Three Part Blends in an open room, via caging, or with tenting as required. Repeat as needed based on response, usually 20 minutes, 3 times a day.
CANINE SUPPORTIVE BLEND: applications as needed based on response, even once to twice a day for acute situations.
ORAL: Copaiba may be helpful for some cases

Single Oils:
Balsam Fir, Black Spruce, Copaiba, Eucalyptus globulus, Eucalyptus radiata, Hyssop, Laurus nobilis, Lavender, Lemon, Lemongrass, Marjoram, Melaleuca alternifolia, Melissa, Myrtle, Oregano, Peppermint, Rosemary, Thyme

CRUCIATE LIGAMENT INJURY
(See also PAIN MANAGEMENT)

A Cruciate injury can generally be categorized into two different types; partial tears and total tears. With a partial tear of the ligament, often natural protocols can result in great healing and pain control. Full tears may still require a surgical correction. Accurate diagnosis is very important. In general, I will allow up to 3 months of natural remedies and treatments before deciding if surgery will be a necessary course of action. For very severe total tears, or for knee injuries with significant cartilage damage, sometimes surgery is best performed right away. Many people who fail at healing this condition, have not used adequate amounts of supplements or oils. Restriction or budgeting of supplements, is greatly discouraged if you would like the best results.

FIRST LINE RECOMMENDATIONS:
ORAL: Copaiba
PETTING: Daily to 3 times a day to knee. With any of the recommended oils, or with diluted Three Part Blends.

Single Oils:
Balsam Fir, Black Spruce, Copaiba, Frankincense, Helichrysum, Lavender, Lemongrass, Marjoram, Peppermint

CRYPTORCHID
(See TESTICLE - UNDESCENDED)

CUSHING'S DISEASE

FIRST LINE RECOMMENDATIONS:
CANINE SUPPORTIVE BLEND: apply as needed, often every 1-7 days. Addition of oils to support the adrenal and endocrine systems are suggested.
WATER DIFFUSION: of Three Part Blends, especially of oils that support hormones, the endocrine system, and stress relief.
ORAL: In the past, Frankincense, Fennel, and Clary Sage in the morning along with Balsam Fir and Copaiba given at night was suggested via oral dosing. While these oils are still recommended, and have great support for Cushing's - oral use is not absolutely necessary. It can be considered for severe and unresponsive cases, but use of these oils within topical blends or through water-based diffusion appears just as effective in most cases, and is more tolerated. Copaiba orally, may be valuable for some cases – and is suggested twice a day in foods when desired.

Single Oils:
Balsam Fir, Black Spruce, Clary Sage, Fennel, Frankincense, Helichrysum, Juniper, Ledum, Myrrh, Nutmeg

CUTS
(See LACERATIONS)

DEMODEX
(See also SKIN INFECTIONS)

Demodex is a mite that lives and reproduces in the hair follicle. It is not contagious, and is largely related to a poor immune system. If secondary skin infections are present, it is very important that they are treated as well. Often secondary infections are overlooked while treating this condition.

FIRST LINE RECOMMENDATIONS:
TOPICAL: diluted Three Part Blends, addition of Three Part Blends to natural ointments and salves. Apply to severely affected areas.
CANINE SUPPORTIVE BLEND: If the skin will tolerate it, generally daily to weekly application with the inclusion of oils such as Melissa, Catnip, and Black Spruce.
BATHING: Add Three Part Blends to natural shampoo.

Single Oils:
Black Spruce, Catnip, Citronella, Clove, Eucalyptus citriodora, Eucalyptus globulus, Eucalyptus radiata, Geranium, Helichrysum, Lavender, Melaleuca alternifolia, Rosemary, Palmarosa, Peppermint

DENTAL DISEASE

FIRST LINE RECOMMENDATIONS:
DRINKING WATER: Copaiba, Peppermint
ORAL: Brushing teeth with toothpastes or wiping with Three Part Blends added to oral care products daily.
TOPICAL: diluted Three Part Blends can be rubbed onto an area of need directly.

Single Oils:
Clove, Copaiba, Helichrysum, Laurus nobilis, Melaleuca alternifolia, Myrrh, Peppermint

DETOXIFICATION
(See VACCINOSIS)

Detoxification from any situation will be similar to the detoxification desired and described within the issue of Vaccinosis.

DEWORMING

FIRST LINE RECOMMENDATIONS:
CANINE SUPPORTIVE BLEND: Support of the body and strong immune system is key in keeping worms under control.
ORAL: diluted Three Part Blends may be considered for some parasitic situations.

Single Oils:
Cinnamon, Clove, Copaiba, Hyssop, Lemon, Lemongrass, Melaleuca alternifolia, Nutmeg, Oregano, Peppermint, Tarragon, Thyme

DIABETES MELLITUS

FIRST LINE RECOMMENDATIONS:
CANINE SUPPORTIVE BLEND: modify including oils such as Spearmint, Dill, or Fennel.

Single Oils:
Black Cumin, Cinnamon, Coriander, Dill, Fennel, Geranium, Myrrh, Spearmint, Ylang Ylang

DIARRHEA
(See also INFLAMMATORY BOWEL DISEASE)

In conditions of diarrhea, a fast is often the recommended starting point. Please consult with a veterinarian, however offering no food (water is generally okay if no vomiting is present) for approximately 24 hours is the best start to ending a cycle of diarrhea. If a dog is lethargic, vomiting, or acting abnormal in any other way, a veterinary exam is suggested immediately. When food is re-introduced after the fast, very small amounts of a bland diet should be given every 1-3 hours. Any food, meals, or supplements that are introduced too quickly to a dog suffering from diarrhea, will only encourage the condition.

FIRST LINE RECOMMENDATIONS:
ORAL: digestive Three Part Blends
PETTING: diluted digestive Three Part Blends

Single Oils:
Anise, Clove, Copaiba, Fennel, Ginger, Lemon, Lemongrass, Marjoram, Oregano, Peppermint, Spearmint, Tarragon, Thyme, Vetiver

DISTEMPER
(See RABIES, VACCINOSIS, and VIRAL CONDITIONS)

DRY EYE
(See also AUTOIMMUNE CONDITIONS, EYE CONDITIONS)

Dry Eye is a condition where not enough tears are produced by the tear glands. This often is related to an autoimmune process within the body. Hydration is of major importance, and adding additional water to every meal the dog eats is suggested. No dry kibble should be fed, without it being completely soaked in water.

FIRST LINE RECOMMENDATIONS:
See recommendations for Autoimmune Conditions, Cornea, and Eye Conditions.

WATER MISTING: Lavender Eye Spritzer as needed for comfort. See Essential Oils & Eyes for more information.
CANINE SUPPORTIVE BLEND: apply at least weekly for full body support and hopeful correction of immune mediated issues.

Single Oils:
Helichrysum, Lavender

DYSTOCIA
(See PREGNANCY & DELIVERY)

EAR INFECTIONS
(See also ALLERGIES)

FIRST LINE RECOMMENDATIONS:

Ear Spray Recipe:
- In a 30 mL glass spray bottle, combine the following:
- 7-8 mL of grain alcohol (Everclear)
- 1 Tablespoon of Fractionated Coconut Oil
- 1 drop of Clove Essential Oil
- 2 drops of Melaleuca alternifolia Essential Oil
- 3 drops of Lemongrass Essential Oil
- 4 drops of Copaiba Essential Oil
- 5 drops of Lavender Essential Oil
- Then fill the rest of the bottle with Distilled Water.

Shake well and spray 1-3 pumps into the ear(s), once to twice a day. You are not attempting to fill the ear with solution, and should be coating the skin and ear canal area with the spray. Monitor the ear tissues for any signs of irritation. If irritation occurs, the solution may be diluted further or discontinued and other methods used. Irritation seems rare with this recipe, however alcohol could always be drying or irritating to sensitive dogs. Discontinue use immediately with any sign of redness or irritation.

Single Oils:
Clove, Copaiba, Geranium, Helichrysum, Lavender, Lemongrass, Melaleuca alternifolia, Oregano, Thyme

EMOTIONAL CLEANSING

Emotional Cleansing is very important for almost every aspect of healing, and especially in cases of cancer. Rotational use of various essential oil blends is incredibly helpful. See the chapters Emotional Work with Oils for more information.

FIRST LINE RECOMMENDATIONS:
PETTING: with diluted Three Part Blends for emotions
WATER DIFFUSION: Rotational diffusion of selected Three Part Blends
CANINE SUPPORTIVE BLEND: The body supportive blends can still carry quite a benefit to emotions. Addition of specific oils for emotional work can be considered. Use as often as dictated by the case and the individual animal.

Single Oils:
Bergamot, Black Spruce, Roman Chamomile, German Chamomile, Geranium, Lavender, Lemon, Melissa, Patchouli, Rose, Vetiver, Ylang Ylang

EPILEPSY
(See SEIZURES)

EPULIS - DENTAL
(See also DENTAL DISEASE)

An Epulis is generally a benign overgrowth of gum tissue in the mouth of a dog. Boxer dogs are particularly prone to this disorder, however it occurs in many breeds. They are difficult to resolve once they are present, but healing after resection and prevention of future occurrence are prime objectives.

FIRST LINE RECOMMENDATIONS:
Use recommendations for Dental Disease as well as:
TOPICAL: diluted Three Part Blends can be applied to the gum and epulis directly.
CANINE SUPPORTIVE BLEND: apply at least weekly to help support normal function of the body

Single Oils:
Copaiba, Frankincense, Helichrysum, Myrrh

EYE CONDITIONS
(See also CORNEA, DRY EYE)

In general, any eye condition can benefit from good nutrition and a broad spectrum use of essential oils The Lavender Eye Spritzer does provide a huge amount of benefits to any eye condition, and is a general starting recommendation.

FIRST LINE RECOMMENDATIONS:
WATER MISTING: Lavender Eye Spritzer. See Essential Oils & Eyes for more information.
WATER DIFFUSION: Any suggested oil diffused via tenting will contact the cornea and eye tissues during diffusion. This is an easy delivery of essential oils to all eye tissues, and generally any essential oil could be considered for use in this way. For an eye infection, mild antibacterial, antiviral, and antifungal oils can be selected for diffusion.

Single Oils:
Copaiba, Frankincense, Helichrysum, Lavender

FALSE PREGNANCY
(See also EQUINE HORMONAL CONDITIONS)

FIRST LINE RECOMMENDATIONS:
CANINE SUPPORTIVE BLEND: add Clary Sage, apply at least weekly
PETTING: diluted topical use of Three Part Blends including Clary Sage
WATER DIFFUSION: of Three Part Blends containing Clary Sage, Ylang Ylang

Single Oils:
Clary Sage, Geranium, Myrtle, Vetiver, Ylang Ylang

FLEAS

Fleas are one of the most difficult parasites to eliminate. Often many multiple layers of prevention are needed. All animals in the household must be treated for fleas, not just one or two.

FIRST LINE RECOMMENDATIONS:
DIFFUSION: See the description for Pepper (Black), for directions for a household Flea Bomb Recipe.
CANINE SUPPORTIVE BLEND: Apply up to once a day in severe situations, and at least weekly for maintenance. Frequency of application can be based on the response and needs of the individual animal. Modifications can be made by including additional insect repelling oils – especially Catnip and Eucalyptus citriodora. Fleas dislike many of the oils within the Canine Supportive Blend, and the blend also strengthens the immune system which makes dogs less attractive to flea infestation.
PETTING: with diluted Three Part Blends. The Feline Supportive Blend can also be used, with modifications to add Catnip and other repellent oils.
BATHING: Bathe with the addition of Three Part Blends to shampoos.

Single Oils:
Catnip, Citronella, Eucalyptus citriodora, Geranium, Lavender, Lemongrass, Melaleuca alternifolia, Melissa, Orange, Oregano, Pepper (Black,) Peppermint, Rosemary

FLU
(See VIRAL CONDITIONS)

FOREIGN BODY - GASTROINTESTINAL

Veterinary attention is very important when a foreign object is suspected within the gastrointestinal system. These suggestions can decrease inflammation and allow the intestinal tract to function more effectively, however should never replace surgery when truly indicated. After a surgical procedure, use of the oils can aid in healing and return to function sooner.

FIRST LINE RECOMMENDATIONS:
PETTING: of diluted digestive Three Part Blends
DIFFUSION: of digestive Three Part Blends
ORAL: digestive Three Part Blends can be considered for oral use when necessary and indicated.

Single Oils:
Anise, Copaiba, Ginger, Helichrysum, Lavender, Marjoram, Peppermint, Vetiver

GALL BLADDER

FIRST LINE RECOMMENDATIONS:
PETTING: diluted Three Part Blends
CANINE SUPPORTIVE BLEND: apply as needed, additional oils stated below may be added.

Single Oils:
Copaiba, Geranium, Helichrysum, Ledum, Lemon, Peppermint, Spearmint

GASTRIC ULCERS

FIRST LINE RECOMMENDATIONS:
ORAL: Copaiba
PETTING: diluted digestive Three Part Blends
CANINE SUPPORTIVE BLEND: support of the entire body is helpful, addition of oils to support ulcers and healing is recommended.

Single Oils:
   Copaiba, Clove, Helichrysum, Nutmeg, Peppermint

GASTRODILITATION VOLVULUS

This is an incredibly serious condition and requires immediate and emergency veterinary attention. Use of the recommendations can aid in supporting the patient, increase circulation to damaged tissues, and speed healing times from surgical procedures. Prevention of the disorder focuses on feeding wet and soaked foods, and providing support and nutrition towards healthy ligaments and connective tissues.

FIRST LINE RECOMMENDATIONS:
   During an Emergency Situation:
   INHALATION: Rose and Frankincense as life force enhancing oils.
   PETTING: Rose, Frankincense, Helichrysum

   For Post-Surgical Healing:
   PETTING: diluted Three Part Blends especially containing Helichrysum
   ORAL: See also Pain Management

   For Prevention Measures:
   CANINE SUPPORTIVE BLEND: use regularly to support health

Single Oils:
   Copaiba, Cypress, Frankincense, Helichrysum, Lavender, Lemongrass, Rose, Tarragon

GDV
   (See GASTRODILITATION VOLVULUS)

GIARDIA
(See also DIARRHEA)

FIRST LINE RECOMMENDATIONS:
CANINE SUPPORTIVE BLEND: with additional digestive supportive oils, apply as needed for response and symptom control.
ORAL: Copaiba, Clove

Single Oils:
Clove, Copaiba, Lemon, Melaleuca alternifolia, Nutmeg, Oregano, Peppermint, Tarragon, Thyme, Vetiver

GLAUCOMA
(See also EYE CONDITIONS)

FIRST LINE RECOMMENDATIONS:
WATER MISTING: Therapeutic Eye Spritzer to general eye area, 2-3 times a day or as needed for individual animal.
PETTING: With any of the suggested oils, diluted within Three Part Blends
CANINE SUPPORTIVE BLEND: apply regularly for health support, consider addition of oils for primary health concerns which may be present

Single Oils:
Copaiba, Helichrysum, Lavender, Ledum

HEAD TILT
(See VESTIBULAR DISEASE, NEUROLOGIC CONDITIONS)

HEART DISEASE

FIRST LINE RECOMMENDATIONS:
PETTING: of diluted Three Part Blends
DIFFUSION: of Three Part Blends
ORAL: Copaiba
CANINE SUPPORTIVE BLEND: apply regularly with additions of oils such as May Chang, Ylang Ylang

Single Oils:
Cistus, Copaiba, Cinnamon, Clove, Helichrysum, Marjoram, May Chang, Nutmeg, Orange, Rose, Spikenard, Thyme, Ylang Ylang

HEARTWORM PREVENTION

It is important to recognize that a healthy immune system, as well as lowering your dogs' exposure to mosquitos, is the best prevention for heartworm that I can recommend. Many essential oils help with both of these aspects, and while there may be some direct evidence that essential oils can kill a variety of parasites, the use of essential oils is not consistent enough to rely on them 100% as a replacement for traditional veterinary medications. While we have documented decreases in microfilaria (baby heartworm) numbers within the blood stream in response to essential oil use, we have not documented full prevention measures.

FIRST LINE RECOMMENDATIONS:
PETTING or TOPICAL: diluted Three Part Blends for insect repelling activity. Use as needed.
CANINE SUPPORTIVE BLEND: apply weekly to monthly for health, immune support, insect repelling properties, as well as potential heartworm control. Consider addition of Catnip.
WATER MISTING: With insect repelling oils added to water or with various bug spray recipes. Use as needed.

Single Oils:
Anise, Balsam Fir, Black Cumin, Catnip, Cinnamon, Copaiba, Eucalyptus citriodora, Fennel, Helichrysum, Melaleuca alternifolia, Nutmeg, Oregano, Sage, Tarragon, Thyme

HEARTWORM DISEASE
(See also HEART DISEASE)

In the past, we had known of several well documented cases of essential oil use helping to eradicate severe heartworm infection in dogs. One such documentation, from a University Veterinary Teaching Hospital, included thorough testing and evaluation, including an echocardiogram. The University had established a very guarded prognosis, where the dog would likely die with or without surgical removal of the heartworms. The dog went home, and proceeded to use a fairly aggressive protocol of essential oil administration. A negative heartworm status was achieved by this dog, and considering the severe nature of the infection, the protocol was far superior to traditional heartworm treatment.

After this book was originally written, I myself rescued a dog from the Oklahoma tornadoes in 2013. Upon bringing her back to Minnesota, we found that she was heartworm positive. It also just so happened at this same time, that the traditional veterinary drug to treat heartworm was unavailable, and only being obtained for severe cases of heartworm. My dog Babe, did not qualify. As Babe had never been treated with any sort of preventive, medication, or even dewormer – I decided that there would be "no time like the present" to embark on my own personal documentation of a slow kill heartworm protocol. Babe did convert totally to a negative status, and what we learned along the way showed that consistent support, in lower concentrations than we thought necessary, were the most effective.

Long term use (4-6 months or more) of essential oil support seems likely to be necessary, and conversion to a negative heartworm test is also not expected for 4-6 months, although it can occur sooner. Slowly killing the heartworm is important. Many times we would treat for a week to a month, and then take 1-3 months off of any oral dosing. Topical applications and mosquito prevention were still used, along with other holistic support including great diet and whole food supplements.

Careful monitoring with a veterinarian is important, and screening and monitoring for microfilaria (via a Knott's Test) within the blood stream during treatment, is suggested to be coordinated with a veterinarian.

FIRST LINE RECOMMENDATIONS:
The following recommendations would be used for most sized dogs.

ORAL HEARTWORM BLEND: Make the recipe for the Feline Supportive Blend, adding the additional oils of Black Cumin, Melaleuca alternifolia, Clove, Cinnamon Leaf, Anise, Fennel, and Sage (also in equal parts). Dilute to a beginning concentration of 5%. The oral use of this blend should be carefully monitored - and used conservatively, with breaks in between.

Week one give one drop of the heartworm solution in food twice a day. Monitor responses with your vet (including microfilaria counts), and decide if week two will be an "off week" with no oils given, or you will increase to two drops twice a day. Based on responses, you and your vet should determine if you will move forward with a higher dose, or take time off. For some very large dogs, your vet may also determine that they would like to stay with more drops twice a day as well. This is where the art of medicine requires your vet's input. Sometimes we determine we want to be more aggressive, and sometimes we determine we should allow the body to take a break.

For Babe, I could distinctly notice a "kill" event within 5 days of starting her oral regimens at certain doses. And for her, continuing topical therapies, oral anti-inflammatory oils, and diffusion (along with supplements and great diet) - but taking a break from oral use of her heartworm active blends - was the most appropriate course of action for her. She often would take a month off in between more aggressive protocols. Oddly enough, our heartworm blends that were more diluted, were generally better absorbed, better tolerated, and more effective than when we administered capsules and "stronger" protocols.

ORAL: for anti-inflammatory support for the heart, Copaiba should be given orally twice a day or as directed by your veterinarian.

CANINE SUPPORTIVE BLEND: topical applications are recommended weekly to monthly for general support and healing, but can be used even daily when indicated by response and need. This blend is also beneficial as an antibacterial agent for the potential Wolbachia bacteria that is potentially released from the dying heartworm. This blend can also aid in repelling insects, as well as in support of heart damage or other symptoms of heartworm "die off." Additional oils to support the heart or insect repellency can be added to the blend – such as Cistus,

May Chang, Catnip, or others. At one point in Babe's therapy, she developed an allergic bronchitis response to "die off" – in this situation the use of this blend with the addition of Melissa for antihistamine type benefits was used.

WATER DIFFUSION: Diffusion of any Three Part Blend you desire can add an additional layer of health support. Symptoms such as cough, or heart disease, can also be supported with the diffusion of oils selected for specific situations and needs.

Single Oils:
Anise, Balsam Fir, Black Cumin, Black Spruce, Catnip, Cistus, Clove, Cinnamon Bark, Cinnamon Leaf, Clove, Copaiba, Fennel, Helichrysum, May Chang, Melaleuca alternifolia, Melissa, Peppermint, Oregano, Sage, Tarragon, Thyme, Ylang Ylang

HEAT STROKE
(See HYPERTHERMIA)

HEMANGIOSARCOMA
(See CANCER – SPLEEN, HEMORRHAGE - INTERNAL)

HEMOABDOMEN
(See HEMORRHAGE - INTERNAL)

HEMORRHAGE - INTERNAL

FIRST LINE RECOMMENDATIONS:
ORAL: Cistus

Single Oils:
Cistus, Geranium, Helichrysum

HISTIOCYTOMA

FIRST LINE RECOMMENDATIONS:
TOPICAL: Frankincense, Copaiba, and Peppermint applied to the lump, sometimes neat. Tumors may look worse before better. Some dogs may require dilution. Apply as frequently as tolerated and indicated by the individual. Usually between every 1-7 days. If the tumor responds well to one application, spacing apart the applications is more likely.
CANINE SUPPORTIVE BLEND: add Frankincense, apply every 1-7 days.

Single Oils:
Copaiba, Frankincense, Lavender, Peppermint, Sandalwood

HORNER'S SYNDROME
(See BELL'S PALSY)

HOT SPOTS
(See also ALLERGIES, SKIN INFECTIONS)

The use of ointments is often discouraged with Hot Spots as they are a moist condition in need of drying. Clipping the wound and using techniques that allow the tissues to dry out is suggested.

FIRST LINE RECOMMENDATIONS:
WATER MISTER: Skin Spray Recipe – Add 8 drops of Copaiba, 14 drops of Lavender, and 10 drops of Melaleuca alternifolia to 4 ounces (120 mL) of distilled water, in a glass spray bottle. Shake well and spray skin as needed, generally 1-4 times a day.
TOPICAL: Hot Spots are usually moist in nature, so essential oils diluted in carrier oils, ointments, or salves may not be indicated when drying actions are desired.
BATHING: Wash the area thoroughly with natural soaps, shampoos or washes containing essential oils.

Single Oils:
Copaiba, Geranium, Helichrysum, Lavender, Myrrh, Palmarosa

HYPERADRENOCORTICISM
(See CUSHING'S DISEASE)

HYPERTHERMIA – EXERCISE INDUCED, HEAT STROKE

FIRST LINE RECOMMENDATIONS:
TOPICAL: diluted Peppermint to ear flaps, foot pads, feet, and over femoral artery – can be used due to severity of the situation. Repeat as needed.
WATER MIST: a water mist containing Peppermint can also be used over the feet or groin and stomach areas to enhance cooling.
ORAL: diluted Peppermint directly into the mouth if needed.
WATER DIFFUSION: of blends containing Peppermint can be cooling.
DRINKING WATER: Peppermint

Single Oils:
Frankincense, Helichrysum, Lavender, Peppermint

HYPOGLYCEMIA

FIRST LINE RECOMMENDATIONS:
Give oral substances containing sugars every 10-15 minutes or as needed to stabilize blood sugar (often recommended is Karo Syrup). Make sure the dog can swallow adequately and seek medical attention.
TOPICAL: Apply diluted Three Part Blends as needed. Blends for nausea may be helpful to stimulate eating.
INHALATION: Whiffs of stimulating, and life force oils such as Peppermint and Rose can stimulate a young dog.

Single Oils:
Dill, Frankincense, Peppermint, Rose

HYPOTHYROIDISM

Elimination of household chemicals and of the drinking of common tap water is highly recommended in cases of Hypothyroidism. Monitoring with a veterinarian is important, and an adjustment of doses based on response is recommended.

FIRST LINE RECOMMENDATIONS:
CANINE SUPPORTIVE BLEND: apply as needed, at least weekly, with additions of thyroid benefiting oils such as Myrtle
WATER DIFFUSION: of Three Part Blends containing thyroid benefiting oils.
PETTING: diluted Three Part Blends containing Myrtle over thyroid area at least daily.
DRINKING WATER: Spearmint

Single Oils:
Lemongrass, Myrrh, Myrtle, Spearmint

IBD
(See INFLAMMATORY BOWEL DISEASE)

IMHA
(See IMMUNE MEDIATED HEMOLYTIC ANEMIA)

IMMUNE MEDIATED HEMOLYTIC ANEMIA
(See also AUTOIMMUNE CONDITIONS)

FIRST LINE RECOMMENDATIONS:
Use the recommendations for Autoimmune Conditions, as well as these specific suggestions.
CANINE SUPPORTIVE BLEND: Modify by adding Black Spruce and Balsam Fir for added cortisone-like benefits, also include Cistus and Helichrysum. Apply up to daily, based on response and need.

Single Oils:
Balsam Fir, Black Spruce, Cistus, Copaiba, Helichrysum

INCONTINENCE - URINARY

FIRST LINE RECOMMENDATIONS:
ORAL: Copaiba
CANINE SUPPORTIVE BLEND: apply regularly; consider addition of Juniper and Clary Sage

Single Oils:
Clary Sage, Copaiba, Helichrysum, Juniper, Lemongrass, Marjoram

INFLAMMATORY BOWEL DISEASE
(See also DIARRHEA)

FIRST LINE RECOMMENDATIONS:
CANINE SUPPORTIVE BLEND: addition of GI supportive oils, apply as needed, at least weekly for full body support
ORAL: The Canine Supportive Blend can be added to food if needed for severe bacterial overgrowth or painful bowels. Start with one drop twice a day per 25 pounds (12 kg).
DRINKING WATER: Copaiba
PETTING: diluted digestive Three Part Blends

Single Oils:
Anise, Balsam Fir, Black Spruce, Copaiba, Fennel, Ginger, Helichrysum, Lemon, Nutmeg, Oregano, Peppermint, Tarragon, Thyme, Vetiver

INFLUENZA
(See VIRAL CONDITIONS)

INTERNAL HEMORRHAGE
(See HEMORRHAGE - INTERNAL)

IVDD
(See INTERVERTEBRAL DISC DISEASE)

INTERVERTEBRAL DISC DISEASE
(See also PAIN MANAGEMENT)

FIRST LINE RECOMMENDATIONS:
CANINE SUPPORTIVE BLEND: addition of Lemongrass, Balsam Fir. Apply up to daily as indicated by the response and individual.
ORAL: See Pain Management for techniques for severe pain. Copaiba is recommended for general use.

Single Oils:
Balsam Fir, Black Spruce, Chamomile (Roman), Copaiba, Helichrysum, Juniper, Laurus nobilis, Lavender, Lemongrass, Marjoram, Nutmeg, Peppermint, Rosemary

INTESTINAL CONDITIONS
(See also DIARRHEA, VOMITING, DEWORMING, INFLAMMATORY BOWEL DISEASE)

KCS
(See DRY EYE)

KENNEL COUGH

FIRST LINE RECOMMENDATIONS:
WATER DIFFUSION: With tenting or caging for 20 minutes, 3-4 times a day. Adjust as needed for individuals. Use respiratory Three Part Blends, especially containing Copaiba.
DIFFUSION: Open Room; up to 24 hours a day with Three Part Blends for respiratory needs. Other oils may be selected for general disinfecting and reduction of transmission.
CANINE SUPPORTIVE BLEND: Up to daily, or as needed. Additional oils may be added.
ORAL: Copaiba may be helpful for additional inflammation reduction
CLEANING: Natural cleaners containing essential oils

Single Oils:
Black Spruce, Eucalyptus globulus, Eucalyptus radiata, Hyssop, Laurus nobilis, Lavender, Lemon, Lemongrass, Marjoram, Melaleuca alternifolia, Melaleuca ericifolia, Melissa, Myrtle, Oregano, Peppermint, Rosemary

KERATOCONJUNCTIVITIS SICCA
(See DRY EYE)

KIDNEY DISEASE

FIRST LINE RECOMMENDATIONS:
CANINE SUPPORTIVE BLEND: apply regularly, at least weekly. Addition of Juniper and Black Cumin.
PETTING: Over Kidney area; diluted Three Part Blends especially containing Juniper, Helichrysum, or any suggested oil.
ORAL: Helichrysum or other suggested oils in severe situations.

Single Oils:
Black Cumin, Copaiba, Grapefruit, Helichrysum, Juniper, Ledum, Lemongrass

KNEE CAP
(See PATELLA - LUXATING)

LACERATIONS

FIRST LINE RECOMMENDATIONS:
TOPICAL: natural ointments or salves can be made, especially with Helichrysum, Lavender, and Myrrh added. If a recipe is recommended for use in or on wounds, then the addition of essential oils in a 1-5% concentration is fine. When stitches are present, direct application of neat oils to the stitch material is generally avoided – however in a water mist, or with dilution the essential oils will not damage the sutures.
WATER MISTING: water mists created including oils such as Helichrysum, Myrrh, and Lavender can aid in healing wounds.

Single Oils:
Cistus, Copaiba, Frankincense, Geranium, Helichrysum, Lavender, Melaleuca alternifolia, Myrrh, Palmarosa, Patchouli

LACTATION

FIRST LINE RECOMMENDATIONS:
CANINE SUPPORTIVE BLEND: use with addition of Fennel
PETTING: With any of the suggested oils, although Fennel is a primary selection. This can begin prior to birthing, or be used when increases in milk supply is desired.
WATER DIFFUSION: Three Part Blends
ORAL: Fennel can also be added to foods to increase milk supply.

Single Oils:
Black Spruce, Celery Seed, Clary Sage, Fennel

LARYNGEAL PARALYSIS
(See also COUGH, NEUROLOGIC CONDITIONS)

FIRST LINE RECOMMENDATIONS:
CANINE SUPPORTIVE BLEND: addition of neurologic and inflammatory supportive oils is suggested, apply as needed, even daily
WATER DIFFUSION: of respiratory, neurologic, and anti-inflammatory oil properties in Three Part Blends
PETTING: diluted Three Part Blends especially containing Helichrysum, Roman Chamomile, Copaiba over throat area daily.
ORAL: Copaiba

Single Oils:
Chamomile (Roman), Copaiba, Geranium, Helichrysum, Juniper, Laurus nobilis, Lemongrass, Marjoram

LENTICULAR SCLEROSIS
(See also CATARACTS, EYE CONDITIONS)

FIRST LINE RECOMMENDATIONS:
CANINE SUPPORTIVE BLEND: with addition of Frankincense. Apply at least weekly.
WATER MISTING: Therapeutic Eye Spritzer; mist face area daily to twice a day. It is not important that this solution contact the inner eye or cornea. Petting applications may be substituted.

Single Oils:
Frankincense, Helichrysum

LICK GRANULOMA
(See also ALLERGIES, SKIN INFECTIONS)

These lesions are incredibly frustrating and can have a variety of reasons for their occurrence. Deep infections (either bacterial or fungal), neuralgia (nerve pain), injury, cancer, arthritis, and many other conditions can promote this disorder. Trying a variety of essential oils to see which provide the best responses is recommended. In some cases, oils can be applied to lesions in their neat form. Mixing with natural ointments can be helpful when applied sparingly, however some animals enjoy the flavor or will lick items off of the wound even more. If licking is increased with applications, discontinue its use, and try a different approach or oil.

FIRST LINE RECOMMENDATIONS:
CANINE SUPPORTIVE BLEND: apply regularly, at least weekly and sometimes daily, as needed. This blend may be applied directly to the wound if needed and helpful. Addition of oils such as Melissa, Myrrh, and Frankincense can be considered as well as others.
TOPICAL: Spikenard, Helichrysum, and any other suggested oil to the lesion 1-4 times a day or as needed. The Ear Spray Recipe featured in Ear Infections is also a wonderful spray for these lesions.
WATER MIST: Some wounds do better with oils diluted within water, and spritzed onto them. This reduces the excess moisture that can be present from ointments or salves.

Single Oils:
Black Spruce, Chamomile (Roman), Frankincense, Geranium, Helichrysum, Juniper, Laurus nobilis, Lavender, Lemongrass, Marjoram, Melaleuca alternifolia, Melaleuca ericifolia, Melissa, Myrrh, Nutmeg, Oregano, Patchouli, Rose, Spikenard, Valerian, Vetiver, Ylang Ylang

LIPOMA

FIRST LINE RECOMMENDATIONS:
CANINE SUPPORTIVE BLEND: regular use of this blend, with addition of oils such as Frankincense, Grapefruit, and Tangerine can help support the body to utilize fats properly. Other oils for metabolism can also be considered. This blend can be used on the lump itself as well as applied along the spine. Both locations are often suggested.
TOPICAL: Massage of the lump daily to four times a day with diluted Three Part Blends especially containing Frankincense, Lemon, and Lemongrass is suggested. Gradually build up in the concentration of oils added to the massage oil based on tolerance. Some owners shave the lump for ease of application. This is a long term problem, and shrinkage of the lump is not expected for several months.
ORAL: Citrus oils have been added to drinking water or foods

Single Oils:
Copaiba, Frankincense, Grapefruit, Ledum, Lemon, Lemongrass, Orange, Tangerine

LIVER DISEASE

FIRST LINE RECOMMENDATIONS:
CANINE SUPPORTIVE BLEND: with addition of Ledum, German Chamomile, apply as needed for symptoms.
ORAL: Helichrysum, Copaiba
PETTING: diluted Three Part Blends, especially containing Ledum and Helichrysum

Single Oils:
Chamomile (German), Chamomile (Roman), Geranium, Grapefruit, Helichrysum, Juniper, Ledum, Myrrh, Myrtle, Nutmeg, Rosemary, Spearmint, Tangerine

LIVER SHUNT
(See also LIVER DISEASE)

FIRST LINE RECOMMENDATIONS:
CANINE SUPPORTIVE BLEND: with addition of Ledum, German Chamomile, apply at least weekly, and as needed for symptoms.
PETTING: diluted Three Part Blends including Helichrysum, Ledum
ORAL: Helichrysum, Copaiba in foods

Single Oils:
Chamomile (Roman), Chamomile (German), Geranium, Grapefruit, Helichrysum, Juniper, Ledum, Lemongrass, Myrtle, Nutmeg, Rosemary, Spearmint, Tangerine

LUPUS
(See AUTOIMMUNE CONDITIONS)

LUXATING PATELLA
(See PATELLA - LUXATING)

LYME DISEASE
(See TICK BORNE DISEASE)

LYMPH NODES - LYMPHADENOPATHY
(See also CANCER - LYMPHOSARCOMA)

FIRST LINE RECOMMENDATIONS:
CANINE SUPPORTIVE BLEND: Apply up to once a day, possibly including application to the Lymph Nodes. Additional oils such as Grapefruit, Frankincense.
TOPICAL: diluted Three Part Blends to lymph nodes
ORAL: Copaiba, Frankincense

Single Oils:
Copaiba, Cypress, Frankincense, Grapefruit, Lemon, Lemongrass, Melissa

LYMPHOMA
(See CANCER - LYMPHOSARCOMA)

LYMPHOSARCOMA
(See CANCER - LYMPHOSARCOMA)

MALDIGESTION
(See also DIARRHEA, INFLAMMATORY BOWEL DISEASE, VOMITING, PANCREATIC INSUFFICIENCY)

FIRST LINE RECOMMENDATIONS:
CANINE SUPPORTIVE BLEND: with addition of Ginger, Anise
ORAL: diluted Three Part Blends
DRINKING WATER: Copaiba

Single Oils:
Anise, Copaiba, Fennel, Geranium, Ginger, Helichrysum, Juniper, Lemon, Peppermint, Tangerine, Tarragon

MAST CELL TUMORS
(See also CANCER)

FIRST LINE RECOMMENDATIONS:
TOPICAL: Neat application of Frankincense to Mast Cell Tumors has been helpful in some situations. Some dogs may require dilution or lesser applications if they are very sensitive. Tumors often look worse before they look better. Frankincense within Three Part Blends of other anti-tumoral oils, is even more synergistic in action.
ORAL: Melissa essential oil can be used for antihistamine effects.
CANINE SUPPORTIVE BLEND: Modify with the addition of Frankincense and Melissa. Apply as indicated for the individual, usually once a week or more. Inclusion of any other indicated oils is suggested, and rotation of oils included is also recommended. This blend can also be applied directly to the Mast Cell Tumors.
WATER DIFFUSION: Diffusion of any of the Three Part Blends for emotion, anti-cancer, or immune support is recommended in rotation.

Single Oils:
Basil, Copaiba, Frankincense, Grapefruit, Helichrysum, Lavender, Lemon, Melissa, Orange, Oregano, Sandalwood, Tangerine, Thyme

MASTICATORY MUSCLE MYOSITIS
(See also AUTOIMMUNE CONDITIONS)

FIRST LINE RECOMMENDATIONS:
CANINE SUPPORTIVE BLEND: Daily to twice daily for 7 days, then every other day for 10 days, then gradually reduce the frequency of applications based on how the individual responds. Including additional oils such as Frankincense, Melissa, and Black Spruce is suggested.
ORAL: Copaiba twice a day in foods

Single Oils:
   Balsam Fir, Black Spruce, Copaiba, Frankincense, Helichrysum, Lavender, Marjoram, Melissa, Vetiver

MASTITIS

FIRST LINE RECOMMENDATIONS:
   TOPICAL: diluted Three Part Blends containing recommended oils can be massaged into the mammary area 1-4 times a day.
   ORAL: Oregano can be considered orally for antibiotic action if needed. Alternately, the Canine Supportive Blend can also be added to foods.
   CANINE SUPPORTIVE BLEND: apply to the entire spine, and can be rubbed as well onto the mammary areas.

Single Oils:
   Copaiba, Cypress, Geranium, Helichrysum, Lavender, Melaleuca alternifolia, Melaleuca ericifolia, Myrrh, Oregano, Thyme

MEGAESOPHAGUS
(See also RESPIRATORY INFECTIONS, COUGH)

FIRST LINE RECOMMENDATIONS:
   CANINE SUPPORTIVE BLEND: with additional gastrointestinal supportive oils. Consider oils such as Ginger, Roman Chamomile - or other selected oils on a rotational basis. Apply as frequently as indicated by the individual, usually weekly to monthly in maintenance situations.
   TOPICAL: diluted applications of digestive Three Part Blends as needed
   WATER DIFFUSION: of digestive Three Part Blends or other indicated oils can also be helpful.
   ORAL: Copaiba, Ginger, Peppermint can be considered for additional aid

Single Oils:
   Anise, Chamomile (Roman), Copaiba, Fennel, Ginger, Helichrysum, Juniper, Laurus nobilis, Lavender, Marjoram, Peppermint, Tarragon

MUSCLE WASTING

Muscle Wasting or Sarcopenia, is common in older dogs and consists of the loss of muscle and condition. Some cases are caused by lack of innervation or from reduced use of the muscles due to pain. Dogs may experience this condition through chronic lack of digestive enzymes, resulting in nutritional deficiency. Digestive enzymes are a mainstay in the repair and prevention of this condition, as can be raw and species appropriate diets.

FIRST LINE RECOMMENDATIONS:
CANINE SUPPORTIVE BLEND: should be applied regularly as a part of balanced health. Additional oils can be added for nerve health or other issues noted with an individual.
PETTING: with diluted Three Part Blends especially containing Lavender, Marjoram

Single Oils:
Copaiba, Helichrysum, Lavender, Marjoram

NEUROLOGIC CONDITIONS

FIRST LINE RECOMMENDATIONS:
CANINE SUPPORTIVE BLEND: apply as needed, consider adding additional supportive oils such as Frankincense and Melissa.
WATER DIFFUSION: of Three Part Blends containing beneficial oils

Single Oils:
Chamomile (Roman), Copaiba, Geranium, Frankincense, Helichrysum, Juniper, Laurus nobilis, Lavender, Melissa, Nutmeg

OBESITY

Obesity can be caused by a lack of nutrients being perceived by the body. When a body perceives that nutrition is lacking, it tried to hold onto any spare energy source (fat) that it can in case of emergency. Digestive enzymes, especially lipase, are also required to "digest away" the fat that is desired to be lost. When animals are in an enzyme deficient state, which is likely occurring in all animals, weight loss is almost impossible to occur.

FIRST LINE RECOMMENDATIONS:
CANINE SUPPORTIVE BLEND: apply at least weekly for full body support. Additional oils may be added as indicated and desired.
WATER DIFFUSION: digestive oils, and those promoting emotional balance or metabolism health can be diffused for additional layers of help.
ORAL: Citrus oils have been added to foods and water
PETTING: diluted Three Part Blends of emotional or indicated oils

Single Oils:
Pepper (Black), Peppermint, Spearmint, Tangerine

OCD
(See BEHAVIORAL CONDITIONS)

ORCHITIS
(See TESTICULAR INFLAMMATION)

OSTEOSARCOMA
(See CANCER - BONE)

PAIN MANAGEMENT

Pain is an important item to address. The presence of pain is not only uncomfortable for an animal, but it will actually suppress the immune system and inhibit healing. All of the recommendations can be used alongside of traditional medications when they are being used. Careful monitoring and care with a veterinarian is recommended to make sure that adequate control of pain is always met.

FIRST LINE RECOMMENDATIONS:
  ORAL: Helichrysum, Copaiba, and Myrrh combination. See oil descriptions for dosing information.
  PETTING: With any oil suggested, as needed.
  CANINE SUPPORTIVE BLEND: apply as needed, for full body support and overall aid in pain support

Single Oils:
  Copaiba, Helichrysum, Lavender, Marjoram, Myrrh, Peppermint

PANCREATIC INSUFFICIENCY
(See also MALDIGESTION)

This disorder is mainly corrected through the supplementation of digestive enzymes, and correct diet. Supporting pancreatic function and the endocrine system is beneficial, as well as is addressing intestinal upset and other underlying issues or conditions.

FIRST LINE RECOMMENDATIONS:
  CANINE SUPPORTIVE BLEND: regular support of the body, including oils to support the digestive system and pancreas is suggested.
  PETTING: diluted Three Part Blends

Single Oils:
  Anise, Copaiba, Geranium, Ginger, Helichrysum, Peppermint, Spearmint, Tarragon

PANCREATITIS
(See also DIARRHEA, PAIN MANAGEMENT, VOMITING)

Pancreatitis is often a severe situation that requires hospital care. Many times dietary change, getting into the garbage, a high fat meal, etc...can cause the pancreas to go into overload, and excrete too many enzymes. The inflammation caused by the enzymes of the pancreas escaping its organ – causes sometimes excruciating pain as the animal's own insides are digested.

FIRST LINE RECOMMENDATIONS:
CANINE SUPPORTIVE BLEND: apply as needed to maintain comfort, addition of digestive supporting oils can be considered.
ORAL: Copaiba, Ginger

Single Oils:
Black Spruce, Copaiba, Geranium, Ginger, Helichrysum, Peppermint, Lavender, Myrrh, Patchouli, Peppermint, Tarragon

PANNUS
(See AUTOIMMUNE CONDITIONS, EYE CONDITIONS)

PANOSTEITIS
(See also BONE CONDITIONS, PAIN MANAGEMENT)

FIRST LINE RECOMMENDATIONS:
PETTING: diluted Three Part Blends especially containing Balsam Fir, Helichrysum, Copaiba over affected area, as needed.
CANINE SUPPORTIVE BLEND: As needed based on response, include additional oils as indicated.
ORAL: Copaiba

Single Oils:
Balsam Fir, Black Spruce, Copaiba, Helichrysum, Lemongrass, Peppermint

PAPILLOMA
(See WARTS)

PARASITES - INTERNAL
(See DEWORMING)

PARVO

(See DIARRHEA, VIRAL CONDITIONS, VOMITING)

Parvo is a virus that causes bloody diarrhea and vomiting, mainly in puppies. Dogs over 1 year of age, generally develop natural immunity. The virus can live in the environment for a very long time, and is resistant to many environmental disinfectants. Parvo often requires hospitalization with intense veterinary care. Do not abandon traditional veterinary treatments, however add in essential oil therapies to increase your outcome. Prevention with these same measures would be wise.

FIRST LINE RECOMMENDATIONS:
CANINE SUPPORTIVE BLEND: Modified by the addition of Melissa, Frankincense, and Ginger. Other oils may be considered and added when needed. Apply daily or more, as indicated by patient.
WATER DIFFUSION: can focus on blends to disinfect the environment, or for gastrointestinal support, anti-viral support, or immune supporting needs. Rotation between several Three Part Blends is a great idea, while continuing diffusion 24 hours a day.
CLEANING: Use of natural cleaners with essential oils added.
PETTING: With diluted Three Part Blends of any of the selected oils, 1-4 times daily. Focus can be placed on gastrointestinal support, immune support, etc. The Canine Supportive Blend is a great way to access all properties.

Single Oils:
Black Spruce, Copaiba, Eucalyptus radiata, Ginger, Hyssop, Lemon, Melaleuca alternifolia, Melissa, Oregano, Patchouli, Peppermint, Tarragon, Thyme

PATELLA - LUXATING

With this condition, the knee cap slips off of its normal position on top of the knee, resulting in abnormal gaits, arthritic pains, as well as degradation of the bone and cartilage. This condition cannot often be reversed from its severe form, due to loss of boney material. Physical Therapy, nutritional supplements, raw diets, and other holistic methods are advancing improvements for dogs diagnosed early in the course of this condition – and essential oils can be a huge synergistic aid. In low grades of luxation, muscles, ligaments, cartilage, and tendons can be improved resulting in less degradation of the condition and less pain. If surgery is necessary, post-surgical healing can be greatly enhanced by the use of essential oils. Even though this condition is not often perceived as painful, I can assure you that inflammation and discomfort are present, and should be addressed.

FIRST LINE RECOMMENDATIONS:
ORAL: Copaiba
PETTING: diluted Three Part Blends over the area of concern as needed, especially containing oils such as Balsam Fir, Copaiba, Lemongrass

Single Oils:
Balsam Fir, Black Spruce, Copaiba, Frankincense, Helichrysum, Lavender, Lemongrass, Marjoram, Peppermint

PEMPHIGUS
(See AUTOIMMUNE CONDITIONS)

PNEUMONIA
(See RESPIRATORY INFECTIONS)

PREGNANCY & DELIVERY

FIRST LINE RECOMMENDATIONS:
WATER DIFFUSION: of Three Part Blends for emotion or delivery. Diffusion can occur in an open room situation from before conception until after birth.
PETTING: of diluted Three Part Blends as needed and indicated, even during delivery.

If painful or stressful birthing occurs, Lavender can be diffused or applied via Petting to relax and reduce stress. After delivery, Frankincense is often used to anoint puppies. See the individual oil description for more information. Myrrh can be applied to umbilical cords as well.

Single Oils:
Chamomile (Roman), Frankincense, Geranium, Helichrysum, Lavender, Myrrh, Rose, Vetiver

PROSTATE CONDITIONS

FIRST LINE RECOMMENDATIONS:
CANINE SUPPORTIVE BLEND: Modify by including other indicated oils. Sage is often considered for prostatic conditions.
ORAL: Copaiba
RECTAL: See Rectal Instillation for more information. Any selected oils could be used in this manner.

Single Oils:
Clary Sage, Copaiba, Frankincense, Helichrysum, Lavender, Myrtle, Oregano, Sage, Thyme, Ylang Ylang

PROSTATITIS
(See PROSTATE CONDITIONS)

Prostatitis is an inflammation of the prostate in male dogs. There are several causes for this condition including bacteria, virus, sexually transmitted diseases, cancer, benign prostatic hyperplasia, and more. If infection is suspected, Oregano or other antibacterial essential oils can be considered orally.

PYOMETRA

Pyometra is a serious bacterial infection of the uterus, that can turn fatal. It is a risk in all unspayed females, especially those who have not given birth. A common form of pyometra is a closed cervix situation, where pus cannot escape the body, and therefore the dog is very ill. The uterus can become very damaged and fragile from the bacterial infection leading to rupture. In an open cervix pyometra, pus can be seen draining from the vulva. The pus can vary in consistency, color, and texture. In most cases, it is very important for the infected uterus to be surgically removed. Only in valuable breeding dogs, are attempts to save the uterus made – often with great difficulty, expense, and poor outcome.

FIRST LINE RECOMMENDATIONS:
    CANINE SUPPORTIVE BLEND: apply as needed, additional oils may be included.
    ORAL: Copaiba
    WATER DIFFUSION: of Three Part Blends or life force oils if situations are critical. Frankincense, Rose, Melissa.

Single Oils:
    Cistus, Copaiba, Eucalyptus radiata, Frankincense, Geranium, Helichrysum, Hyssop, Laurus nobilis, Lavender, Lemon, Lemongrass, Marjoram, Melaleuca alternifolia, Myrrh, Myrtle, Oregano, Thyme

RABIES
(See also VACCINOSIS, VIRAL CONDITIONS)

An entire book could certainly be written on the subject of Rabies, Rabies vaccinations, and the holistic approach to all of these subjects. In brief, we are often held to legal requirements within our communities as to whether or not we are obligated to vaccinate our animals. There are more and more holistic veterinarians consenting to the fact that vaccinations are less and less necessary. When health concerns are noted, many holistic veterinarians will now write a letter of recommendation to your community heads, that future vaccinations (of all sorts) are no longer recommended for your animal. Titers for vaccinations are also more widely accepted, so make sure you do your due diligence and research, and hold your ground if you feel you are being forced or encouraged into a situation which you feel is unhealthy for the animals in your care.

Certainly the decision will have to be a personal one, hopefully guided by a realistic holistic veterinarian by your side. However, if vaccination is deemed necessary, support of the body and "detoxification" from the vaccination is important. The use of a vaccination which is Thimerosal-free (Merial IMRAB 3 TF) is highly recommended.

For animals who are not vaccinated for a variety of diseases, the focus would be creating a competent and healthy immune system. Good nutrition, regular exposure to essential oils, quality supplementation, and regular applications of blends such as the Canine Supportive Blend is recommended.

Symptomatic forms of Rabies will not be discussed due to the controversial nature of the disease, and the nearly almost fatal implications to both animals and humans. What can be said is what I would do for a suspected exposure to Rabies in an animal, or for an animal who was placed under a quarantine situation.

FIRST LINE RECOMMENDATIONS:
For suspected Rabies Exposure:
- CANINE SUPPORTIVE BLEND: With additional oils of Spikenard, Melissa, and Frankincense applied up to daily. Other oils can be considered or added as desired.
- WATER DIFFUSION: of Three Part Blends containing immune supportive, and anti-viral oils. Rotation through several versions of blends is suggested.

Single Oils:
Copaiba, Frankincense, Helichrysum, Hyssop, Melissa, Oregano, Spikenard, Thyme

RESPIRATORY INFECTIONS
(See also KENNEL COUGH, MEGAESOPHAGUS)

Respiratory infections can have many causes – bacterial, fungal, viral. Even allergies, parasitic infections, and cancer can cause the appearance of a lung infection. Having an accurate diagnosis is important in addressing the specific cause of a lung condition. However, the most assuring fact is that a holistic approach to health will truly benefit any lung condition, regardless of the cause.

FIRST LINE RECOMMENDATIONS:
CANINE SUPPORTIVE BLEND: Apply up to daily as needed by the individual. Additional oils can be added as desired.
WATER DIFFUSION: of Three Part Blends for respiratory needs, up to 24 hours a day. Tenting and caging methods can also be utilized with Water Diffusion.

Single Oils:
Balsam Fir, Black Spruce, Cinnamon, Clove, Copaiba, Eucalyptus globulus, Eucalyptus radiata, Hyssop, Laurus nobilis, Lavender, Lemon, Lemongrass, Marjoram, Melaleuca alternifolia, Melaleuca ericifolia, Myrtle, Oregano, Rosemary, Thyme

RINGWORM

FIRST LINE RECOMMENDATIONS:
TOPICAL: Neat Lavender has been applied to lesions once to twice a day. Oils can also be mixed into natural ointments for application. Diluted applications of Three Part Blends is most suggested.
BATHING: With natural shampoo containing essential oils. Most antifungal shampoos are desired at approximately 2% concentration of essential oil.
CANINE SUPPORTIVE BLEND: Apply at least weekly, include other oils as desired. This blend can also be applied to focal lesions.
CLEANING: Wash bedding and other areas and materials in contact with infected individuals often with detergents including essential oils.
WATER MISTING: Can be used on the animal, or on the environment for aide in disinfection.

Single Oils:
Eucalyptus radiata, Geranium, Lavender, Lemongrass, Marjoram, Melaleuca alternifolia, Melaleuca ericifolia, Myrrh, Oregano, Rosemary, Thyme

ROCKY MOUNTAIN SPOTTED FEVER
(See TICK BORNE DISEASE)

SARCOPTIC MANGE
(See also SKIN INFECTIONS)

Sarcoptic Mange is a contagious mite that lives in the skin of dogs. It is often very itchy, and can have secondary skin infections present. Traditional treatments with injectable Ivermectin are often quite effective, and are not associated with as many side effects as the high dose treatments used for

Demodex Mange. Dips and other various forms of treatment are highly toxic, and are not recommended at all. All dogs in contact with an affected dog should be treated, whether or not they show symptoms.

FIRST LINE RECOMMENDATIONS:
CANINE SUPPORTIVE BLEND: Include oils such as Catnip, Eucalyptus citriodora, and Geranium. Apply at least weekly, often daily use may be used initially.
BATHING: add anti-parasitic Three Part Blends to natural shampoos.
PETTING: with diluted topical Three Part Blends
WATER MISTS: can be soothing and calming to the skin, as well as anti-parasitic.

Single Oils:
Black Spruce, Catnip, Citronella, Eucalyptus citriodora, Geranium, Helichrysum, Lavender, Palmarosa, Peppermint

SEBACEOUS CYSTS

FIRST LINE RECOMMENDATIONS:
CANINE SUPPORTIVE BLEND: including oils such as Frankincense and Melissa. Apply at least weekly. This blend may be dripped onto large cysts as well, or the Feline Supportive Blend may also be applied to the cysts.
WATER MISTS: Soothing and supportive water mists containing Copaiba, Lavender, Myrrh, or other skin supportive oils can be used.

Single Oils:
Copaiba, Frankincense, Geranium, Grapefruit, Lavender, Lemon, Myrrh, Myrtle, Orange, Palmarosa, Patchouli, Vetiver

SEBORRHEA - OLEOSA

FIRST LINE RECOMMENDATIONS:
BATHING: add oils to natural shampoos, especially Lavender, Lemon, and other selections that reduce sebum.

Single Oils:
Geranium, Grapefruit, Lavender, Lemon, Myrtle, Orange, Palmarosa, Vetiver

CANINE CONDITIONS

SEIZURES

FIRST LINE RECOMMENDATIONS:
WATER DIFFUSION: rotation between various Three Part Blends including oils for neurologic benefits, especially including Balsam Fir, Helichrysum, and Copaiba up to 24 hours a day.
CANINE SUPPORTIVE BLEND: apply at least weekly for general health, and up to daily when indicated. Include other oils to benefit the neurologic system.
ORAL: Copaiba can be used on a regular basis.
INHALATION: Some find help and relief from a seizure by having the animal sniff an oil directly from the bottle, or very via strong applications on the hands of the human.
PETTING: with diluted Three Part Blends made with suggested oils, or emotional supportive oils

Single Oils:
Balsam Fir, Chamomile (Roman), Copaiba, Frankincense, Helichrysum, Juniper, Laurus nobilis, Lavender, Melissa, Valerian

CAUTIONS:
These oils have general recommendations to avoid in people with epilepsy. Please see the single oil comments for more information: Basil, Fennel, Hyssop, Rosemary, Sage, Tarragon, Wintergreen.

SENILITY
(See COGNITIVE DYSFUNCTION)

SKIN INFECTIONS
(See also ALLERGIES, HOT SPOTS)

FIRST LINE RECOMMENDATIONS:
TOPICAL: The Ear Spray Recipe can be used on yeast feet infections and other sites of need. See Ear Infections.
WATER MISTS: Water misting can be very helpful, Three Part Blends especially including Copaiba, Lavender
PETTING: with diluted Three Part Blends
BATHING: essential oils added to natural shampoos

Single Oils:
Laurus nobilis, Lavender, Lemongrass, Marjoram, Melaleuca alternifolia, Melaleuca ericifolia, Myrrh, Myrtle, Oregano, Patchouli, Spikenard

SKIN TAGS

FIRST LINE RECOMMENDATIONS:
TOPICAL: Oregano applied neat to the skin tag, up to multiple times daily or as tolerated. The skin tag will look worse and may become crusty and scabbed prior to falling off.

OTHER: Addressing liver health is helpful in reducing the formation of skin tags. See information and oil suggestions for liver support.

Single Oils:
Frankincense, Oregano

SNAKE BITE

Naturally, veterinary attention is the most important recommendation when a snake bite has occurred. All traditional methods and recommendations should be followed. Essential oils can help to support all that we do with a snake bite situation. You can use one recommendation, or layer multiple to fit the severity and needs of the case.

FIRST LINE RECOMMENDATIONS:
TOPICAL: To the wound itself, essential oils can be applied. Most often diluted Three Part Blends are suggested, but any essential oil in an urgent case can be applied as soon as possible. Oils such as Helichrysum, Basil, and Hyssop have been indicated. Water-mists, essential oils in flush solutions, or within ointments or salves can be used.
CANINE SUPPORTIVE BLEND: This is most likely my preferred application. I apply this blend to the spine of the animal, as well as to the bite wound itself. Addition of oils such as Ledum, additional Helichrysum, and Melissa are often advised.
ORAL: Copaiba, Helichrysum

Single Oils:
Basil, Copaiba, Cypress, Frankincense, Helichrysum, Hyssop, Ledum, Oregano, Thyme

SPINAL CONDITIONS
(See also INTERVERTEBRAL DISC DISEASE)

FIRST LINE RECOMMENDATIONS:
PETTING: diluted Three Part Blends, especially with Black Spruce, Copaiba, Helichrysum
CANINE SUPPORTIVE BLEND: Apply as needed for individual, include additional oils as desired.

Single Oils:
Balsam Fir, Black Spruce, Copaiba, Geranium, Helichrysum, Juniper, Laurus nobilis, Lavender, Lemongrass, Marjoram, Peppermint

SPLEEN
(See also CANCER - SPLEEN)

SPONDYLOSIS
(See also SPINAL CONDITIONS, ARTHRITIS)

FIRST LINE RECOMMENDATIONS:
CANINE SUPPORTIVE BLEND: Apply as often as indicated by response, usually weekly. Include oils such as Balsam Fir, Black Spruce.
PETTING: diluted Three Part Blends for bone and inflammation.
ORAL: Copaiba

Single Oils:
Balsam Fir, Black Spruce, Copaiba, Helichrysum, Juniper, Laurus nobilis, Lavender, Lemongrass, Marjoram, Myrrh, Nutmeg, Peppermint, Thyme

STAPH INFECTIONS
(See SKIN INFECTIONS)

STEROIDS - REPLACEMENT

When steroids have been indicated or are being used for a condition, I have most commonly found that the Drip & Rub Techniques or Canine Supportive Blend can replace the use of, or reduce the use of these harmful drugs. Starting with a higher frequency of administration (often daily) and gradually reducing to every other day, every third day, every week, every month, and so forth is suggested. The administration must be adjusted to the individual response and needs of the animal.

FIRST LINE RECOMMENDATIONS:
CANINE SUPPORTIVE BLEND: include oils such as Black Spruce, Melissa, and Frankincense. Apply as needed initially, then you may find less often is necessary for maintenance.
WATER DIFFUSION: is always helpful to support full health. Oils such as Clove – also appear to reduce allergic responses.
ORAL: Copaiba twice daily in food, combined with other topical applications and water-based diffusion

Single Oils:
Balsam Fir, Black Spruce, Copaiba, Oregano, Thyme

STOOL EATING
(See COPROPHAGIA)

SYSTEMIC LUPUS ERYTHEMATOSIS
(See AUTOIMMUNE CONDITIONS)

TAIL CHASING
(See BEHAVIORAL CONDITIONS)

TESTICULAR INFLAMMATION

FIRST LINE RECOMMENDATIONS:
ORAL: Copaiba
CANINE SUPPORTIVE BLEND: Up to daily or as needed.
WATER MISTS: water mists of Three Part Blends of the recommended oils can be soothing and helpful to inflammation

Single Oils:
Black Spruce, Chamomile (German), Copaiba, Frankincense, Helichrysum, Lavender

TESTICLE - UNDESCENDED

FIRST LINE RECOMMENDATIONS:
CANINE SUPPORTIVE BLEND: with addition of Clary Sage. Regular body support, with support of normal hormone function is recommended.
PETTING: diluted Three Part Blends

Single Oils:
Clary Sage, Lemongrass

THROMBOCYTOPENIA
(See AUTOIMMUNE CONDITIONS)

THYROID - LOW
(See HYPOTHYROIDISM)

TICK BITES

It is important to recognize that information regarding Ticks and essential oils has greatly advanced. Many people may recommend applying essential oils directly onto the offending insect, to force it to withdraw from a body. This is not recommended. Even the human medical community greatly discourages any sort of irritation to be made to a tick that is embedded. The reason for this is that when an insect is irritated, being by alcohol, a match, or an essential oil, they generally secrete (or inject) more of their saliva into the body they are attached to. What this means is that if the tick embedded in your dog is carrying Lyme Disease, an "angry" tick is all the more likely to inject even more of the disease agent (Borrelia burgdorferi) into your dog (or cat, or horse, or human).

The application of essential oils has likely still been a "safer" form of irritation, because at least the area is also being flooded with an agent that most likely carries antibacterial properties. But, this relationship is like mopping your floor before you have picked up the dog poop. It's just messier. We are far better off to gently remove the tick with traction, and then apply an essential oil to the extraction site. In this way, we have less "tick vomit" to deal with – and a much healthier situation in the end.

FIRST LINE RECOMMENDATIONS:
TOPICAL: Apply any essential oil to a tick bite as soon as possible (often diluted, but neat can be considered for some oils and situations). The Canine Supportive Blend is a wonderful blend to apply to the bite area, however any oil should be used if the oils listed below are not available.
CANINE SUPPORTIVE BLEND: apply this blend in general to a dog for tick bites. Not only can it support the immune system, but it may have actions against the pathogen itself. This blend also has some insect repelling properties, so is a win-win situation.

Single Oils:
Catnip, Eucalyptus citriodora, Hyssop, Lavender, Melaleuca alternifolia, Oregano, Thyme

TICK BORNE DISEASE

FIRST LINE RECOMMENDATIONS:
ORAL: Oregano and Copaiba can be considered
CANINE SUPPORTIVE BLEND: Daily to every other day depending on response of individual. Inclusion of other oils can be considered.

Single Oils:
Catnip, Eucalyptus citriodora, Copaiba, Helichrysum, Hyssop, Melissa, Oregano, Thyme

TICK PARALYSIS
(See also TICK BORNE DISEASE)

FIRST LINE RECOMMENDATIONS:
ORAL: Helichrysum, Copaiba
CANINE SUPPORTIVE BLEND: Up to daily, include Hyssop, Melissa.

Single Oils:
Copaiba, Helichrysum, Hyssop, Juniper, Melissa, Oregano, Thyme

ULCERS - GASTRIC
(See GASTRIC ULCERS)

URINARY INCONTINENCE
(See INCONTINENCE - URINARY)

VACCINATION
(See VACCINOSIS)

VACCINOSIS

FIRST LINE RECOMMENDATIONS:
CANINE SUPPORTIVE BLEND: At least monthly, include oils such as Ledum. Rotation through inserted oils is suggested.
ORAL: Helichrysum

Single Oils:
Chamomile (German), Chamomile (Roman), Copaiba, Geranium, Grapefruit, Helichrysum, Hyssop, Juniper, Ledum, Lemon, Oregano, Thyme

VAGINITIS

FIRST LINE RECOMMENDATIONS:
CANINE SUPPORTIVE BLEND: Apply weekly or as indicated by the individual response.
WATER MISTS: to the vaginal area to reduce inflammation and decrease infection; Copaiba, Lavender is suggested.
TOPICAL: diluted Three Part Blends
ORAL: Copaiba

Single Oils:
Clary Sage, Copaiba, Eucalyptus radiata, Helichrysum, Lavender, Lemon, Lemongrass, Melaleuca alternifolia, Melaleuca ericifolia, Myrtle, Oregano, Thyme

VERTIGO
(See VESTIBULAR DISEASE)

VESTIBULAR DISEASE
(See also NEUROLOGIC CONDITIONS)

FIRST LINE RECOMMENDATIONS:
CANINE SUPPORTIVE BLEND: Include additional oils such as Melissa. Apply up to daily.
ORAL: Copaiba
PETTING: with diluted Three Part Blends made with suggested oils

Single Oils:
Chamomile (German), Chamomile (Roman), Copaiba, Frankincense, Geranium, Helichrysum, Juniper, Laurus nobilis, Lavender, Melissa, Valerian, Vitex

VIRAL CONDITIONS

FIRST LINE RECOMMENDATIONS:
CANINE SUPPORTIVE BLEND: Apply up to daily. Insertion of other antiviral oils is also suggested, especially Melissa.
WATER DIFFUSION: rotation through various Three Part Blends including disinfecting oils and anti-viral oils, up to 24 hours a day. Tenting and Caging diffusion can be used when needed (see Respiratory recommendations).
PETTING: of diluted Three Part blends of indicated oils
CLEANING: natural cleaners with essential oils
ORAL: Melissa, Copaiba

Single Oils:
Eucalyptus globulus, Geranium, Helichrysum, Hyssop, Laurus nobilis, Melissa, Oregano, Peppermint, Sandalwood, Thyme

VOMITING

(See also DIARRHEA)

An accurate diagnosis with a veterinarian is mandatory for cases of vomiting. Using recommendations specific to the cause of the vomiting is advised. Fasting during the initial phases of vomiting is important, and often water will have to be withheld as well. Consult with a veterinarian to determine if fasting is appropriate for your situation, and for how long. See the description within Diarrhea for more information regarding fasting.

FIRST LINE RECOMMENDATIONS:
CANINE SUPPORTIVE BLEND: can be applied for full body support of whatever condition may be causing the vomiting. Additional oils for digestive concerns can be added.
PETTING: diluted digestive Three Part Blends
ORAL: if vomiting is occurring, buccal absorption of oils is indicated. Diluted Three Part Blends of Ginger, Peppermint, and Copaiba can be considered and rubbed onto gums.

Single Oils:
Anise, Copaiba, Ginger, Helichrysum, Lemon, Marjoram, Nutmeg, Patchouli, Peppermint, Spearmint, Tarragon

WARTS

FIRST LINE RECOMMENDATIONS:
TOPICAL: Clove or Oregano, up to daily depending on how the dog tolerates it. Neat application is often used. Warts may look worse before resolving.
CANINE SUPPORTIVE BLEND: add oils such as Frankincense, Melissa
ORAL: Melissa (for viral concerns)

Single Oils:
Blue Cypress, Cinnamon, Clove, Frankincense, Melissa, Oregano, Peppermint, Sandalwood

WORMS - INTESTINAL
(See DEWORMING)

YEAST INFECTIONS
(See SKIN INFECTIONS)

EQUINE SUPPORTIVE BLEND

Please see the chapters on the Drip & Rub Techniques as well as the Body Supportive Blends. The Large Animal Supportive Blend will be the mainstay of support for most Equids and large animals.

Modifications of this blend, are generally achieved by adding additional oils of interest to the base blend, then diluting the base to the desired end concentration.

Just as described previously – this blend is more appropriate for horses and larger animals. While other animals can still use this blend, it was mainly created with the needs of horses and other livestock in mind. In general this blend is used between a 20-50% concentration.

To create a neat base blend; combine equal parts Oregano, Thyme, Basil, Cypress, Marjoram, Lavender, Black Spruce, Copaiba, Helichrysum, Ginger, and Peppermint. Add to carrier oil to create the desired concentration. Additional oils often considered to add to the base blend include Frankincense, Melissa, Catnip, Balsam Fir, German Chamomile, Ledum, or additional portions of Copaiba, Helichrysum or Marjoram.

Alternately, add 25 drops each of Oregano, Thyme, Basil, Cypress, Marjoram, Lavender, Black Spruce, Copaiba, Helichrysum, Ginger, and Peppermint to 25mL of Fractionated Coconut Oil. Apply 12-15 drops of this solution up the back, and stroke in. This blend may also be applied using the Petting Technique.

See the Chapter on Drip & Rub Techniques for more information on balancing and energy work prior to applications.

In some situations, Drip & Rub Recipes will be applied in serial applications for a stronger effect. For serious conditions, or where the Large Animal Supportive Blend has not been powerful enough, please feel free to create several Drip & Rub Recipes to apply as instructed within that chapter. Each Drip & Rub Recipe, should be diluted to the 20-50% concentration, prior to dripping along the spine. Many Drip & Rub Recipes, may start with a Three Part Blend as their base. Any of the listed oils for a condition, can be considered for use in your Three Part Blends or in the Drip & Rub Recipes.

EQUINE CONDITIONS

ABSCESS
(See also STRANGLES, HOOF ABSCESS)

An abscess in a horse can have many different causes and many different locations; from a contagious bacteria which causes "Strangles" to an abscess related to a snake bite wound. No matter what the cause, the basic care of these pus filled pockets can be addressed in a similar manner.

It is important to note, that there are forms of sterile abscesses as well – which are not related to bacterial infection at all. No matter what, the body is still "misbehaving" and the immune system is attempting to "eject" a substance from the body. Essential oils can be tremendously helpful as they support multiple levels of health; providing antibacterial, antifungal, and antiviral actions, immune system support, and aiding in tissue healing and regeneration. Accurate diagnosis can aide in supporting animals with a more exact approach to the origin of the condition.

FIRST LINE RECOMMENDATIONS:
TOPICAL: Apply "hot oils" within Three Part Blends (often neat) to the abscess head, up to twice a day. Hot pack the abscess with a very warm, damp wash cloth to help bring the abscess to a "head" or to drain. Once the "head" has opened and drainage is occurring, flush the wound with solutions containing essential oils.
ORAL: Copaiba,
LARGE ANIMAL SUPPORTIVE BLEND: Apply up to once per day. This blend can also be applied to the abscess itself. Additional oils can be added as desired.

Single Oils:
Cassia, Cinnamon, Laurus nobilis, Lavender, Lemon, Lemongrass, Melaleuca alternifolia, Oregano, Spikenard, Thyme

ANESTHESIA DETOXIFICATION

FIRST LINE RECOMMENDATIONS:
LARGE ANIMAL SUPPORTIVE BLEND: Applied up to once per day.
PETTING: diluted Three Part Blends, especially focused on digestive blends, or liver support
ORAL: Copaiba, Helichrysum

Single Oils:
Chamomile (Roman), Geranium, Ginger, Grapefruit, Helichrysum, Hyssop, Juniper, Ledum, Lemon, Peppermint

ARTHRITIS
(See also LAMENESS, NAVICULAR DISEASE)

Arthritis is an inflammatory condition of the joint by definition. However many owners will describe general stiffness, gait abnormalities, and other related changes as arthritis. Holistically we focus on supporting joint health, decreasing inflammation, and supporting health. With this approach, no matter what the cause of the perceived arthritis, the body will generally benefit and improvements will be seen. When possible, an accurate veterinary diagnosis is important.

FIRST LINE RECOMMENDATIONS:
ORAL: Copaiba
PETTING: Any selected oil. Diluted Three Part Blends as needed.
LARGE ANIMAL SUPPORTIVE BLEND: Apply up to once per day.
WATER MISTING: Add 20 drops of desired essential oil(s) to 4 ounces of distilled water. Shake well, mist over arthritic area.

Single Oils:
Balsam Fir, Black Spruce, Clove, Copaiba, Frankincense, Helichrysum, Lavender, Lemongrass, Marjoram, Myrrh, Nutmeg, Pepper (Black), Peppermint, Thyme, Vetiver

AUTOIMMUNE DISORDERS

Any condition in which the immune system is malfunctioning can benefit from the following suggestions. Whether the immune system is overactive or underactive, the same supportive measures will allow the immune system to function appropriately.

FIRST LINE RECOMMENDATIONS:
LARGE ANIMAL SUPPORTIVE BLEND: Modify by including Frankincense, Melissa, Balsam Fir. Apply up to once a day.
ORAL: Copaiba

Single Oils:
Balsam Fir, Basil, Black Spruce, Copaiba, Frankincense, Helichrysum, Melissa, Oregano, Thyme

BACK, SPINAL CONDITIONS
(See also ARTHRITIS)

There can be many situations in which a condition is considered back related in a horse. Arthritis will also relate to many conditions that feature back discomfort. An accurate diagnosis is important with a qualified veterinarian as something as simple as a poor fitting saddle – to something as severe as a fracture – could fall into the category of a "back problem". The methods below are indicated and helpful for any form of back discomfort. It is important to keep in mind that a kidney infection (which is widely unrelated to the spine itself) can manifest as a back condition.

FIRST LINE RECOMMENDATIONS:
LARGE ANIMAL SUPPORTIVE BLEND: up to once a day. Modify by including Balsam Fir, Lemongrass, Black Spruce.
ORAL: Copaiba
PETTING: With any selected oil, up to multiple times daily.
SPRAYING: 20 drops or more of essential oil(s) can be added to 4 ounces of distilled water or carrier oil to be misted over the back area.

Single Oils:
Balsam Fir, Bergamot, Black Spruce, Copaiba, Frankincense, Helichrysum, Juniper, Laurus nobilis, Lavender, Lemongrass, Marjoram, Oregano, Peppermint, Thyme, Vetiver

BEHAVIORAL CONDITIONS
(See also HORMONAL CONDITIONS)

FIRST LINE RECOMMENDATIONS:
See Emotional Work with Oils.
LARGE ANIMAL SUPPORTIVE BLEND: Apply as needed, including other emotional oils as indicated.
PETTING: Any selected oil, or diluted Three Part Blend multiple times a day or as needed.

Single Oils:
Bergamot, Black Spruce, Chamomile (German), Chamomile (Roman), Clary Sage, Geranium, Grapefruit, Lavender, Lemon, Marjoram, Melissa, Myrtle, Orange, Patchouli, Rose, Spikenard, Tangerine, Valerian, Vetiver, Ylang Ylang

BIRTHING AND DELIVERY

FIRST LINE RECOMMENDATIONS:
DIFFUSION: This may happen via Air-Diffusion in a barn, Indirect Diffusion, or even Water-Misting when needed. Use Three Part Blends made with recommended oils.
PETTING: diluted Three Part Blends of recommended oils, especially Frankincense

Single Oils:
Bergamot, Chamomile (Roman), Clary Sage, Frankincense, Geranium, Lavender, Marjoram, Myrrh, Orange, Rose, Vetiver

BONE CONDITIONS

FIRST LINE RECOMMENDATIONS:
PETTING: With any selected oil, multiple times per day.
LARGE ANIMAL SUPPORTIVE BLEND: apply as needed for full body support. This blend can be applied to locations of need as well, and additional oils can be added as indicated.

Single Oils:
Balsam Fir, Black Spruce, Copaiba, Thyme

BOWED TENDON
(See TENDON CONDITIONS)

BRUISED SOLES

Also known as Corns, the condition is the bruising of the bottom of the horse hoof. This is a condition mainly caused by improper trimming or shoeing of the horse. Generally the heel is found to be too long and/or horse shoes too small. Although the recommendations can aid in healing, the underlying issue that caused the bruising to begin with needs to be addressed first and foremost.

FIRST LINE RECOMMENDATIONS:
TOPICAL: Direct neat application of Balsam Fir, Helichrysum, and/or Cypress to the bruised area. Several drops, multiple times a day can be applied.

Single Oils:
Balsam Fir, Cypress, Frankincense, Geranium, Helichrysum

BRUISING

Any trauma can result in a bruising of tissues, from surgery to a kick by another horse. All bruising will respond to these general methods. An important note is that certain essential oils carry blood thinning or anti-coagulant properties. If bruising continues, does not improve, or worsens – omitting the oral use or excessive topical use of oils such as Cinnamon or Clove is suggested.

FIRST LINE RECOMMENDATIONS:
TOPICAL: Direct application or Petting of Balsam Fir, Helichrysum, and/or Cypress to the bruised area, up to several times a day. The method chosen may depend more on location and size of the injury.
WATER MISTING: Place 20 or more drops of the selected essential oil(s) into 4 ounces (120 mL) of distilled water or carrier oil and mist onto bruised area.
OINTMENT: Mix desired essential oil(s) into ointment and massage onto location.

LARGE ANIMAL SUPPORTIVE BLEND: application of this blend can help with all aspects of bruising. Additional oils can be added as desired.

Single Oils:
Cypress, Helichrysum, Balsam Fir, Frankincense, Geranium, Lavender

CANCER

(See also CANCER in Feline and Canine descriptions)

It is very important in conditions such as cancer, to incorporate as many layers of care as possible. This is one situation, where starting with small amounts of items, in low amounts, but building up to using many, many items and in relatively high amounts (sometimes quickly) is fully warranted.

FIRST LINE RECOMMENDATIONS:
DIET: Eliminate items such as sweet feed, corn, or high carbohydrate diets. Purified or spring water should be provided if possible.
ELIMINATE TOXINS: For horses this often consists of cleaners, bug sprays, or shampoos.
SUPPLEMENTS: Whole Food Supplements are available for horses through Standard Process. Equine Immune Support is suggested.
DIFFUSION: Rotational diffusion of emotional oils is recommended if possible. See also the chapter on Emotional Work with Oils for more information. Diffuse any anti-cancer oils up to 24 hours a day. Rotation through a variety of oils is recommended. Alternate methods of exposure to emotional oils is fine – be creative and expose the horse through water-mists, human diffusion, passive diffusion, or any method you see fit.
LARGE ANIMAL SUPPORTIVE BLEND: Use this blend up to twice a day, and often in between more complex Drip & Rub applications. Modify by including oils such as Frankincense, Melissa, and Balsam Fir to the mixture.
DRIP & RUB TECHNIQUE: At least once a week, I recommend an application that is more in line with what is described in the Drip & Rub chapter. Think of this as a "Five Course Meal" of essential oil application. This can be an episode to address emotional health and clearance, or for specific physical effects. Most of the Drip & Rub Recipes should be based in Three Part Blends, and diluted prior to use.

Read more at the beginning of the Equine chapter – Equine Supportive Blend for more information. If you find this application more beneficial than a basic Supportive Blend application, then I suggest you repeat the Drip & Rub more often.

PETTING: Applying any essential oil desired (often within diluted Three Part Blends) up to twice a day or more.

ORAL: Frankincense, Copaiba. Frankincense has been given orally in quite high doses for cancer. Unfortunately, the benefits of high oral amounts of Frankincense, have not been as clinically promising as presented in marketing.

DRINKING WATER: Frankincense, Copaiba, Orange, Tangerine, or other desired oils may be added.

Single Oils:
Balsam Fir, Black Spruce, Blue Cypress, Clove, Copaiba, Frankincense, Grapefruit, Lemon, Melissa, Orange, Oregano, Sandalwood, Sandalwood, Tangerine, Thyme

CANKER

Canker is a horrible condition which acts somewhat like a cancerous wart-like tumor in horses. Affecting the foot of the horse, it has resulted in permanent lameness and club foot deformities in many horses. Often a condition of the "well-kept horse" there are many cases documented of profound response to the use of essential oils. Traditionally, this condition is treated with various forms of surgery, all which are quite bloody in nature. It is not surprising that treatment with essential oils, can also bring forth some bleeding in this condition.

Supporting the immune system and providing for good nutritional support is also vital in this condition. Outlined below are recommendations for the canker lesion itself - care of the immune system is an important layer as well.

FIRST LINE RECOMMENDATIONS:
TOPICAL: Neat application of Oregano, Cassia, Cinnamon, Frankincense, and Copaiba essential oils to the canker. Bleeding may start or increase temporarily, due to the "cauterizing" sort of action we desire on this lesion. Repeat several times per day.
ORAL: Copaiba
LARGE ANIMAL SUPPORTIVE BLEND: apply as needed to support full body health.

Single Oils:
　　Cassia, Cinnamon, Clove, Copaiba, Frankincense, Copaiba, Lemongrass, Oregano, Thyme

CASTRATION
(See also PAIN MANAGEMENT)

FIRST LINE RECOMMENDATIONS:
　　TOPICAL: diluted Myrrh (especially within Three Part Blends) applied to castration site prior to the surgical procedure is helpful.
　　OINTMENT: Selected oils can be mixed into natural ointments or salves and applied to the site of the castration as needed.
　　SURGICAL SCRUB: Cleansing the castration site with essential oils within shampoo, soaps, or surgical scrub
　　WATER MISTING: 10-20 drops of Helichrysum, Myrrh, Melaleuca alternifolia or other desired oil(s) within a Three Part Blend, can be added to 4 ounces (120 mL) of distilled water and misted onto the castration site several times a day, or as needed.
　　ORAL: see Pain Management, Copaiba

Single Oils:
　　Cistus, Copaiba, Helichrysum, Laurus nobilis, Lavender, Lemon, Melaleuca alternifolia, Myrrh

CHOKE

FIRST LINE RECOMMENDATIONS:
　　PETTING: application of a diluted calming Three Part Blend can be helpful to the situation.
　　ORAL: Give 20 drops of Three Part Blends for digestion, especially including Marjoram, Peppermint, and Ginger into the bottom lip. Repeat if needed.

Single Oils:
　　Anise, Copaiba, Ginger, Marjoram, Peppermint, Vetiver, Ylang Ylang

CHRONIC OBSTRUCTIVE PULMONARY DISEASE
(See HEAVES)

CLUB FOOT

Club foot is a crippling condition in which contraction of the tendons and ligaments surrounding the hoof and foot are tight and result in abnormal structure of the foot of the horse. The condition can arise secondary to injury, infection, surgery or other forms of trauma. A proactive preventive approach to this condition is ideal, as once the condition has set in, it is very difficult to correct. A natural, barefoot farrier with experience in the condition is mandatory. This condition has commonly occurred after Canker surgery in many horses.

FIRST LINE RECOMMENDATIONS:
TOPICAL: diluted applications of Three Part Blends containing indicated oils, applied to the affected leg up to multiple times per day.
LARGE ANIMAL SUPPORTIVE BLEND: applied as needed, and can also be applied to the affected leg. Include other oils within blend as indicated or desired.
ORAL: Copaiba

Single Oils:
Balsam Fir, Black Spruce, Copaiba, Lavender, Lemongrass, Marjoram, Thyme

COLD & FLU
(See also EQUINE HERPES VIRUS, RESPIRATORY CONDITIONS, STRANGLES, HEAVES)

Cold and flu-like symptoms can have many causes in horses. From viral infections such as Equine Herpes Virus, bacterial infections such as Strangles, inflammatory conditions such as Heaves, many conditions affect the respiratory system of horses. Although it is ideal to be able to use essential oils that are specifically directed toward viruses or bacteria – the broad spectrum activity of essential oils, as well as their tremendous support to the immune system and body as a whole – we are often able to effectively benefit the entire respiratory system when an exact contributing factor has not been identified.

FIRST LINE RECOMMENDATIONS:
LARGE ANIMAL SUPPORTIVE BLEND: Apply up to twice a day, or as needed. For severe cases, consider Drip & Rub applications.
ORAL: Oregano, Copaiba
DIFFUSION: if possible, Three Part Blends for respiratory needs

Single Oils:
Balsam Fir, Black Spruce, Copaiba, Eucalyptus globulus, Eucalyptus radiata, Hyssop, Laurus nobilis, Lavender, Lemon, Marjoram, Melissa, Myrtle, Oregano, Peppermint, Rosemary, Sandalwood, Thyme

COLIC

Colic is the leading cause of death in horses. It is defined as any condition that causes intestinal or abdominal pain or discomfort in a horse or equid. There are many causes for the condition including impaction of intestinal material, parasites, twisted intestinal tracts, tumors and more. Symptoms of colic can vary from just being "off" to pawing at the ground, kicking at the belly, sweating, going off feed, and also full out rolling on the ground. This situation is certainly an emergency, and an accurate diagnosis from a veterinarian is imperative to accurately deal with the cause of the colic.

It is recommended that you call your equine veterinarian first, but while they are on their way – you use the following recommendations to support your horse. It is not uncommon that you will not need your veterinarian once they arrive to your farm.

FIRST LINE RECOMMENDATIONS:
The following recommendations are for an average sized horse. Smaller amounts may be indicated for miniature horses, ponies, or smaller equids. First - call your veterinarian.
PETTING: Calm the horse and owner by petting diluted Three Part Blends for emotions and calming onto the chest area of the horse. Applications to the belly can be considered if it is safe for the human to reach that location. Repeat this step every 20 minutes or as needed.

ORAL: Administer 20 drops of a digestive Three Part Blend orally, generally within the lip pocket (buccal absorption). Ginger, Marjoram, and Peppermint oil are common recommendations, and you could also include Copaiba in addition. Placing these oils into a 2 mL Essential Oil Sample Bottle is a great way to have a pre-measured and convenient way to dispense the oils into the mouth. Having several of these small bottles ready and waiting in your equine emergency kit is wise.

TOPICAL: Next apply 20 drops of the digestive Three Part Blend to the abdomen, in the location near the umbilicus. This can often be applied as a neat (undiluted application). In general, Ginger and Peppermint have a priority to be included within your digestive blend.

Repeat the calming, oral, and topical applications every 20 minutes until symptoms have improved. There has not appeared to be a maximum dose reached in this therapy, and many horses have consumed entire bottles of essential oils during difficult colic situations. If the colic does not respond within 1 hours' time, generally it is found that the colic situation will require surgery. Never neglect veterinary attention.

Single Oils:
Anise, Copaiba, Fennel, Frankincense, Ginger, Helichrysum, Lavender, Marjoram, Peppermint, Tarragon, Valerian, Vetiver, Ylang Ylang

COLIC, IMPACTION

This protocol was originally created by Sara Kenney, and modified slightly for current use. This protocol can be quite useful, especially for mini horses, who tend to experience impaction more often.

FIRST LINE RECOMMENDATIONS:
RECTAL INSTILLATION: Mix 20 drops of a digestive Three Part Blend within 4 cups of warm water. This solution is inserted rectally and/or orally every 15 minutes for 4 doses. A Turkey Baster or large syringe can be used for the rectal enema. When available, digestive enzymes can be added to this solution as well. Blends especially containing Ginger, Peppermint, and Marjoram are suggested.

Single Oils:
Anise, Copaiba, Ginger, Juniper, Lavender, Marjoram, Peppermint, Valerian, Tarragon, Valerian, Vetiver, Ylang Ylang

CONTRACTED TENDONS
(See also CLUB FOOT)

FIRST LINE RECOMMENDATIONS:
TOPICAL: diluted applications of Three Part Blends of the recommended oils can be massaged onto tendon area multiple times per day. The blend can also be added to natural ointments or salves as desired.

Single Oils:
Copaiba, Lavender, Lemongrass, Marjoram

COPD
(See HEAVES)

CORNEA
(See CORNEA in CANINE CONDITIONS)

CORNS
(See BRUISED SOLES)

COUGH
(See HEAVES, RESPIRATORY CONDITIONS, COLD & FLU)

EQUINE CONDITIONS

CRIBBING
(See also BEHAVIORAL CONDITIONS)

FIRST LINE RECOMMENDATIONS:
PETTING: With any selected oil, diluted within Three Part Blends.
DIFFUSION: If possible, with any selected oil, especially within Three Part Blends.
EMOTIONAL TECHNIQUES: See Emotional Work with Oils for more information.
LARGE ANIMAL SUPPORTIVE BLEND: Can be applied for full body support. Some horses may crib in response to physical conditions or pain.
ORAL: Copaiba

Single Oils:
Bergamot, Black Spruce, Chamomile (Roman), Copaiba, Geranium, Grapefruit, Lavender, Lemon, Melissa, Orange, Patchouli, Spikenard, Tangerine, Valerian, Vetiver, Ylang Ylang

CUSHING'S

FIRST LINE RECOMMENDATIONS:
PETTING: diluted Three Part Blends including Nutmeg, Clove, Rosemary over adrenal gland area, up to twice a day or as needed. Diluted Three Part Blends containing Cedarwood, Frankincense, and Black Spruce can be applied to the brainstem. Any other suggested oils may be used.
ORAL: Balsam Fir and Lavender in the evening has been used in efforts to reduce cortisol levels. Dill, Spearmint, or Fennel can be used for blood sugar handling.
LARGE ANIMAL SUPPORTIVE BLEND: Full body support is always indicated. Consider addition of oils such as Nutmeg and Balsam Fir.

Single Oils:
Balsam Fir, Black Spruce, Cedarwood, Cinnamon, Clove, Copaiba, Coriander, Dill, Fennel, Frankincense, Helichrysum, Lavender, Ledum, Lemon, Nutmeg, Rosemary

CUTS
(See LACERATIONS)

CYSTIC OVARY
(See LARGE ANIMAL CONDITIONS)

DEWORMING
(See also PARASITES, GASTROINTESTINAL CONDITIONS, DIARRHEA)

Deworming holistically is a frustrating predicament for many veterinarians. On one hand, a protocol will have complete success when even traditional remedies have failed, and then for the next animal – we will see no response at all. This is the way of the parasite. They are incredibly deceptive and have a strong will to live and survive in their host. It is important to recognize that no "one" remedy will be effective for every situation, and screening and checking stool samples with a veterinarian will often be helpful in determining the results of your efforts.

FIRST LINE RECOMMENDATIONS:
LARGE ANIMAL SUPPORTIVE BLEND: apply as needed for whole body health benefits, add additional anti-parasitic oils as desired.
ORAL: occasionally administration of diluted Three Part Blends of anti-parasitic oils has helped to purge worms from the body. Oils such as Tarragon, Anise, and Cinnamon are often helpful.

Single Oils:
Anise, Cinnamon, Eucalyptus globulus, Ginger, Hyssop, Lemon, Lemongrass, Melaleuca alternifolia, Nutmeg, Oregano, Peppermint, Sage, Tarragon, Thyme, Ylang Ylang

DIARRHEA

(See also DEWORMING, GASTROINTESTINAL CONDITIONS)

FIRST LINE RECOMMENDATIONS:
ORAL: digestive Three Part Blends, Copaiba, Peppermint
ORAL: For severe diarrhea with bacterial components Oregano, Clove, Ginger
PETTING: diluted digestive Three Part Blends, Copaiba, Peppermint
LARGE ANIMAL SUPPORTIVE BLEND: Up to daily or as needed.

Single Oils:
Anise, Clove, Copaiba, Fennel, Ginger, Lemon, Lemongrass, Melaleuca alternifolia, Melissa, Oregano, Peppermint, Tarragon, Thyme, Vetiver

EDEMA, PERIPHERAL

FIRST LINE RECOMMENDATIONS:
PETTING: diluted Three Part Blend, especially containing Cypress
LARGE ANIMAL SUPPORTIVE BLEND: Up to daily or as needed, can also be massaged into the affected limbs.
DRINKING WATER: Citrus oils, Copaiba

Single Oils:
Black Pepper, Copaiba, Cypress, Grapefruit, Tangerine

EHRLICHIA
(See TICK BORNE DISEASES)

EHV
(See EQUINE HERPES VIRUS)

ENCEPHALITIS
(See also WEST NILE VIRUS, VIRAL CONDITIONS)

FIRST LINE RECOMMENDATIONS:
LARGE ANIMAL SUPPORTIVE BLEND: Modify by including Roman Chamomile, additional Helichrysum, and Melissa. Apply up to daily.
TOPICAL: diluted Three Part Blends of any selected oils for underlying condition, especially apply to brainstem area.
ORAL: Copaiba

Single Oils:
Chamomile (Roman), Copaiba, Helichrysum, Juniper, Laurus nobilis, Melissa, Oregano, Thyme

EPM
(See EQUINE PROTOZOAL MYELOENCEPHALITIS)

EQUINE HERPES VIRUS
(See also VIRAL CONDITIONS)

FIRST LINE RECOMMENDATIONS:
LARGE ANIMAL SUPPORTIVE BLEND: Modify by including Melissa
ORAL: Melissa

Single Oils:
Geranium, Helichrysum, Laurus nobilis, Marjoram, Melaleuca ericifolia, Melissa, Oregano, Peppermint, Rose, Sandalwood, Thyme

EQUINE PROTOZOAL MYELOENCEPHALITIS

FIRST LINE RECOMMENDATIONS:
LARGE ANIMAL SUPPORTIVE BLEND: Modify by including additional Helichrysum, as well as Melissa, Clove. Apply up to daily, rotation of inserted oils is suggested.
ORAL: Clove, Copaiba, Helichrysum
PETTING: diluted Three Part Blends over brain stem area.

Single Oils:
Chamomile (Roman), Clove, Copaiba, Helichrysum, Juniper, Laurus nobilis, Oregano, Thyme

EYE CONDITIONS
(See also UVEITIS)

FIRST LINE RECOMMENDATIONS:
WATER MISTING: Lavender or Therapeutic Eye Spritzer
LARGE ANIMAL SUPPORTIVE BLEND: apply as needed for full body support, include additional oils as indicated for underlying issue.
ORAL: Copaiba

Single Oils:
Copaiba, Frankincense, Helichrysum, Lavender

FEVER

FIRST LINE RECOMMENDATIONS:
LARGE ANIMAL SUPPORTIVE BLEND: Apply as needed, up to once a day.
PETTING: Peppermint
ORAL: Peppermint, Copaiba
DRINKING WATER: Peppermint
DIFFUSION: Any selected oil

Single Oils:
Eucalyptus globulus, Helichrysum, Lavender, Melaleuca alternifolia, Melissa, Oregano, Peppermint, Thyme

FLOAT RIDES
(See TRANSPORTATION)

FLU
(See COLD & FLU, RESPIRATORY CONDITIONS)

FOUNDER
(See LAMINITIS)

GASTRIC ULCERS
(See ULCERS, GASTRIC)

GELDING
(See CASTRATION)

GIRTH GALLS
(See SADDLE SORES)

GREASY HEEL
(See SCRATCHES, SKIN CONDITIONS)

HEAVES
(See also RESPIRATORY CONDITIONS)

FIRST LINE RECOMMENDATIONS:
DIFFUSION: any indicated oil within respiratory Three Part Blend if possible.
ORAL: Oregano, Copaiba
TOPICAL: diluted Three Part Blends, especially with small amounts of Oregano, or other selected oils to throat and chest area, multiple times a day.
LARGE ANIMAL SUPPORTIVE BLEND: Apply as needed. Include additional indicated oils as desired.

Single Oils:
Balsam Fir, Black Spruce, Cedarwood, Cinnamon, Clove, Copaiba, Eucalyptus globulus, Eucalyptus radiata, Hyssop, Laurus nobilis, Lavender, Lemon, Lemongrass, Marjoram, Melissa, Myrtle, Oregano, Peppermint, Rosemary

HENDRA VIRUS
(See also VIRAL CONDITIONS)

FIRST LINE RECOMMENDATIONS:
DRINKING WATER: addition of essential oils within Three Part Blends can aid in disinfection of the water source.
LARGE ANIMAL SUPPORTIVE BLEND: Weekly to monthly for prevention. Up to daily for at risk horses or symptomatic horses. Include Melissa, Spikenard, Eucalyptus globulus, Hyssop.
ORAL: Copaiba, Melissa
CLEANING: use essential oils within cleaning products

Single Oils:
Blue Cypress, Clove, Copaiba, Eucalyptus globulus, Frankincense, Helichrysum, Hyssop, Laurus nobilis, Melissa, Spikenard

HIVES

FIRST LINE RECOMMENDATIONS:
ORAL: Basil or Melissa for antihistamine actions.
LARGE ANIMAL SUPPORTIVE BLEND: apply as needed, include oils such as Melissa and German Chamomile.

Single Oils:
Basil, Black Spruce, Chamomile (German), Copaiba, Geranium, Patchouli, Lavender, Melissa, Myrrh

HOOF ABSCESS
(See also PAIN MANAGEMENT)

FIRST LINE RECOMMENDATIONS:
TOPICAL: Three Part Blends made with "hot" oils such as Cinnamon, Clove, and Oregano. Apply to abscess area or hoof three or more times a day.
ORAL: Clove, Copaiba, Oregano.
LARGE ANIMAL SUPPORTIVE BLEND: As needed, can be applied to abscess area and affected hoof and leg as well.

Single Oils:
Cassia, Cinnamon, Clove, Helichrysum, Laurus nobilis, Lavender, Lemongrass, Melaleuca alternifolia, Oregano, Thyme

HORMONAL CONDITIONS

FIRST LINE RECOMMENDATIONS:
LARGE ANIMAL SUPPORTIVE BLEND: apply at least weekly, include oil additions such as Clary Sage, Ylang Ylang
DIFFUSION: Ylang Ylang, Clary Sage
PETTING: with diluted Three Part Blends of indicated oils

Single Oils:
Black Spruce, Clary Sage, Geranium, Lavender, Marjoram, Myrrh, Myrtle, Spikenard, Tarragon, Vetiver, Ylang Ylang

HYPERADRENOCORTISICM
(See CUSHING'S)

IMPACTION COLIC
(See COLIC, IMPACTION)

INSECT BITES

FIRST LINE RECOMMENDATIONS:
TOPICAL: diluted Three Part Blends applied to area of concern. Oils can be selected to ease the sting (Basil, Peppermint) or to repel insect bites (Catnip)
LARGE ANIMAL SUPPORTIVE BLEND: This blend not only carries insect repelling properties, but will also aid in comforting bites, infections, or irritations. Animals in greater health, are often less attractive to insects. Addition of oils such as Melissa can be helpful for insect bite reactions, where Catnip and Eucalyptus citriodora can be added for additional repelling actions.

Single Oils:
Basil, Catnip, Eucalyptus citriodora, Eucalyptus globulus, Geranium, Hyssop, Lavender, Lemongrass, Melissa, Patchouli, Peppermint

INSULIN RESISTANCE
(See also METABOLIC SYNDROME, CUSHING'S)

FIRST LINE RECOMMENDATIONS:
ORAL: Black Cumin, Dill
LARGE ANIMAL SUPPORTIVE BLEND: apply as needed, including oils for sugar handling

Single Oils:
Black Cumin, Cinnamon, Dill, Fennel, Pepper (Black), Spearmint, Ylang Ylang

KIDNEY CONDITIONS

FIRST LINE RECOMMENDATIONS:
TOPICAL: Juniper, Geranium within diluted Three Part Blends over the Kidney area.
LARGE ANIMAL SUPPORTIVE BLEND: apply as needed, including oils such as Juniper

Single Oils:
Geranium, Grapefruit, Helichrysum, Juniper, Ledum, Marjoram

LACERATIONS

FIRST LINE RECOMMENDATIONS:
TOPICAL: Three Part Blends for skin can be mixed into natural ointments (approximately 5 drops of each into 1 tablespoon) and salves. Repeat applications as needed, generally once or twice a day.

WATER MISTING: add recommended oils for skin care into water mists and spritz over laceration. Water mists in proper concentrations are safe for suture materials.

Single Oils:
Copaiba, Geranium, Helichrysum, Lavender, Melaleuca alternifolia, Myrrh, Palmarosa

LAMINITIS
(See also PAIN MANAGEMENT)

FIRST LINE RECOMMENDATIONS:
LARGE ANIMAL SUPPORTIVE BLEND: Up to once a day, including application to legs and corinet band. Include additional oils as desired, especially additional Cypress and Black Pepper.
TOPICAL: diluted Three Part Blends can be applied at the heels for vasodilation. Especially oils of Clove, Cypress, Copaiba.
ORAL: Copaiba (see also Pain Management)

Single Oils:
Balsam Fir, Black Pepper, Black Spruce, Clove, Copaiba, Cypress, Helichrysum, Lavender, Lemongrass, Marjoram, Peppermint

LICE
(See also INSECT BITES)

FIRST LINE RECOMMENDATIONS:
BATHING: With Three Part Blends for insects added to natural shampoo.
OIL SPRITZER: Mix large amounts (20 or more drops each) of Catnip, Eucalyptus citriodora, Peppermint, and Eucalyptus globulus per 1 ounce (30 mL) of Fractionated Coconut Oil and spray heavily. Repeat daily or as needed.
WATER MISTING: Selected oils can also be made into water mists.
LARGE ANIMAL SUPPORTIVE BLEND: This blend is also anti-bug in nature. Animals in poor health, are often more inclined to have lice infestations. Supporting full health is important.

Single Oils:
Catnip, Clove, Eucalyptus citriodora, Eucalyptus globulus, Geranium, Lavender, Lemon, Lemongrass, Orange, Oregano, Peppermint

LIVER DISEASE

FIRST LINE RECOMMENDATIONS:
ORAL: Helichrysum
LARGE ANIMAL SUPPORTIVE BLEND: apply as needed, especially including additions of Ledum, German Chamomile or other indicated oils for liver health
PETTING: diluted Three Part Blends especially containing Ledum

Single Oils:
Celery Seed, Chamomile (German), Geranium, Grapefruit, Helichrysum, Juniper, Ledum, Myrrh, Myrtle, Nutmeg, Rosemary, Spearmint, Tangerine

LYME DISEASE
(See TICK BORNE DISEASE)

MANGE
(See also INSECT BITES, SKIN CONDITIONS)

FIRST LINE RECOMMENDATIONS:
BATHING: With Three Part Blends for insects added to natural shampoo.
LARGE ANIMAL SUPPORTIVE BLEND: with additional insect oils, apply as needed, and to support full body health.
TOPICAL: diluted Three Part Blends for insects, or to soothe skin. Water-mists can also be used.
ORAL: Copaiba for inflammation. Melissa or Basil for antihistamine action. Vetiver for severe itching.

Single Oils:
Basil, Black Spruce, Chamomile (Roman), Eucalyptus globulus, Geranium, Helichrysum, Lavender, Melissa, Myrrh, Oregano, Palmarosa, Patchouli, Peppermint, Thyme, Vetiver

METABOLIC SYNDROME
(See also CUSHING'S, INSULIN RESISTANCE)

FIRST LINE RECOMMENDATIONS:
Use recommendations for Cushing's and Insulin Resistance.

Single Oils:
Cinnamon, Dill, Geranium, Grapefruit, Lavender, Ledum, Myrrh, Myrtle, Nutmeg, Pepper (Black), Spearmint, Ylang Ylang

MITES
(See MANGE)

MOON BLINDNESS
(See UVEITIS, EYE CONDITIONS)

MUSCULAR CONDITIONS

FIRST LINE RECOMMENDATIONS:
PETTING: diluted Three Part Blends especially including Marjoram, Lavender
LARGE ANIMAL SUPPORTIVE BLEND: Applied at least weekly. Additional oils for muscular concerns or primary issues can be included.

Single Oils:
Cedarwood, Copaiba, Cypress, Helichrysum, Lavender, Lemongrass, Marjoram, Pepper (Black), Peppermint

NAVICULAR DISEASE

FIRST LINE RECOMMENDATIONS:
LARGE ANIMAL SUPPORTIVE BLEND: Up to daily, including application to legs, frog, corinet band, etc. Include additional oils as desired.
ORAL: Copaiba. Clove may also be used for severe pain, see Pain Management for more in information.
PETTING: Any recommended oils within diluted Three Part Blends as needed, usually 3-4 times a day for severe cases. Lemongrass is suggested.

Single Oils:
Balsam Fir, Black Pepper, Black Spruce, Clove, Copaiba, Helichrysum, Lavender, Lemongrass, Marjoram, Peppermint, Pine, Thyme

NEUROLOGIC CONDITIONS

FIRST LINE RECOMMENDATIONS:
LARGE ANIMAL SUPPORTIVE BLEND: Including additional oils for neurologic health. Apply as needed for symptom relief, even twice a day. Can be applied to brainstem area as well.
PETTING: diluted Three Part Blends of indicated oils to brain stem area 3 times a day or as needed.
ORAL: Copaiba, Helichrysum

Single Oils:
Chamomile (Roman), Copaiba, Frankincense, Geranium, Helichrysum, Juniper, Laurus nobilis, Nutmeg, Valerian

OBSCESSIVE COMPULSIVE CONDITIONS
(See BEHAVIORAL CONDITIONS, CRIBBING)

OCD
(See BEHAVIORAL CONDITIONS, CRIBBING)

PAIN MANAGEMENT

FIRST LINE RECOMMENDATIONS:
ORAL: Clove, Copaiba, Helichrysum, and Myrrh 5 drops of each, repeat as needed. This mixture has been given neat, within the buccal pocket of the lip. Dilution may be desired for some horses.
PETTING: diluted Three Part Blends of indicated oils.
LARGE ANIMAL SUPPORTIVE BLEND: include additional indicated oils as desired (for muscular or bone needs or other primary conditions). Apply as needed.

Single Oils:
Balsam Fir, Clove, Copaiba, Helichrysum, Myrrh, Peppermint, Valerian, Vetiver

PAPILLOMA VIRUS
(See WARTS)

PARASITES
(See DEWORMING, LICE, INSECT BITES, MANGE)

PERFORMANCE TESTING
(See WINTERGREEN)

Please see the discussion of essential oils and performance testing within the Single Essential Oils chapter, under Wintergreen.

PHOTOSENSITIVITY
(See also LIVER DISEASE)

Causes of Photosensitivity often include ingestion of plants such as Alsike Clover, Vetch, Alfalfa, or St. John's Wort. Liver Disease and the use of medications such as Tetracycline can also cause this disorder. Sunburns are not a normal occurrence for horses, no matter how white or fair skinned they are, and veterinary diagnosis should always be explored.

FIRST LINE RECOMMENDATIONS:
TOPICAL: Myrrh, Helichrysum, Patchouli, Lavender added to Coconut Oil and applied topically.

Single Oils:
Chamomile (Roman), Geranium, Helichrysum, Lavender, Ledum, Myrrh, Patchouli

PIGEON FEVER
(See STRANGLES)

Pigeon Fever is similar in nature to Strangles infection. Recommendations for this disease are the same as for Strangles.

POTOMAC FEVER
(See also UVEITIS)

FIRST LINE RECOMMENDATIONS:
LARGE ANIMAL SUPPORTIVE BLEND: Apply up to twice daily. Include other oils as indicated.
ORAL: Oregano, Copaiba

Single Oils:
Copaiba, Helichrysum, Mountain Savory, Oregano, Thyme

PROUD FLESH

FIRST LINE RECOMMENDATIONS:
TOPICAL: Helichrysum, Copaiba, Palmarosa especially. Apply various oils via Water Misting or by mixing into natural ointment.
LARGE ANIMAL SUPPORTIVE BLEND: full body support is valuable.

Single Oils:
Chamomile (German), Chamomile (Roman), Copaiba, Geranium, Helichrysum, Lavender, Melaleuca alternifolia, Melaleuca ericifolia, Myrrh, Palmarosa, Patchouli, Rose, Sandalwood, Spikenard

QUEENSLAND ITCH (QLD ITCH)
(See SUMMER ITCH, INSECT BITES)

RABIES
(See RABIES in CANINE CONDITIONS)

RAIN ROT
(See also SKIN CONDITIONS)

FIRST LINE RECOMMENDATIONS:
BATHING: With Three Part Blends within natural shampoos.
LARGE ANIMAL SUPPORTIVE BLEND: Apply as possible, avoiding broken and irritated skin. Additional oils can be added as desired.
WATER MISTING: with Three Part Blends of indicated oils, can be a gentle soothing and healing method of application.

Single Oils:
Copaiba, Eucalyptus globulus, Geranium, Helichrysum, Laurus nobilis, Lavender, Lemongrass, Marjoram, Melaleuca alternifolia, Melaleuca ericifolia, Myrrh, Oregano, Patchouli, Rose, Rosemary, Sandalwood, Spikenard, Thyme

"RAINDROP" WELTS

It is hopeful that this occurrence will no longer happen, now that proper dilution is suggested prior to oil applications for horses. Please see the chapter on Previous Techniques for more in depth discussion on welts. Generally when these occur it is best to just apply additional Fractionated Coconut Oil to the sites, and leave the welts alone. They will generally resolve in around 24 hours. If severe irritation is noted, contact your veterinarian for additional help. While we can treat these much like Hives, they are in fact, different – and a direct irritation from inappropriate oil application.

FIRST LINE RECOMMENDATIONS:
TOPICAL: dilution with further carrier oil

Single Oils:
Lavender, Melissa, Myrrh, Patchouli

RASHES
(See SKIN CONDITIONS)

RESPIRATORY CONDITIONS
(See also HEAVES)

FIRST LINE RECOMMENDATIONS:
DIFFUSION: Any selected oil within a Three Part Blend. Tenting can be achieved by hanging a piece of painting plastic over the stall door or shelter entrance, for severe situations. Ideally water-based diffusion could be used, but in barn situations air-style may be necessary. Water-mists of the essential oils can also be used near the horse or in a confined area.
LARGE ANIMAL SUPPORTIVE BLEND: Apply up to twice daily. Additional oils can be included as desired.
PETTING: With any indicated oil, diluted within Three Part Blends, up to multiple times per day. Applying onto the chest area, in a stronger (50%) concentration can provide some sort of diffusion and inhalation actions.

Single Oils:
Balsam Fir, Black Spruce, Clove, Copaiba, Eucalyptus globulus, Hyssop, Laurus nobilis, Lavender, Lemon, Lemongrass, Marjoram, Melaleuca alternifolia, Melaleuca ericifolia, Oregano, Peppermint, Rosemary

RETAINED PLACENTA

FIRST LINE RECOMMENDATIONS:
INSTILLATION: Place 20-30 drops each of Myrrh and Copaiba into a syringe with 30-60 mL of water or carrier oil. Instill into uterus. If infection is suspected, oils for microbes can be selected to instill as well (Melaleuca alternifolia).

Single Oils:
Copaiba, Lavender, Marjoram, Myrrh, Sage

RHINO
(See EQUINE HERPES VIRUS, VIRAL CONDITIONS)

RHODOCOCCAL PNEUMONIA
(See also RESPIRATORY CONDITIONS)

Rhodococcus equi is a bacteria that causes pneumonia in immune compromised and susceptible foals, generally between 3 weeks and 6 months of age.

FIRST LINE RECOMMENDATIONS:
DIFFUSION: If possible in the barn setting (see Heaves). Three Part Blends for respiratory concerns.
LARGE ANIMAL SUPPORTIVE BLEND: Up to twice daily, include other oils as indicated.
ORAL: Oregano

Single Oils:
Black Spruce, Laurus nobilis, Lavender, Lemongrass, Marjoram, Melaleuca alternifolia, Melaleuca ericifolia, Myrtle, Oregano, Peppermint, Rosemary, Thyme

EQUINE CONDITIONS

RINGBONE
(See also PAIN MANAGEMENT)

FIRST LINE RECOMMENDATIONS:
TOPICAL: Any of the indicated oils, especially Balsam Fir, Lemongrass, and Thyme applied within diluted Three Part Blends multiple times per day.
LARGE ANIMAL SUPPORTIVE BLEND: Apply to spine as well as to frog and bulb area up to daily.
ORAL: Balsam Fir and Clove, Copaiba.

Single Oils:
Balsam Fir, Black Spruce, Clove, Copaiba, Frankincense, Helichrysum, Lemongrass, Myrrh, Oregano, Peppermint, Thyme

RINGWORM

FIRST LINE RECOMMENDATIONS:
BATHING: with antifungal essential oils within natural shampoo
TOPICAL: Neat oils may be considered for focal lesions, such as Lavender, Melaleuca alternifolia, or any selected oils to the lesion multiple times per day. Diluted Three Part Blends can also be applied.
OINTMENT: Mix several indicated oils into a natural ointment. This can be made very strong in concentration. Apply to lesions as needed, usually 1-2 times per day.
LARGE ANIMAL SUPPORTIVE BLEND: Full body support is wise, and this blend contains many healing and antifungal essential oils. Application in general to the spine, as well as to lesions is suggested. This blend could also be added to ointments, shampoos, or salves.

Single Oils:
Geranium, Laurus nobilis, Lavender, Lemongrass, Marjoram, Melaleuca alternifolia, Melaleuca ericifolia, Myrrh, Oregano, Pepper (Black), Peppermint, Rosemary, Thyme

ROTAVIRUS DIARRHEA

FIRST LINE RECOMMENDATIONS:
ORAL: Three Part Blends for digestion can be given orally, also see diarrhea for more options.
LARGE ANIMAL SUPPORTIVE BLEND: Apply up to twice daily. Include other oils as desired.
DIFFUSION: of Three Part Blends when possible. Oils to disinfect or stimulate immune function.
CLEANING: Essential oils within natural cleaners.

Single Oils:
Copaiba, Ginger, Melissa, Oregano, Peppermint, Tarragon, Thyme

SADDLE SORES

FIRST LINE RECOMMENDATIONS:
TOPICAL: diluted Three Part Blends of indicated oils, several drops applied at least daily.
OINTMENT: Various indicated oils can be mixed into natural ointment or salve and applied once to twice per day.
LARGE ANIMAL SUPPORTIVE BLEND: This blend serves multiple functions, and you will find many whole body healing oils within. Apply as needed, include additional oils as desired.

Single Oils:
Balsam Fir, Chamomile (Roman), Copaiba, Geranium, Helichrysum, Lavender, Myrrh, Palmarosa, Patchouli, Rose, Sandalwood, Spikenard

SARCOIDS

FIRST LINE RECOMMENDATIONS:
LARGE ANIMAL SUPPORTIVE BLEND: Up to twice daily, and including application to the sarcoid when possible and tolerated. Include oils such as Sandalwood, Frankincense, and Melissa.
TOPICAL: Oregano, Frankincense applied to sarcoid neat several times a day. Other oils may be applied as well, selections should be based on responses. Usually, the sarcoid will look much worse and crusty before getting better.

ORAL: Copaiba, Melissa

Single Oils:
Blue Cypress, Cinnamon, Clove, Copaiba, Frankincense, Grapefruit, Helichrysum, Lavender, Melissa, Orange, Oregano, Peppermint, Sandalwood, Tangerine, Thyme

SCRATCHES

FIRST LINE RECOMMENDATIONS:
Clip the area if necessary.
BATHING: Wash the area gently but thoroughly with Three Part Blends added to natural shampoos. Select oils with strong actions for the underlying cause (bacteria, parasites, fungus…)
TOPICAL: natural toothpaste is a wonderful poultice to apply to the washed and dried area. Additional oils such as the base for the Large Animal Supportive Blend or other desired Three Part Blends (Melaleuca alternifolia, Helichrysum, and Copaiba) may be mixed into the toothpaste.
LARGE ANIMAL SUPPORTIVE BLEND: This blend can be used to support the entire body, and can be applied to areas of concern as well. The neat version of this blend, prior to being diluted, can be added to shampoos and poultices as well.

Single Oils:
Catnip, Clove, Copaiba, Geranium, Helichrysum, Lavender, Lemongrass, Marjoram, Melaleuca alternifolia, Melaleuca ericifolia, Myrrh, Oregano, Patchouli, Rosemary, Thyme

SEEDY TOE
(See WHITE LINE DISEASE)

SKIN CONDITIONS

FIRST LINE RECOMMENDATIONS:
BATHING: With essential oils within natural shampoo. Oils can be selected for your particular needs (soothing, anti-parasitic, antibacterial, anti-fungal, etc…)
WATER MISTING: This can be helpful to apply oils to a broad area. Place 10-20 drops of any selected oils into 4 ounces (120 mL) of distilled water and mist the area of concern several times a day or as needed.
TOPICAL: Oils can also be added to natural ointments or salves for additional care and support.
LARGE ANIMAL SUPPORTIVE BLEND: Full body support and care is always indicated.

Single Oils:
Basil, Black Spruce, Chamomile (Roman), Copaiba, Geranium, Helichrysum, Juniper, Lavender, Ledum, Lemon, Lemongrass, Melaleuca alternifolia, Melaleuca ericifolia, Melissa, Myrrh, Oregano, Patchouli, Rose, Rosemary, Sandalwood, Spikenard, Thyme, Vetiver

SPLINTS
(See also BONE CONDITIONS)

FIRST LINE RECOMMENDATIONS:
TOPICAL: diluted applications of Three Part Blends especially containing Balsam Fir, Helichrysum (or other indicated oils) can be applied over the splint area, at least daily.
LARGE ANIMAL SUPPORTIVE BLEND: This can be helpful as well, and should be given to include application over the affected legs.

Single Oils:
Balsam Fir, Black Spruce, Copaiba, Cypress, Frankincense, Helichrysum, Lemongrass, Peppermint, Thyme

STOCKING UP
(See EDEMA, PERIPHERAL)

STRANGLES

FIRST LINE RECOMMENDATIONS:
See the information in ABSCESS as well.
CLEANING: Essential oils within natural cleaning recipes, or in foot bath solutions and quarantine stations.
LARGE ANIMAL SUPPORTIVE BLEND: Applied up to twice daily. Oils can also be applied to large abscesses if they are in locations that are amenable to it.
ORAL: Oregano, Thyme, Copaiba.
TOPICAL: Any of the suggested oils applied up to 4 times per day to the abscess, generally diluted in Three Part Blends.

Single Oils:
Cassia, Cinnamon, Helichrysum, Laurus nobilis, Lavender, Lemongrass, Melaleuca alternifolia, Mountain Savory, Oregano, Thyme

STREPTOCOCCUS EQUI
(See STRANGLES)

SUMMER ITCH
(See also INSECT BITES)

FIRST LINE RECOMMENDATIONS:
LARGE ANIMAL SUPPORTIVE BLEND: Use caution around irritated skin, however many insects dislike this blend. Apply as often as indicated by the individual.
PETTING: With diluted Three Part Blends or other indicated oils to repel insects. Occasionally, neat oils may be used.
OIL SPRITZER: Adding additional oils such as Oregano, Catnip, and Eucalyptus citriodora into Fractionated Coconut Oil and using as a bug spray works well. Other oils can be selected or used.
WATER MIST: Oils can be applied through a water mist as well.
ORAL: Melissa, Copaiba

Single Oils:
Basil, Catnip, Chamomile (Roman), Citronella, Copaiba, Eucalyptus citriodora, Eucalyptus globulus, Geranium, Helichrysum, Lavender, Lemongrass, Melissa, Myrrh, Orange, Oregano, Patchouli, Vetiver

SUNBURN
(See PHOTOSENSITIVITY)

SWABBING
(See PERFORMANCE TESTING)

SWEET ITCH
(See SUMMER ITCH, INSECT BITES)

TENDON CONDITIONS

FIRST LINE RECOMMENDATIONS:
PETTING: Apply diluted Three Part Blends of selected oils to the tendon area up to 4 times a day.
OINTMENT: Mix any selected oils into a natural ointment or salve and rub into the tendon area for a long lasting application.
LARGE ANIMAL SUPPORTIVE BLEND: Apply as needed along the spine, and also to the tendon area. Additional oils can be included such as Lemongrass and Balsam Fir.

Single Oils:
Balsam Fir, Black Spruce, Copaiba, Helichrysum, Lavender, Lemongrass, Marjoram

TETANUS
(See LARGE ANIMAL CONDITIONS)

THRUSH

FIRST LINE RECOMMENDATIONS:
TOPICAL: Apply Three Part Blends neat to the affected hoof area, 2-4 times a day or as needed.

Single Oils:
Cassia, Cinnamon, Eucalyptus globulus, Lavender, Lemongrass, Marjoram, Melaleuca alternifolia, Mountain Savory, Oregano, Pepper (Black), Thyme

TICK BITES

There has been a common recommendation within the aromatherapy world, to apply essential oils to a tick to force it to withdraw. Please see further information in the Canine section regarding Ticks and essential oils – to learn more about why this is not recommended. Remember, while some essential oils may be ideal, almost any essential oil can be used on a tick bite location.

FIRST LINE RECOMMENDATIONS:
TOPICAL: As soon as a bite is detected or a tick is removed, apply any of the recommended oils to the bite site AFTER removal of the tick. Neat application is generally tolerated, but may be inappropriate based on the location of the bite. Diluted Three Part Blends or a Supportive Blend is ideal, however any oil can be used early in the course of a bite, for the best protective effects.
LARGE ANIMAL SUPPORTIVE BLEND: Applying this blend to the animal in general, is recommended as soon as tick exposure is known. In these ways, we hope for prevention of transmission of tick borne disease. This blend also carries insect repelling properties as well. This blend is ideal for application to a tick bite, after removal of the tick. Repeat once to twice a day, as indicated by the appearance of the tick bite.

Single Oils:
Cinnamon, Clove, Copaiba, Hyssop, Lavender, Melaleuca alternifolia, Oregano, Thyme

TICK BORNE DISEASE

FIRST LINE RECOMMENDATIONS:
ORAL: Oregano, Copaiba
LARGE ANIMAL SUPPORTIVE BLEND: Up to twice daily depending on response of individual. Inclusion of other oils as indicated. In severe or symptomatic cases, Drip & Rub Techniques may be used instead or alternating with Supportive Blend applications.

Single Oils:
Black Spruce, Copaiba, Helichrysum, Melaleuca alternifolia, Oregano, Thyme

TRAILER RIDES
(See TRANSPORTING)

TRANSPORTING

FIRST LINE RECOMMENDATIONS:
PETTING: diluted Three Part Blends for emotions, calming, and grounding
INDIRECT DIFFUSION: Drip oils such as Lavender within Three Part Blends into the manger or other area where the horse can inhale them.
ORAL: digestive Three Part Blends may be helpful to prevent motion sickness and keep the intestinal tract happy and healthy while traveling.

Single Oils:
Bergamot, Black Spruce, Blue Cypress, Cedarwood, Chamomile (German), Chamomile (Roman), Frankincense, Lavender, Rose, Valerian, Vetiver, Ylang Ylang

TUMORS
(See CANCER, CANKER, PROUD FLESH, SARCOIDS, WARTS)

TYING UP
(See also MUSCULAR CONDITIONS)

FIRST LINE RECOMMENDATIONS:
TOPICAL: diluted applications of Three Part Blends especially containing Marjoram, Copaiba, Balsam Fir
ORAL: Balsam Fir, Cypress, Lavender, Copaiba
LARGE ANIMAL SUPPORTIVE BLEND: full body support is quite helpful. Include additional oils as desired.
DIFFUSION: if possible with Three Part Blends for emotional support, as well as physical including Balsam Fir, Cypress, Lavender, and/or Marjoram on a rotational schedule.

Single Oils:
Balsam Fir, Black Spruce, Cedarwood, Copaiba, Cypress, Frankincense, Helichrysum, Lavender, Lemongrass, Marjoram, Nutmeg, Peppermint, Valerian, Vetiver, Ylang Ylang

ULCERS, GASTRIC

FIRST LINE RECOMMENDATIONS:
ORAL: Copaiba, digestive Three Part Blends
DIFFUSION: Oils to reduce stress such as Lavender or Three Part Blends for emotional calming
LARGE ANIMAL SUPPORTIVE BLEND: Full body support is always suggested, additional amounts of Copaiba, and other digestive oils can be added. Apply as needed.

Single Oils:
Anise, Copaiba, Clove, Ginger, Helichrysum, Melissa, Nutmeg, Patchouli, Peppermint, Rose, Valerian, Ylang Ylang

UMBILICAL INFECTION

FIRST LINE RECOMMENDATIONS:
TOPICAL: Oils such as Myrrh, or other indicated oils within Three Part Blends can be applied directly to the site of infection several times a day. For application to the umbilical stump, often neat oils can be used. On the skin location, dilution is suggested.
LARGE ANIMAL SUPPORTIVE BLEND: Apply up to twice daily as needed. This blend can also be applied to the area of concern.
WATER MISTING: Three Part Blends of suggested oils can be misted onto the area of concern as needed, often twice a day.
ORAL: Oregano, Copaiba

Single Oils:
Cassia, Cinnamon, Clove, Copaiba, Laurus nobilis, Lavender, Lemon, Lemongrass, Melaleuca alternifolia, Myrrh, Oregano, Thyme

UVEITIS

FIRST LINE RECOMMENDATIONS:
ORAL: Copaiba
LARGE ANIMAL SUPPORTIVE BLEND: With additional oils included as desired, apply up to twice daily or as needed.
WATER MISTING: With Therapeutic Eye Spritzer twice a day. This spray does not need to contact the cornea, the presence of the oils around the eye area is beneficial.

Single Oils:
Copaiba, Frankincense, Helichrysum, Lavender

VACCINATION DETOXIFICATION

FIRST LINE RECOMMENDATIONS:
LARGE ANIMAL SUPPORTIVE BLEND: Given on a regular basis, weekly to monthly depending on need. Inclusion of Ledum, additional Helichrysum, and other liver supporting oils are suggested.
ORAL: Helichrysum, Copaiba if needed.

Single Oils:
Chamomile (German), Chamomile (Roman), Copaiba, Geranium, Grapefruit, Helichrysum, Hyssop, Juniper, Ledum, Lemon

VIRAL CONDITIONS

FIRST LINE RECOMMENDATIONS:
LARGE ANIMAL SUPPORTIVE BLEND: Up to twice daily with additional oils Melissa, Frankincense, and other indicated oils.
ORAL: Melissa, Copaiba if necessary
DIFFUSION: if possible, with Three Part Blends

Single Oils:
Blue Cypress, Geranium, Helichrysum, Hyssop, Laurus nobilis, Melaleuca ericifolia, Melissa, Oregano, Peppermint, Rose, Sandalwood, Thyme

WARTS

FIRST LINE RECOMMENDATIONS:
LARGE ANIMAL SUPPORTIVE BLEND: at least weekly applications, oils such as Clove, Blue Cypress, Frankincense, or other indicated oils can be included. Overall body support is suggested, but this blend can also be applied to the wart itself.
TOPICAL: Clove or Oregano applied neat, directly to warts located in areas that can tolerate it.

Single Oils:
Blue Cypress, Cinnamon, Clove, Frankincense, Lemon, Melissa, Oregano, Peppermint, Sandalwood, Thyme

WEST NILE VIRUS
(See VIRAL CONDITIONS, ENCEPHALITIS)

FIRST LINE RECOMMENDATIONS:
ORAL: Oregano, Copaiba
LARGE ANIMAL SUPPORTIVE BLEND: Apply up to twice a day for severe situations. Modify with addition of Melissa and other anti-viral oils.
TOPICAL: diluted Three Part Blends for neurologic needs, to brain stem area, once or more per day.
PETTING: With any of the selected oils, diluted in a Three Part Blend, multiple times a day.

Single Oils:
Chamomile (Roman), Copaiba, Helichrysum, Hyssop, Melissa, Oregano, Thyme

WHITE LINE DISEASE

FIRST LINE RECOMMENDATIONS:
TOPICAL: Apply 3-4 drops of strong anti-microbial Three Part Blends, directly to the hoof wall 3-4 times a day. Hoof wall resection is not necessary, however if a small groove has been made for diagnosis, drip the oil directly into the area. Treatment for 2 or more weeks is recommended, until confirmation of the condition being resolved.

Single Oils:
Black Pepper, Cassian, Cinnamon, Copaiba, Cypress, Eucalyptus globulus, Lavender, Lemongrass, Melaleuca alternifolia, Mountain Savory, Oregano, Thyme

WINDGALLS

FIRST LINE RECOMMENDATIONS:
LARGE ANIMAL SUPPORTIVE BLEND: Apply at least weekly, including leg applications.
TOPICAL: Any of the suggested oils can be applied as needed, generally within diluted Three Part Blends.

Single Oils:
Balsam Fir, Basil, Black Spruce, Copaiba, Cypress, Helichrysum, Lemongrass, Marjoram

WOUNDS
(See LARGE ANIMAL CONDITIONS)

LARGE ANIMAL TECHNIQUES

For the majority of Large Animals, the techniques and application methods will be similar to those used for dogs and for horses. Animals such as goats and pigs, tend to follow the dog recommendations. And larger animals such as Cattle, Alpaca, Llama, and other hoof stock, tend to follow the horse recommendations. Supportive Blends and Drip & Rub Recipes for these animals should follow the descriptions and recommendations made within the dog and horse section, as well as the respective chapters.

ABSCESS
(See discussion in EQUINE CONDITIONS)

ARTHRITIS
(See discussion in EQUINE CONDITIONS)

BIRTHING & DELIVERY
(See also discussion in EQUINE CONDITIONS)

FIRST LINE RECOMMENDATIONS:
TOPICAL: Apply Myrrh or other essential oils to the umbilical cord upon birth.
DIFFUSION: Three Part Blends
PETTING: diluted Three Part Blends

Single Oils:
Frankincense, Geranium, Lavender, Marjoram, Myrrh, Orange, Rose

BLOAT

FIRST LINE RECOMMENDATIONS:
ORAL: Tarragon for its anti-fermentation action. Also digestive Three Part Blends or Peppermint may be given.
TOPICAL: Apply diluted Three Part Blends for digestion to abdomen area.
PETTING: Any suggested oils, multiple times per day or as needed.

Single Oils:
Anise, Copaiba, Fennel, Ginger, Juniper, Lavender, Marjoram, Peppermint, Tarragon, Vetiver, Ylang Ylang

CAE
(See CAPRINE ARTHRITIS ENCEPHALITIS)

CANCER
(See discussion in EQUINE CONDITIONS)

CAPRINE ARTHRITIS ENCEPHALITIS
(See also MASTITIS, and VIRAL CONDITIONS in EQUINE)

Caprine Arthritis Encephalitis is caused by an RNA virus and affects goats. Symptoms include arthritis, encephalitis, hard udder, mastitis, poor milk production, pneumonia, and weight loss.

FIRST LINE RECOMMENDATIONS:
LARGE ANIMAL SUPPORTIVE BLEND: Apply up to twice daily. Include oils such as Melissa or other recommended oils.
ORAL: Oregano, Copaiba may be indicated for some cases.
DIFFUSION: Three Part Blends if possible

Single Oils:
Copaiba, Helichrysum, Laurus nobilis, Lavender, Melissa, Mountain Savory, Oregano, Thyme

CASEOUS LYMPHADENITIS

Caseous Lymphadenitis is also known as CLA, Cheesy Gland, Lympho, or Thin Ewe Syndrome. It is caused by the bacteria Corynebacterium pseudotuberculosis, and affects sheep and goats. The bacteria can survive for several months in the environment. The bacteria have a thick lipid wall, making essential oils a perfect tool to penetrate and destroy the otherwise difficult bacteria.

FIRST LINE RECOMMENDATIONS:
CLEANING: Spray farm, especially shady areas, with cleaning solutions containing essential oils.
LARGE ANIMAL SUPPORTIVE BLEND: Apply up to twice a day, drip oils onto the abscess sites when possible. Include additional oils as desired.
ORAL: Oregano, Copaiba may be indicated for some cases.

Single Oils:
Copaiba, Grapefruit, Laurus nobilis, Lavender, Lemon, Lemongrass, Mountain Savory, Oregano, Rosemary, Thyme

CASTRATION
(See discussion in EQUINE CONDITIONS)

CLA
(See CASEOUS LYMPHADENITIS)

COCCIDIA
(See also DIARRHEA)

FIRST LINE RECOMMENDATIONS:
ORAL: Oregano, Clove may be indicated for some cases.
LARGE ANIMAL SUPPORTIVE BLEND: Applied as needed, at least weekly. Addition of digestive oils may be desired.

Single Oils:
Anise, Clove, Lemon, Melaleuca alternifolia, Mountain Savory, Nutmeg, Oregano, Tarragon, Thyme

CRYPTOSPORIDIA

FIRST LINE RECOMMENDATIONS:
ORAL: Oregano up to four times per day. Three Part Blends (digestive)
LARGE ANIMAL SUPPORTIVE BLEND: Apply as needed, up to twice per day in severe situations. Include additional oils as desired.
DRINKING WATER: For some animals addition of essential oils to drinking water may be of benefit.

Single Oils:
Anise, Copaiba, Ginger, Lemon, Lemongrass, Marjoram, Melaleuca alternifolia, Mountain Savory, Oregano, Patchouli, Peppermint, Tarragon, Thyme

CYSTIC OVARY

FIRST LINE RECOMMENDATIONS:
LARGE ANIMAL SUPPORTIVE BLEND: Apply as needed, weekly or more often. Include oils such as Clary Sage, Frankincense, and Myrrh.
INSTILLATION: This method would only be used in last resort cases. The strength can be doubled if no effects are noted. Work closely with your veterinarian to determine proper course of action for your animal. Add 1-2 drops each of Myrrh, Lavender, Frankincense, and Myrtle to 10 mL of carrier. Instill into the uterus, twice a day for 5-7 days.

Single Oils:
Clary Sage, Copaiba, Frankincense, Lavender, Marjoram, Myrrh, Myrtle, Orange

DEHORNING
(See also PAIN MANAGEMENT in EQUINE CONDITIONS)

Just as with declawing cats, this procedure is not necessary for most livestock. Please do your due research, as there are many fallacies surrounding the need to dehorn goats, cattle, and others.

FIRST LINE RECOMMENDATIONS:
   TOPICAL: Apply any essential oil to the site of dehorning immediately. Mix oils into natural ointments or salves for longer lasting applications. In this situation, quite strong concentrations can be used.
   LARGE ANIMAL SUPPORTIVE BLEND: General support for inflammation and infections is provided through this blend.
   PETTING: diluted Three Part Blends for emotions and trauma.

Single Oils:
   Copaiba, Geranium, Helichrysum, Lavender, Lemongrass, Melaleuca alternifolia, Myrrh, Palmarosa, Valerian

DEWORMING
   (See discussion in EQUINE CONDITIONS)

DIARRHEA

FIRST LINE RECOMMENDATIONS:
   ORAL: digestive Three Part Blends, Copaiba, Peppermint
   LARGE ANIMAL SUPPORTIVE BLEND: Apply as needed. Additional digestive oils can be added.
   PETTING: diluted digestive Three Part Blends as needed.

Single Oils:
   Anise, Copaiba, Fennel, Ginger, Lemon, Lemongrass, Melaleuca alternifolia, Melissa, Mountain Savory, Oregano, Peppermint, Tarragon, Thyme, Vetiver, Ylang Ylang

LICE
   (See discussion in EQUINE CONDITIONS)

LIVER DISEASE
   (See discussion in EQUINE CONDITIONS)

MANGE
(See discussion in EQUINE CONDITIONS)

MASTITIS

FIRST LINE RECOMMENDATIONS:
ORAL: Oregano, Copaiba
TOPICAL: Oregano and other indicated oils, can be added to natural ointments, salves, or carrier oils to be applied to the udder. Many oils can be incorporated into an "udder rub", and the solution can be made very strong when needed. Occasionally, neat oils are applied to the udder.
LARGE ANIMAL SUPPORTIVE BLEND: This blend can be applied up to twice a day (or as needed), and can be utilized as an udder rub as well.

Single Oils:
Cinnamon Bark, Cinnamon Leaf, Copaiba, Cypress, Helichrysum, Laurus nobilis, Lavender, Lemongrass, Melaleuca alternifolia, Melaleuca ericifolia, Mountain Savory, Oregano, Thyme

MILK PRODUCTION

FIRST LINE RECOMMENDATIONS:
ORAL: Fennel
PETTING: Fennel
LARGE ANIMAL SUPPORTIVE BLEND: Apply at least every 3 days, with additional Fennel added to the blend.

Single Oils:
Fennel, Celery Seed

PAIN MANAGEMENT
(See discussion in EQUINE CONDITIONS)

POLIOENCEPHALOMYELITIS

FIRST LINE RECOMMENDATIONS:
LARGE ANIMAL SUPPORTIVE BLEND: Apply as needed. Include additional oils as desired.
PETTING: with diluted Three Part Blends
ORAL: Copaiba

Single Oils:
Chamomile (German), Chamomile (Roman), Copaiba, Frankincense, Helichrysum, Juniper, Laurus nobilis, Melissa, Oregano, Thyme

RINGWORM
(See discussion in EQUINE CONDITIONS)

SCOURS
(See DIARRHEA)

SCRAPIE
(See also VIRAL CONDITIONS, NEUROLOGIC CONDITIONS in EQUINE CONDITIONS)

Scrapie is a condition mainly of sheep, and rarely of goats, which is similar in nature to Mad Cow Disease, and caused by a prion. It affects the central nervous system and is a reportable disease. Positive animals are quarantined and often destroyed. Protocols will mainly focus on prevention of the disease. It is unknown if the disease can be cleared, as most positive animals are slaughtered. Certainly, the protocols could be used more aggressively in attempts to clear positive animals, however cooperation with your state and government agencies regarding this disease, must be followed.

FIRST LINE RECOMMENDATIONS:
LARGE ANIMAL SUPPORTIVE BLEND: Apply up to twice daily or as needed. Inclusion of oils such as Melissa and Hyssop are suggested.
ORAL: Oregano, Copaiba

Single Oils:
Helichrysum, Hyssop, Melissa, Oregano, Thyme

TEAT DIP, TEAT WASH

FIRST LINE RECOMMENDATIONS:

Use natural organic shampoos or soaps to make a teat wash solution. The addition of Vegetable Glycerin to the solution can help to condition the skin. Additional oils may be added to the wash solution to create custom benefits or preventive measures. For example, cows prone to mastitis could have Oregano, Melaleuca alternifolia, and Copaiba added to their teat wash, to be regularly exposed to their effects. The addition of Fennel, can be an easy way to increase milk supply through absorption within the teat wash or dip. In many cases Three Part Blends can be used, but for many udder situations, I may include multiple Three Part Blends within the following recipes, or more than three individual oils total as needs dictate.

Udder Wash Recipe:
1/2 Gallon of Water
1/2 Tablespoon or more of Liquid Castile Soap
   (like Dr. Bronner's Baby Mild) or another natural soap.
1/2 Tablespoon of Vegetable Glycerin
30-50 drops of selected essential oils

I will usually mix the essential oils into the soap first, then add it to the water along with the glycerin. You can add more or less essential oil to the mixture depending on your needs. Rock the mixture before each use.

You should not have to rinse the udder after washing, however if large amounts of essential oils remain on the teats, and you hand milk or contaminate milk with the left over wash residue, flavors could transfer into your milk. However, we have not noticed milk flavor change due to essential oil use or absorption alone.

After milking, the use of a natural and therapeutic teat dip is strongly suggested. My favorite is to use a natural ointment applied by hand, instead of a liquid dip per se.

LARGE ANIMAL CONDITIONS

DIY Udder Salve Recipe:
1/2 cup Coconut Oil (Raw, Organic; often solid at room temperature)
1 ounce (1 bar) of Beeswax
40-50 drops of selected essential oils

Melt the Coconut Oil over low heat, and add the Beeswax. I like to use a glass pan, as it is inert and does not react with any essential oil. Stir often until the Beeswax is melted fully into the Coconut Oil. Allow the mixture to cool, and add the essential oils before it starts to solidify too much. Mix well, and transfer into a glass canning jar to store. If you need to make a stronger salve, you can gently reheat it to aid in the mixing, or if your salve is pliable enough, mix it into the cold mixture.

The limiting "freshness" factor of this preparation is how clean you are - we have used jars for 3-6 months without spoiling or rancid concerns. However, if you dip dirty fingers into the mix (as we often do on a farm) - just be sure to smell and evaluate your salve to make sure you have not overly contaminated it. In general, the essential oils help to naturally preserve it - but it is a good idea to double check things along the way.

I often use this salve as a replacement for a Post-Milking Teat Dip. We often leave our calves on the mother, and share our milk supply. I find that the calves suckle the teat with the essential oils on them very well, and are probably gleaning health benefits all the while!

For those who like a more liquid teat dip, various essential oils can be added to a liquid carrier oil or other natural recipes, and these solutions can be applied via a teat dip cup.

Single Oils:
Copaiba, Fennel, Frankincense, Geranium, Lavender, Melaleuca alternifolia, Melaleuca ericifolia, Mountain Savory, Oregano

TETANUS
(See also NEUROLOGIC CONDITIONS in EQUINE CONDITIONS)

FIRST LINE RECOMMENDATIONS:
Prevention of Tetanus is the wisest approach. Application of ANY essential oil to any wound or surgical site should occur immediately.

Selection of an antibacterial essential oil can be applied neat, diluted, or within a natural ointment or salve.

ORAL: Copaiba, Helichrysum. For active infection and symptoms, oral administration of additional oils can be considered. Copaiba, Laurus nobilis, and Spikenard have been given orally in past reports. Never neglect veterinary care and attention, additional oils can be considered for oral use when indicated, such as Oregano and Helichrysum.

LARGE ANIMAL SUPPORTIVE BLEND: apply as needed, often up to twice a day. Additional oils such as Melissa and Frankincense are suggested.

TOPICAL: to any wound, Three Part Blends can be applied. This may include neat applications for some situations. Water-mists, natural ointments, and salves can also be utilized.

Single Oils:
Copaiba, Helichrysum, Juniper, Laurus nobilis, Lavender, Melaleuca alternifolia, Melissa, Mountain Savory, Oregano, Spikenard, Thyme

WOUNDS

FIRST LINE RECOMMENDATIONS:
TOPICAL: Mix Three Part Blends especially containing Helichrysum into natural ointments (approximately 15 drops into 1 tablespoon) and apply to wound. Repeat as needed, generally once or twice a day. Neat oils can also be applied to wounds as indicated, and if needed.

WATER MISTING: Selected essential oils can easily be applied over a larger area via misting. Generally this can be a fairly strong concentration, 20 or more drops of each oil added to 4 ounces (120 mL) of distilled water. Apply multiple times a day or according to response.

Single Oils:
Copaiba, Frankincense, Geranium, Helichrysum, Lavender, Lemongrass, Melaleuca alternifolia, Melaleuca ericifolia, Myrrh, Palmarosa, Spikenard

REFERENCES

Recommended Books

Aromatica: A Clinical Guide to Essential Oil Therapeutics. Volume I: Principles And Profiles. Peter Holmes Lac, MH. Singing Dragon Publishing 2016.

Clinical Aromatherapy: Essential Oils in Healthcare. 3rd Edition. Jane Buckle PhD, RN. Elsevier publishing 2015.

Essential Oil Safety. 2nd Edition. Robert Tisserand & Rodney Young. Churchill Livingstone Elsevier publishing 2014.

The Essential Oils. Volumes I – VI. Ernest Guenther. First Published in the 1940's – these volumes are now available in reprint, and considered the "must have" of many in the industry.

Essential Oils: A Handbook for Aromatherapy Practice. 2nd Edition. Jennifer Peace Rhind. Singing Dragon publishing 2012.

Medicinal Essential Oils: The Science and Practice of Evidence-Based Essential Oil Therapy. Dr. Scott A. Johnson. Scott A. Johnson Professional Writing Services, LLC 2017.

Power of the Seed. Susan M. Parker. Process Media 2014.

Supercritical Essential Oils: A Companion Resource to Medicinal Essential Oils. Dr. Scott A. Johnson. Scott A. Johnson Professional Writing Services, LLC 2017.

Find a Holistic Vet

American Holistic Veterinary Medical Association
www.AHVMA.org

Evaluation of Essential Oils

Essential Oil Analysis Foundation
www.essentialoilanalysis.com

The Essential Oil University
www.essentialoils.org

Phytochemia
www.phytochemia.com

Books on Carrier Oils

Power of the Seed. Susan M. Parker. Process Media 2014.

Veterinary Screened Essential Oils

animalEO Essential Oils for Animals
www.animalEO.info

Information on Ketogenic Diets

KetoPet Sanctuary
www.KetoPetSanctuary.com

Resource for Natural Pet Care, Longevity, and Cancer Research

Planet Paws – Rodney Habib
www.PlanetPaws.ca

Holistic Information for Cats

Lisa A. Pierson, DVM
www.catinfo.org

INDEX

1,8-cineole cautions	141
Abscess, canine	446
Abscess, equine	519
Abscess, feline	405
Abscess, hoof	537
Absolutes	96
Absorption	62
Acai Oil	78
Acne, feline	406
Acupressure	214
Acupuncture, use of oils with	215
Addison's Disease	447
Adrenal tumors, Ferrets	372
Agarwood	224
Air Freshening Recipes	338
Ajowain	224
Alcohols	27
Aldehydes	27
Alkenes	26
Allergies to essential oils	71
Allergies, canine	447
Allergies, feline	406
Allspice	225
Allspice Berry	224
Almond oil	78
Aloe Vera	78
Alopecia X	448
Amphibians	382
Amyloidosis	448
Amyris	225
Anal Glands	449
Anaplasma	See Tick Borne Disease
Andiroba Oil	78
Anemia, feline	407
Anesthesia, equine	520
Angelica	225
Anise	225
Anise, Star	226
Aniseed Myrtle	226
Anorexia, canine	450
Anorexia, feline	408
Antihistamine	450
Anti-Inflammatory Recipes	342
Antimicrobial Recipes	341
Anxiety, canine	451
Aortic Thromboembolism	See Saddle Thrombus
Application, frequency	193
Application, quantity	193
Apricot Oil	78
Aquariums	180, 386
Argan Oil	78
AromaBoost	196
aromatic plant species	19
AromaTouch	196
Arthritis, Avian	348
Arthritis, canine	451
Arthritis, equine	520
Arthritis, feline	408
Ascites	452
Asian Beetles	314
Aspergillosis	348
Asthma, feline	408
Atopy	See Allergies
Aural Hematoma	452
Australian Sandalwood	319
Autoimmune, canine	453
Autoimmune, equine	521
Autoimmune, feline	409
aversions	144
Avian respiratory system	65
Avian, essential oils	343
Avocado Oil	79
Babassu Oil	79
Back conditions, equine	521
Bacteria, resistant	280
baking soda	180

Balancing	199
Balancing Recipes	337
Balsam Fir	226
Baobab Oil	79
Basil	228
Basil, Holy	227
Basil, Lemon	227
Basil, linalool	228
Basil, sweet	228
bathing with essential oils	180
Bay Laurel	273
Bay Rum	229
Bee Balm	290
Beeswax	93
Behavior, canine	453
Behavior, equine	522
Behavior, feline	409
Behavior, hormonal equine	538
Behavioral conditions, Avian	349
Bell's Palsy	454
Benign Prostatic Hypertrophy	*See* Prostate
Benzoin	229
Bergamot	229
Bergamot, mint	230
Bilious Vomiting	455
bioavailability	66
Birch	230
Birds, essential oils	343
Birds, respiratory system	65
Birth & Delivery Recipes	342
Birthing, equine	522
Birthing, large animals	561
Bitter Orange	230
Black Cumin	230
Black Cumin Oil	79
Black Cumin Seed Oil	230
Black Currant Seed Oil	79
Black Pepper	305
Black Seed oil	79
Black Spruce	322
Blackberry Seed Oil	79
Bladder Infections	*See* Urinary Infection
Bladder Stones, canine	455
Blastomycosis	456
Bleeding, Avian	350
Blending Log	171
Blends, mixing	208
Bloat	*See* Gastrodilitation Volvulus
Bloat, canine	477
Bloat, large animals	562
Blocked, feline	410
Blood Clot	*See* Saddle Thrombus
Blood Feather	350
Blue Cypress	247
Blue Tansy	324
Blueberry Seed Oil	80
Body Supportive Blends	204
Bois de rose	316
Bone, broken	457
Bone, conditions	457
Bones, Broken, Avian	350
Bones, equine	522
Borage Seed Oil	80
Borna Virus	351
Boswellia carterii	256
Boswellia frereana	261
Boswellia sacra	261
Boswellia serrata	261
Box Elder Bugs	314
BPH	*See* Prostate
Brazil Nut Oil	80
Breeding, Rabbits	375
Broadleaf Eucalyptus	252
Broad-leaf Paperbark	287
Broccoli Seed Oil	80
Brucella Canis	458
Brucellosis	458
Bruised sole, equine	523
Bruising, equine	523
Buccal absorption	67
Bumblefoot	351
Buriti Oil	80
Butterflies	389
CAE	562
Cajeput	231
Callus	458
Calming Recipes	337
Camelina Oil	80
Camellia Oil	80
Cancer, Avian	352
Cancer, bone	461
Cancer, canine	459
Cancer, equine	524

INDEX

Cancer, feline 411
Cancer, liver 461
Cancer, lung 461
Cancer, lymph 462
Cancer, mammary 462
Cancer, spleen 462
Candelilla Wax 93
Canine Influenza .... *See* Virus, canine
Canine Supportive Blend 206, 445
Canker 525
Canola Oil 80
capric triglyceride 82
Caprine Arthritis Encephalitis 562
caprylic triglyceride 82
Caraway Seed 231
Carboxylic Acids 28
Carboxylic Esters 28
Cardamom 231
Cardiomyopathy, canine 463
Cardiomyopathy, feline*See* Heart Disease
carrier oil application, timing 202
Carrier Oils 77
Carrot Root Oil 81
Carrot Seed 231
Carrot Seed Oil 80
Caseous Lymphadenitis 563
Cassia 231
Castor Oil 81
Castration, large animal 526
Cat metabolism 36
Cataract 463
Catnip 232
Catnip, lemon 233
Cats 397
Cats, citrus toxicity 47
Cats, enzyme deficiency 34
Cats, exotic 383
Cats, large 383
Cats, limonene toxicity 47
Cats, linalool toxicity 48
Cats, phenol toxicity 50
Cats, pine toxicity 51
Cats, scientific references 38
Cats, toxicity 35
Cavity*See* Feline Odontoclastic Resporptive Lesion

CBD oil 85
Cedar, Western Red 233
Cedarwood 233
Celery Seed 234
Cervical Line, feline*See* Feline Odontoclastic Resorptive Lesion
Chakra, oil techniques 210
Chamomile, German 234
Chamomile, Roman 235
Chaste Berry 332
Chaste Tree 332
Cheesy Gland 563
Cherry Kernel Oil 81
Cheyletiella 376
Chia Seed Oil 81
children, breathing problems 142
Chilean Hazelnut 85
Chinchillas 383
Chiropractic 215
Choke 526
Chronic Obstructive Pulmonary Disease
 .... *See* Heaves
Cilantro 235
Cinnamon Bark 236
Cinnamon Leaf 237
Cistus 237
Citronella 238
CLA 563
Clary Sage 239
Cleaning Recipes 338
Clove 240
Club foot 527
CO_2 Extracts 30, 96
Coccidia 563
Cocoa Butter 82
Coconut Oil 82
Coffee Oil 84
Cognitive dysfunction 464
Cognitive Recipes 338
Cold and flu, equine 527
Colic 528
Colic, impaction 529
Collapsing Trachea 464
Common Tansy 325
Competition testing 333
concentration charts 121
Concentration, for use 117

Concentrations, for species 119
Conjugation Pathways 55
Conjunctivitis, feline 414
Constipation 465
Constituent categories 21
Constituents, essential oil 24
Contracted tendons 530
Copaiba 241
Copaiba, beta-caryophyllene content .. 25
Copaiba, differences 25
Copaiba, diterpenes 25
Copaiba, oleoresin 244
Copal 241
COPD .... 536, See Heaves
Coprophagia 466
Coriander 245
Coriander Leaf 235
Corn Oil 84
Cornea 466
Cornmint 246
Corns, canine 458
Corns, equine 523
Corynebacterium 563
Cougars 383
Cough, canine 467
Cranberry Seed Oil 84
Cribbing 531
Crop Infection 352
Crop Stasis 353
Cruciate injury 467
Cryptorchid ...... See Testicle, undescended
Cryptosporidia 564
Crystals, feline .... See Urinary, feline
Cucumber Seed Oil 84
Cumin 246
Curcumin 330
Cushing's, canine 468
Cushing's, equine 531
Cuterebra 376
Cuts .... See Laceration
Cypress 247
Cypress, Blue 247
Cypress, White 333
Cystitis, feline .... See FLUTD
Cytochrome p450 398
Cytochrome pathways 34

Daikon Radish Seed Oil 84
Dalmatian Sage 317
Davana 248
Declaw, feline 415
DEET 251
Dehorning 565
Demodex 469
Dental Disease, canine 469
Dental, feline 416
Dermal absorption 67
Detoxification .... 58, See Vaccinosis
Deworming, equine 532
Deworming, feline 416
Diabetes, canine 470
Diabetes, feline 417
Diarrhea, Avian 353
Diarrhea, canine 471
Diarrhea, equine 533
Diarrhea, feline 417
Diarrhea, Ferrets 372
Diarrhea, large animal 565
Diarrhea, Rabbits 376
Diffusion 147
Diffusion, air 150
Diffusion, as topical application 182
Diffusion, avian/birds 344
Diffusion, caging 149
Diffusion, Cats 400
Diffusion, monitoring 151
Diffusion, open room 149
Diffusion, tenting 150
Diffusion, water-based 147
Digestive Recipes 339
Dill 248
Dill Seed 248
Dill Weed 248
dilution of oils 117
Dilution Rates 117
Dilution, forms of 130
dimethyl sulfoxide 94
Direct application 174
Dispersing agents 180
Dispersment 131
Distemper, feline .... See Viral, feline
Diterpene 25
DMSO 94

INDEX

Dorado Azul	249
Douglas Fir	250
Drinking water, adding oils	157
Drip & Rub Recipe, Ferret	374
Drip & Rub Technique, equine	518
Drip & Rub Techniques	199
Drip & Rub, Avian	345
Drip & Rub, Rabbit	378
Drop size	133
Drug Interactions	74
Dry Eye	471
Dystocia	See Pregnancy & Delivery, See Pregnancy & Delivery
Ear cleaning recipe	190
Ear Infections	472
Ear Mites, feline	418
Ear Spray Recipe	189
Ears, applying oils to	176
Ears, use of essential oils	187
Edema, equine	533
Egg binding	354
Egg laying, excessive	354
Egg laying, inadequate	354
Ehrlichia	See Tick Borne Disease
EHV	534
Elemi	250
Elephants	384
Elimination, inappropriate	429
Emotional Cleansing	473
Emotional Cleansing Recipes	341
Emotional work with oils	207
emulsifiers	131
Emulsions	131
Endocrine Recipes	341
Epilepsy	See Seizures
EPM	534
EPO	84
Epsom salt	180
Epulis	473
Equine Herpes Virus	534
Equine Protozal Myeloencephalitis	534
Equine Supportive Blend	206
Equine Supportive Blends	518
Essences, flower	96
Essential oil creation	19
Essential oil toxicity	53
Essential oils, toxic	51
Esters	28
Ethers	28
Eucalyptus Blue	251
Eucalyptus citriodora	251
Eucalyptus dives	252
Eucalyptus globulus	252
Eucalyptus polybractea	253
Eucalyptus radiata	254
Eucalyptus Radiata	254
Evening Primrose Oil	84
Excretion	60
Eye spritzer, therapeutic	186
Eyes, canine	474
Eyes, equine	535
Eyes, use of essential oils	184
Fading Kitten Syndrome	418
False pregnancy	474
Fatty Liver Disease, feline	419
Fatty Liver, Avian	355
Fatty tumor	491
FCO	83
FDA concerns	219
Feather loss	355
Feather picking	356
Feather Spray Recipe	344
Feet, applying to	176
Feline Acne	406
Feline Infectious Peritonitis	420
Feline Leukemia	See Viral, feline
Feline Odontoclastic Resorptive Lesions	421
Feline Supportive Blend	205, 402
Feline, metabolism	36
FELV	See Viral, feline
Fennel	255
Ferrets	371
Fever, equine	535
Fever, feline	421
FIP	420
First Pass Metabolism	66
Fish	386
FIV	See Viral, feline
Flax Seed Oil	84
Flea Bomb Recipe	306
Fleas, canine	475
Fleas, feline	422

Float rides 556
Float Rides .... *See* Transportation
Flower Essences 96
Flu .... *See* Virus
Flu, equine 527
FLUTD 423
Folding, term meaning 26
Foods, adding oils to 162
Foraha Oil 92
Foreign body, canine 476
FORL 421
Founder .... *See* Laminitis
Fractionated Coconut Oil 82, 83
Frankincense 256
Frankincense, carterii 256
Frankincense, frereana 261
Frankincense, Sacred 261
Frankincense, serrata 261
Frequency of application 193
Frogs 382
Function, essential oils 20
Functional groups 26
FUO .... *See* Fever, feline
Furanocoumarins 29
Future research 222
Galangal 262
Galbanum 262
Gall Bladder 476
gamma linolenic acid 84
Garlic oil 262
Gas Chromatograph 115
Gastric Ulcers, canine 476
Gastrodilatation Volvulus 477
Gastrointestinal, Avian 357
GC analysis 115
GC/MS 115
GDV 477
Gelding .... *See* Castration
Generally Recognized As Safe 112
Geranium 262
Gerbils 391
German Chamomile 234
Gevuina Oil 85
GI Recipes 339
Giardia, Avian 357
Ginger 264

Girth Galls .... *See* Saddle Sores
GLA 84
Glaucoma, canine 478
Glucosidation 50
Glucuronidation 36
Glucuronyltransferase 36
Glutathione 55
Glutathione S-transferase 55
Goldenrod 265
Gout, Avian 358
Grape Seed Oil 85
Grape toxicity 85
Grapefruit 266
Grapefruit & medications 55
Grapefruit, and medications 266
GRAS status 112
Greasy Heel .... 551, *See* Scratches
Grounding Recipes 337
Guinea Pigs 387
hair follicles 63
Hair follicles 140
Hair loss, from essential oils 327
Hairballs, feline 424
half-life 60
Hamsters 391
Hazelnut Oil 85
Head tilt .... *See* Vestibular disease
Head trauma, Avian 358
Heart, feline 425
Heartworm disease 480
Heartworm, prevention 479
Heat Stroke .... *See* Hyperthermia
Heaves 536
Heavy Metals, Avian 359
Hedgehogs 387
Helichrysum 267
Helicobacter, Ferrets 372
Hemangiosarcoma 462
Hemlock 329
Hemorrhage, internal 482
Hemp 270
Hemp Seed oil 85
Hendra Virus 537
Hermit Crabs 389
Herpes, feline 426
Hinoki 270

INDEX

Hippopotamus 388
Histiocytoma 483
Hit by Car 426
Hives, equine 537
Holy Basil 270
Honey Bees 389
Hoof abscess 537
Hops 270
Hormonal conditions, Avian 359
Hormonal Recipes 341
Hormones, equine 538
Horner's Syndrome .... 427, See Bell's Palsy
Hot Spots 483
Hydrocarbons 24
Hydro-distillation 95
Hydrosols 97
Hyperesthesia 427
Hypersensitivity response 71
Hypertension 428
Hyperthermia 484
Hyperthyroidism 428
Hypoglycemia 484
Hypothyroid 485
Hyssop 271
IBD, canine 486
IBD, feline 430
IMHA 485
Immune Mediated Anemia 485
Incontinence, urinary 486
Indirect application 183
Inflammation Recipes 339
Inflammatory Bowel, feline 430
Influenza, canine .... See Virus, canine
Ingestion of essential oils 68
Ingestion of oils 152
Inhalation absorption 64
Injections of oils 217
Insect Bites, equine 538
Insects, pets 389
Insulin resistance, equine 539
Insulin, use with 76
Insulinoma, Ferrets 373
Intravenous use of oils 217
Ironbark, lemon-scented 279
Ishpingo 297
Isomers 22

Isoprene unit 24
Jackson Galaxy 96
Jasmine 272
Jojoba 85
Juniper 272
Kennel Cough 488
Ketones 28
Kidney Disease, Avian 360
Kidney, canine 488
Kidney, equine 539
Kidney, feline 430
Kiwi Seed Oil 86
Knee injury, canine 467
Koi 386
Kukui Nut Oil 86
Labdanum 237
Lacerations, canine 489
Lacerations, equine 539
Lactation and oils 136
Lactation, canine 489
Lactones 29
Laminitis 540
Lanolin 93
Lard 92
Large Animal Supportive Blend 206
Large Animals 561
Laryngeal paralysis 490
Laurus Nobilis 273
Lavandin 274
Lavender 274
Lavender Eye Spritzer 186
Lavender Tea Tree 287
Lavender, spike 276
Lead Poisoning .... See Heavy Metals
Ledum 276
Lemon 277
Lemon Balm 288
Lemon Catnip 233
Lemon Eucalyptus 251
Lemon Myrtle 279
Lemon Tea Tree 280
Lemongrass 280
Lemon-Scented Gum 251
Lemon-Scented Ironbark 279
Lenticular sclerosis 490
Lice 540

579

Lick granuloma	490
Life Force Oils	313
Lime	282
Limping Kitten Syndrome	431
Lions	383
Lipoma	491
Litter Box Recipes	398
Litter box, not using	429
Liver Disease, Avian	360
Liver metabolism, cats	398
Liver Shunt, canine	492
Liver Support Recipes	342
Liver, canine	492
Liver, equine	541
Liver, feline	431
Lizards	390
Lupus	See Autoimmune
Luxating Patella	See Patella
Lyme Disease	See Tick Borne Disease
Lymph nodes, canine	493
Lympho	563
Lymphoma, Ferrets	373
Lymphosarcoma	462
Macadamia Nut oil	86
Macaw Wasting Disease	See Proventricular Dilatation Disease
Maldigestion, canine	493
Malnutrition, Avian	361
Mandarin	282
Mange, equine	541
Mange, sarcoptic	505
Mango Butter	86
Manuka	283
Marigold	323
Marjoram	283
Mass Spectrometry	115
massage	215
Mast Cell Tumors	494
Masticatory Myositis	494
Mastitis, canine	495
Mastitis, large animal	566
May Chang	284
MCT	82
Meadowfoam Seed Oil	86
measurement conversions	121
measurement of oils	133
Megaesophagus	495
Melaleuca alternifolia	285
Melaleuca Ericifolia	287
Melaleuca Quinquenervia	287
Melaleuca, Cats	397
Melatonin	448
Melissa	288
Metabolic Bone Disease	390
Metabolic Pathways	54
Metabolic syndrome, equine	542
Metabolism	34
Metabolism enzymes	54
Methicillin Resistant Staph. aureus	280
Methyl Salicylate	333
Mevalonate pathway	19
Mice	391
Milk production	566
Milk Thistle Seed Oil	86
milligram measurements	134
Mineral Oil	87
Mite, demodex	469
Mites, equine	541
Mites, Rabbits	376
Mites, sarcoptic	505
Modifications, recipes	203
Monarda	290
Monkeys	390
Monoterpene	24
Moon Blindness	558, See Uveitis
Moringa Oil	87
Morphine in cats	104
Mountain Savory	290
MQV	287
MRSA	280
Mugwort	291
Muscle Wasting	496
Muscular conditions, equine	542
Mustard	291
Mutilation, Avian	361
Myrrh	291
Myrtle	294
Myrtle, Lemon	279
Mysore Sandalwood	318
Natrasorb Bath	180
Navicular Disease	543
Neat oils, use of	127

INDEX

Neem oil	87
Neroli	295
Nerolina	288
Nerve Recipes	338
Neurologic conditions, Avian	362
Neurologic, canine	496
Neurologic, equine	543
Neurologic, feline	432
New Animal Recipes	341
Newts	382
Niaouli	287
Nigella	79, 230
Nursing animals	136
Nutmeg	296
Oat Seed Oil	88
Obesity, canine	496
OCD	See Behavior, See Behavior
Ocotea	297
Odor Elimination Recipes	342
Oil Misting	182
Ointment, adding oils to	181
Olive Oil	88
Opoponax	298
Optical rotation	22
Oral administration	68
Oral Administration, Cats	401
Oral use of oils	165
Orange Blossom	295
Orange essential oil	298
Orange, bitter	230
Orange, sweet	298
Orchitis	See Testicle
Oregano	300
Oregano & pregnancy	139
Oregano, onites	302
Organic oils	106
Organoleptics	110
Osteosarcoma	See Cancer, bone
Ovary, cystic	564
Paclitaxel	85
Pain Control, feline	432
Pain management, Avian	363
Pain Recipes	339
Pain, canine	497
Pain, equine	544
Pain, Physical recipes	339
Palm Fruit oil	88
Palm Kernel Oil	88
Palmarosa	302
Palo Santo	303
Pancreatic insufficiency	498
Pancreatitis	433
Pancreatitis, canine	498
Pannus	See Autoimmune
Panosteitis, canine	499
Papaya Seed Oil	88
Papilloma, Avian	363
Papilloma, canine	516
Papilloma, Rabbits	380
Parasites	See Deworming
Parasites, Rabbits	376
Parrot Fever	See Psittacosis
Parvo, canine	500
Passion Fruit Seed Oil	89
Pasteurella, Rabbits	377
Patchouli	304
Patella, luxating	500
PBFD	See Psittacine Beak and Feather Disease
PDD	..See Proventricular Dilatation Disease
Peach Kernel Oil	89
Peanut oil	89
Pecan oil	89
Pemphigus	See Autoimmune
Pennyroyal	305
Pepper, Black	305
Peppermint	307
Peppermint Eucalyptus	252
Pequi Oil	89
Performance testing 333,	See Wintergreen
Perilla Seed Oil	89
Peru Balsam	310
Petitgrain	310
Petroleum Jelly	89
Petting	175
Petting, Cats	401
Phenols	27
Photosensitivity	544
Pigeon Fever	545
Pillow Paw	See Autoimmune, feline
Pine	310
Pistachio Nut Oil	89
Placenta, retained	548
Plai	312

Plum Kernel Oil 89
PMD (p-Menthane-3,8-diol) 251
Pneumonia .... *See* Respiratory
Pneumonia, aspiration .... *See* Cough
Polioencephalomyelitis 567
Pomegranate Seed Oil 90
Ponds 180, 386
Poppy Seed Oil 90
Potomac Fever 545
Poultry 347
Pracaxi Oil 90
Pregnancy 136
Pregnancy & Delivery, canine 501
Pregnancy, feline 434
Primates 390
Prostate, Ferrets 374
Prostatitis, canine 502
Proud Flesh 545
Proventricular Dilatation Disease 364
Psittacine Beak and Feather Disease .. 365
Psittacosis 366
Pulmonary contusions 268
Pumpkin Seed Oil 90
Punicic acid 90
Pyometra 502
Pyruvate pathway 19
Queensland Itch .... *See* Summer itch
Rabbits 375
Rabies 503
Rain Rot 546
Raindrop Technique 196
Rapeseed Oil 80
Raspberry Seed Oil, red 90
Rats 391
Ravensara 312
Ravintsara 312
Rectal administration 70
Rectal, use of oils 191
reflexology 214
Regurgitation, Avian 366
Reiki 216
Reproduction and oils 136
Reptiles 390
Respiratory infections, canine 504
Respiratory Recipes 338
Respiratory, Avian 367

Respiratory, equine 547
Respiratory, feline 441
Rhino 534
Rhodococcus equi 548
Rice Bran Oil 90
Ringbone 549
Ringworm, canine 505
Ringworm, feline 436
Ringworm, large animal 549
Rock Rose 237
Rocky Mountain Spotted Fever *See* Tick Borne Disease
Rodents 391
Roman Chamomile 235
Rosalina 287
Rose 313
Rose Geranium 262
Rose Hip Seed Oil 90
Rose of Sharon 237
Rose Otto 313
Rosemary 314
Rosemary, Verbenone 316
Rosewood 316
Rotavirus 550
Rue 317
Rue oil toxicity 137
Sacha Inchi Oil 90
Sacred Frankincense 261
Saddle Sores 550
Saddle Thrombus 437
Safe use of oils 102
Safflower oil 91
Sage 317
Salamanders 382
Sandalwood 318
Sandalwood, Australian 319
Santanol 318
Sarcoids 550
Sarcoma, feline 438
Sarcoma, vaccine 438
Sarcoptic Mange 505
Saro 319
Scaly face mites 367
Scotch pine 310
Scrapie 567
Scratches 551

INDEX

Screening of oils	106
Sea Buckthorn Oil	91
Sebaceous cyst	506
Seborrhea	506
secondary metabolites	20
Seedy Toe	560, *See* White Line Disease
Seizures, Avian	368
Seizures, canine	507
Seizures, feline	438
Select CO_2	31
Selection of oils	106
Self-mutilation, Avian	361
Senility	*See* Cognitive dysfunction
Sensitization	71
Sesame Seed Oil	91
Sesquiterpene	25
Shampoo, adding oils to	181
Shea Butter	91
Shea Oil	91
Shikimate Pathway	19
Shikimic Acid pathway	19
Shope Papilloma, Rabbits	380
Shortening	92
silymarin	86
Sinus infection, Avian	368
Skin Conditions, equine	552
Skin infections, canine	507
Skin Recipes	342
Skin tags	508
Small Animal Supportive Blend	205
Smell, sense of	140
Snake Bite	508
Snakes	390
Snuffles, Rabbits	377
Soaking water	180
Solubol	180
Solvents	131
Soybean Oil	92
Spearmint	320
Spike Lavender	276
Spikenard	321
Spinal, equine	521
Spine, canine	509
Splints, equine	552
Spondylosis	509
Spritzers	178
Spruce	322
Spruce, Black	322
Squalene	92
Squamous Cell Carcinoma	439
St. John's Wort	318
Staph infections	*See* Skin Infections
Star Anise	226
steam distillation	95
Steroids	510
Stocking up, equine	533
Stomatitis	440
Stool eating	*See* Coprophagia
Strangles	553
Streptococcus equi	553
Subcritical extracts	31
Sugar Gliders	392
Sulfation	55
Summer Itch	553
Sunburn	*See* Photosensitivity
Sunflower Oil	92
Supercritical extracts	30
Suppositories	191
surfactants	130
Swabbing	*See* Wintergreen
Sweet Birch	230
Sweet Itch	553
Sweet Myrrh	298
Swimming pools	180
Synergy, drugs	75
Syphilis, Rabbits	379
Tagetes	323
Tamanu Oil	92
Tangerine	323
Tansy	325
Tansy, Blue	324
Tarantulas	389
Tarragon	325
Tauntauns	393
Tea Tree Oil	285
Tea Tree Oil, Cats	397
Tea Tree, lavender	287
Tea Tree, Lemon	280
Teat dip	568
Teat wash	568
Tendons, equine	554
Testicle, inflammation	511
Testicle, undescended	511

Tetanus 569
Therapeutic Eye Spritzer 186
Therapeutic Mucus..............................65
Thin Ewe Syndrome............................563
Three Part Blends 167
Thrombocytopenia *See* Autoimmune, *See* Autoimmune
Thrush 554
Thyme 326
Thymoquinone..............................230, 290
Tick bites, canine 512
Tick bites, equine 555
Tick Borne Disease, canine...................513
Tick Borne Disease, equine 555
Tick Paralysis 513
Tigers..383
Toads 382
Tomato Seed Oil...................................92
Topical application..............................174
Torticollis, Rabbits...............................377
Tortoises...394
Total CO_2..31
Toxoplasmosis.....................................441
Trailer rides 556
transdermal absorption 63
Transporting...556
Treponema, Rabbits 379
Tritrichomonas....................................441
Tsuga 329
Tumor, canine 454
Tumor, fatty...491
Turmeric...330
Turtles 394
Tying up..556
Udder care 568
Ulcers, canine gastric 476
Ulcers, equine......................................557
Umbilical infection, large animal 557
Unicorns...395
Upper Respiratory Infections 441
Urethra, blocked 410
URI, feline 441
Urinary Disease, feline........................423
Uveitis, equine 558
Vaccination Detox, feline....................443
Vaccine Detox, equine 558

Vaccinosis 514
Vaginitis, canine 514
Valerian..330
Vanilla 331
Vaseline..89
Vent, Rabbits 379
Vestibular disease, canine 515
Veterinary Aromatic Medicine 18
Vetiver..331
Viral, feline 444
Virus, equine 558
Vitex...332
Vomiting, canine..................................516
Vomiting, feline 444
Walnut Oil 92
Warts, Avian ....*See* Papillomatosis
Warts, canine.......................................516
Warts, equine.......................................559
Warts, Rabbits 380
Wasting Disease, Avian *See* Proventricular Dilatation Disease
Water misting.......................................178
Water, adding oils to............................157
Waterfall Technique 196
Water-Misting, birds 344
Welts, equine.......................................547
Welts, Raindrop...................................547
West Nile Virus...................................559
Western Red Cedar 233, 332
Wheat Germ Oil 93
White Cypress 333
White Line Disease.............................560
Windgalls...560
Winter Savory 290
Wintergreen...333
witch hazel..180
WNV..559
Worms ....*See* Deworming
Wormwood 291, 334
Wounds, Avian 370
Wounds, large animal..........................570
Wry Neck, Rabbits..............................377
Yarrow...334
Yeast infections ....*See* Skin infections
Ylang Ylang 334
Yuzu 335
Zdravetz...336

INDEX

Zinc Poisoning, Avian *See* Heavy Metals, Avian
Zinziba 336
Zoo Animals 396
Zoopharmacognosy 212

Made in the USA
Las Vegas, NV
24 November 2023

81457364R00321